The Encyclopedia of Bodywork

From Acupressure to Zone Therapy

Elaine Stillerman, L.M.T.

Facts On File, Inc.

This book is dedicated to my mother and father.

Facts On File, Inc.
11 Penn Plaza
New York NY 10001

Library of Congress Cataloging-in-Publication Data

Stillerman, Elaine.
   The encyclopedia of bodywork / Elaine Stillerman. -- New York: Facts on File, Inc.) 1996.
   320 p. : cm. ill
   Includes bibliographical references and index.
   ISBN 0-8160-3187-8 (alk. paper)
   1. Mind and body therapies—Encyclopedias.   I. Titles.
RZ999.S82   1996
615.5′03=dc20   95-45829

R
615.503
STI

Cover design by Leah Lococo
Illustrations by Jeremy Eagle, Marc Green, and Dale Williams

This book is printed on acid-free paper.

Printed in the United States of America

TT RRD 10 9 8 7 6 5 4 3 2 1

. . . There are more things in heaven and earth,
Than are dreamt of in your philosophy.

—William Shakespeare
Hamlet

CONTENTS

ACKNOWLEDGMENTS

This book could not have been written without the cooperation of hundreds of bodyworkers who provided me with information and fact-checking about their systems. If I have overlooked mentioning any of them, it does not reflect that their tremendous help was any less significant.

With admiration and gratitude, I want to thank Barb Baun of the Desert Institute of the Healing Arts, Elisabeth F. Benitah (Electrical Current Therapy), Russell Borner (Chair Massage), Margaret Ann Case (Reiki), Bonnie Eichar (Reiki), Steven Goldstone (Hypnotherapy), Kathryn Hansman (Fascial Kinetics), Peggy Horan of the Esalen Institute, Florence Horn (Spiritual Healing), George Kousaleos (Core Bodywork), Jon Levy (Massage For AIDS), Patricia Liantonio (A.O.B.T.A.), Dietrich W. Miesler (Geriatric Massage), Keith Miller (A.M.T.A.), Eolani Negri (Lomilomi), Neil Olson, Pacific Institute of Oriental Medicine (Kevin Ergil, Marni Ergil and Kate Martin), Gary Peterson (Polarity Therapy), Kamala Renner (Alchemical Synergy), Mary Alice Roche (Sensory Awareness), Victoria Ross (Thérèse Primmer Method of Deep Muscle Therapy), Anita and Samuel Strauss (Reiki), Caroline Sutton and Dr. John Upledger, D.O. (Upledger Institute).

I particularly want to thank the following professionals who took the time and care to make sure that their respective bodywork systems were accurately explained: Carolyn Bengston, Lic. Ac.; Emil Grancagnolo, L.M.T.; Susan Krieger; Dr. Paul Nissman, D.C.; and Moe Slotin, L.M.T., P.T.

On a personal note, many thanks to Harold Abrams, Steve Helfand, Barbara Messing and Maura Spiegel.

Finally, to Paul Solotaroff, my husband, for his constant love and support.

INTRODUCTION

The 1990 study by the investigators from Harvard Medical School revealed that an estimated one fourth of the American population sought the help of alternative health care practitioners and paid more visits to them than all primary care medical doctors nationwide.[1] In addition, most of these people paid for these holistic providers out of their own pockets, without the benefit of insurance reimbursement.

This growing trend of choosing, and in many cases preferring, unconventional therapies necessitates a reference work, which details what these therapies are. This information may help make appropriate alternative health care choices easier.

I intend *The Encyclopedia of Bodywork: From Acupressure to Zone Therapy* to serve two functions. Primarily, it provides in-depth descriptions, explanations and historical backgrounds of common, esoteric and sacred bodywork systems to people who are unfamiliar with them.

Secondly, this text presents professional bodyworkers, students of the healing arts and their schools with the most comprehensive, up-to-date resource list of holistic health in the United States and Canada in the event they want to further their education.

I have expanded the term **bodywork** to include all the hands-on therapies, movement reeducation systems, psychological techniques and metaphysical and energetic modalities, which recognize the unity of the **body/mind/spirit/emotions**. Throughout the book, the words body/mind/spirit/emotions appear joined to express the idea that an individual is an integrated being. Alternative health care workers uphold this philosophy and it is reflected in the work they do.

In order to be included in this book, these systems had to conform to certain guidelines: that they offer natural, noninvasive approaches to healing, and the goal of the work promotes a salubrious change in the condition of an individual's body/mind/spirit/emotions, or the whole person.

Many of the bodywork systems in this book were developed and thrived when conventional medicine failed. Repeatedly, innovators of these techniques, some of whom had survived near-death experiences, "incurable" diseases or physical disabilities, were able to cure themselves and, subsequently, others, with self-discovered techniques. Several of these systems might appear to be far-fetched and difficult to understand, but that does not undermine their relevance nor the fact that they work for some people. Scientific rules are not the only means to measure the efficacy of these bodywork systems.

Many of these systems have to be experienced in order to be understood. The proof for the individual, however, is in the result, and each person must decide if a system is appropriate for himself/herself.

In researching this book, I made every attempt to contact the respective authorities for accuracy in the description and representation of their work. In the absence of any texts, this was the only way to provide a factual account of the technique.

The pronouns he/she are used interchangeably. When the practitioner is described as a woman, the client, or recipient, is male, and vice versa. Generally, professionals, those who need a license to practice, are called therapists, while unlicensed bodyworkers are referred to as practitioners, providers or facilitators.

To find a specific bodywork system, look under the appropriate letter. Within an entry, cross-references to other systems are printed in SMALL CAPITAL letters. Terms relevant to the entry word appear in **boldface**.

This book, which has taken the better part of two years to research, compile and write, has been, indeed, a labor of love. It has given me a rare opportunity to meet and get to know many extraordinary, talented bodyworkers and provided me with an incredible education.

Health care choices are personal ones. I hope that this book helps you to make clear and proper decisions.

—Elaine Stillerman, L.M.T.

Notes

[1] Eisenberg, David M., M.D., et al., "Unconventional Medicine in the United States," *The New England Journal of Medicine*, 328, no. 4 (January 1993): 251.

FOREWORD

Many of the procedures and techniques that today are considered to be standard medical practice were once seen by the physician and patient alike as curious, whimsical and unconventional therapies. Even those treatments that over time met with observed clinical improvements in the patients for whom they were prescribed were often misunderstood, and sometimes distrusted, by the medical community. As worldwide travel and immigration has effected a melding of many cultures and societies, the commonplace medicinals, practices and local folklore of one people have become adopted, and adapted, by another.

Such therapies as manual massage and acupuncture date centuries across the world. Were these techniques harmful or without any apparent benefit they likely would have fallen from favor and would have been long forgotten. Newer techniques must yet stand years of application before judgment may be made regarding their efficacies.

The medical consumer of today is faced with a wide variety of available treatments. To adequately choose the proper one, information must be gathered regarding the philosophies of potentially suitable techniques, the methods of administration and the claimed benefits. The task of collecting all this information seems dizzying at best, and downright formidable at worst.

In encyclopedic form, Elaine Stillerman, L.M.T., has presented a wonderful summary of today's most popular bodywork systems. Although many of these practices lie outside the boundaries of "accepted" medical standards and may not necessarily be advocated by myself or other physicians, the service that Ms. Stillerman provides her readers by explaining in detail the subtleties and meanings of these practices (with their often imposing names) is considerable. Patients and physicians will better understand techniques and modalities that are increasingly touted by the media and advertisement.

In years to come, some of these treatments may prove ineffective and be quickly dismissed; others may be found to have real and unquestioned worth. Time and experience will be the final judges for these methods. Thankfully, *The Encyclopedia of Bodywork: From Acupressure to Zone Therapy* is available now, to those of us too impatient to wait or too curious to remain uninformed.

—Willibald Nagler, M.D.
Physiatrist-in-Chief, The New York Hospital
Professor of Rehabilitation Medicine,
Cornell University Medical Center

LIST OF ENTRIES

A Alpha Calm Therapy®
Actinotherapy
Acu-points (see Tsubo Therapy)
Acupressure
Acupuncture
Acu-yoga
Alchemia Heart Breath
Alchemical Synergy®
Alexander Technique™
Alignment
AMMA Therapy®
Ampaku Therapy
Applied Kinesiology
Applied Physiology
Appropriate Touch
Aromatherapy
Aston-Patterning®
Aura Therapy
Autogenic Training
Avatar®
Ayurvedic Medicine

Barefoot Shiatsu (see Macrobiotic Shiatsu)
Bartenieff Fundamentals℠
Bates Method of Vision Training
Benjamin System of Muscular Therapy
Bindegewebsmassage
Bioenergetics
Biofeedback
Biomagnetics (see Magnetic Therapy)
Bladder Meridian
Body-centered Transformation
Body-Enlightenment®
Body-Mind Centering®
Bodymind Integration
Body Mind Integrative Therapy™
Bodywork for the Childbearing Year℠
Body Wraps
Bowen Body Balancing (see Fascial Kinetics)
Breath Therapy
Breema
Barbara Brennan Healing Science

Cayce/Reilly Massage
Chair Massage
Chakra Balancing
Chi (Ki) (Qi)
Chi Nei Tsang
Chinese Massage (see Tui-Na)
Chinese Medicine
Chiropractic
Chua Ka℠
Bonnie Bainbridge Cohen System (see Body-Mind Centering®)
Color Therapy
Conception Vessel (Meridian)
Connective Tissue
Connective Tissue Massage
Constitutional Massage℠ (also called Holistic Massage℠)
CORE Bodywork℠
Core Energetics®
CranioSacral Therapy℠
Cross-Fiber Friction (see Cyriax Massage)
Cryotherapy (see Ice Therapy)
Crystal Healing
Cupping
Cyriax Massage

Dance Injury Massage
Dance Therapy
Deep Massage
Deep Tissue Massage
Dō-In
Drama Therapy

Ear Therapy
Effleurage
Egoscue Method®
Electrical Current Therapy
Electromagnetics
Embodyment Training
Emotional-Kinesthetic Psychotherapy
Emotional Release
Energy Bio-field Work
Ericksonian Hypnotherapy

A

A Alpha Calm Therapy® an integrated system that uses ERICKSONIAN HYPNOTHERAPY, breathing exercises, meditation, Jacobson's progressive relaxation exercises (contraction/ release), GUIDED IMAGERY and self-hypnosis to reach the unconscious mind and change harmful behavior patterns.

The trance state can be a pleasant and rich experience for the client who, during a session, is encouraged to breathe deeply and regularly. She may experience personal insight, self-empowerment, a clear sense of direction and control of her life. Some people feel the effects after only one session, others after a few sessions.

Developed in 1991 by psychotherapist Hal Brickman, C.S.W., A Alpha Calm Therapy takes distorted messages from the unconscious mind and replaces them with healthy choices. Bad habits, such as overeating, and addictions, such as smoking or drug dependency, can be relieved through this personalized work.

actinotherapy (see ELECTROTHERAPY) harnesses the radiant energy, such as from the sun, to produce chemical changes. INFRARED RADIATION, a luminous form of actinotherapy, and ULTRAVIOLET RADIATION, a nonluminous form, are two types of radiant energy used for therapeutic purposes.

acu-points another term for TSUBO THERAPY, which treats the client by stimulating the ACUPUNCTURE points. Each point has a specific relationship with a body part or organ. Pressure on this point, in the form of finger, knuckle or elbow activation, promotes the free flow of healing energy to that region.

acupressure a Chinese massage system that dates back at least 4,000 years. This technique is documented in the oldest extant Chinese medical text, *Huangdi Nei Jing* (The Yellow Emperor's Classic of Internal Medicine) written between 300 B.C. and 100 B.C. by unknown authors. The Yellow Emperor, who may be a mythological figure, was said to have lived around 2697 B.C.–2596 B.C.

Acupressure theory is based on the precepts of CHINESE MEDICINE, a venerable and complex art and science that describes the physiology, pathology, diagnosis and treatment of the human body in intricate and mutually related, energetic terms. According to this theory, illness is caused by blockages or interruptions in the natural flow of vital energy, *qi* or CHI in Chinese, through the MERIDIANS, or energy pathways. These meridians make up a complex system of energy channels that circulate life's energy, blood and essence throughout the body. Meridians are associated with specific internal organs and body systems.

Acupressure stimulates specific points along the meridians, using thumb, finger or knuckle pressure, or with a blunt instrument called *tei shin*. This instrument is a small wooden knob with a rounded tip. Acupressure, which can often be self-administered, was developed to treat diseases, such as arthritis, release the blocked energy pathways to restore the normal flow of vital energy, and maintain health.

The terms acupressure (which is translated from the Chinese *zhi zhen liao fa* describing the finger movements) and SHIATSU, an ancient Japanese massage system that means finger (*shi*) pressure (*atsu*), are often used interchangeably, although there are some important distinctions between the two. Both systems are used to improve the flow of *qi* energy,[1] but acupressure uses all the pressure points of acupuncture (there are currently 365 acupuncture points, with this number growing as more of them are discovered), while shiatsu treats almost 660 points, called TSUBOS. Another distinction is the amount of pressure and stroke duration, with acupressure being somewhat softer in touch and longer in point-holding time. In contrast, shiatsu is more vigorous with firm pressure held for only three to five seconds.

The muscular system is directly involved in acupressure treatments. Accumulated muscle tension causes contractions around the points, which inhibit energy and blood flow. Pressure on these points releases the underlying tightness as well as stimulating the related organ systems along the particular meridian. By promoting the free flow of blood and *qi* energy, the body's innate ability to seek and maintain HOMEOSTATIC balance is enhanced. This is what is known as the body healing itself.

Acupressure is used to restore balance to the energy flow within the meridians, relieve pain, increase blood circulation, remove toxins from the tissues and treat many physical conditions such as sinus congestion, headaches, menstrual difficulties, the discomforts of pregnancy and labor, muscular aches and many others.

There are many explanations for acupressure's success. Acupressure stimulates the release of endorphins, those "feel-good" compounds, which mollify pain and promote a sense of well-being. During a treatment, there is an elongation of the muscle fibers, which contributes to the release of toxins and waste materials within the tissues, an increase in the circulation of oxygenated blood thereby promoting cellular nutrition, and a stronger resistance to disease. Through acupressure, the body is rebalanced, which also prompts a reduction in emotional and psychological tensions. As with most bodywork, there is a stronger sense of body awareness after an acupressure treatment.

The effects of acupressure are cumulative. Benefits from individual sessions can last as long as two to three days, with more regular, or weekly treatments, producing more long-lasting results.

The acupuncture points used in acupressure are sites on and near the surface of the skin that are sensitive to bioelectrical impulses. Western scientists have verified the existence of this bio-

energy through the use of sophisticated electrical devices that measure the electrical output of each pressure point. Yet it was through a painstaking evolution of trial and error that the ancient Chinese developed this complex system.

Acupressure achieves its results through local stimulation to points as well as through *referred,* or *trigger point,* relief, which produces a far-reaching effect elsewhere along the meridian. Pressure points are located by the use of anatomical references, such as their proximity to bone, and have Chinese names, which describe their nature, such as gall bladder 41, found in the depression between the fourth and fifth toes, means "almost crying," location, such as triple heater 14 found on the top of the shoulder and translates to "top of the shoulder," or benefit, such as spleen 10, or "ocean of blood," and helps release suppressed menses.

Traditional acupressure techniques are made up of pressing, pinching, pushing and rolling, friction, rubbing and stretching strokes. Pressing (*dian qia*) is done with the pad of the thumb pressed perpendicularly on a point. The pressure can be either gentle or strong, depending upon the desired effect. Pressing with the tips of several fingers (*dian kou*) covers a larger surface. In order to stimulate deep nerves, tendons, muscles or symmetrical points, a pressing and picking-up movement (*an ban*) is used. One finger presses on a point and another finger picks up the muscle in the opposite direction. Another deep technique is pinching (*nie na*), which pinches the skin between the thumb, index and middle fingers.

Short applications of pressure, under 10 seconds, will have a stimulating effect while longer pressure, from 10 seconds up to 3 minutes, will sedate.

The Chinese massage system of TUI-NA (*tui* means push and *na* means grasp or roll) is a type of acupressure massage. The pushing and rolling technique (*nie ji liao fa*) is performed by rolling the tissues on either side of the spine. This *tui-na* technique is beneficial to the circulation of energy within the channels, invigorates the blood by increasing the oxygen level and balances the digestive tract.

The friction techniques of acupressure (*gua sha liao fa*) are done briskly across the muscle fibers to unblock the stagnated energy. Rubbing is performed with a coin or smooth-edged spoon dipped in water and coated with tiger balm, a topical analgesic made of camphor and menthol, which brings heat and blood to an area. The acupuncture point is rubbed in only one direction.

Stretching the point, or contracting it, is done by holding the edges of an area with the fingertips of the left hand and curling the four fingers (the thumb is excluded from this stroke) of the right hand into the shape of a hook. The right hand is dipped into cold water and then pushed down repeatedly away from the left hand, stretching the skin.

Acupressure can be self-administered on those points that are accessible. Those which are difficult to reach can be stimulated by placing a soft ball on the point and rolling on it. Older or infirm people can lean against the ball while seated. The pressure should produce a "good hurt" in order to be deep enough to have an effect.

It is advisable to avoid acupressure when acute infections are present, immediately after meals or strenuous activity or in cases of skin diseases, ulcerations or inflammations near a point.

Notes
[1] *Qi* may also be spelled as *chi* or *ki*.

Further Reading
Bauer, Cathryn, *Acupressure for Everybody,* Owl Books, Henry Holt and Co., N.Y., 1991. This easy-to-understand book explains the history and philosophy of acupressure. Points for specific problems are provided.

———— , *Acupressure for Women,* Crossing Press, Freedom, Calif., 1987. Women's specific needs are addressed in this book, including menstruation, PMS, pregnancy, birthing, nursing and treatments for menopause. The book is clear and easy to understand, especially for women who are interested in taking care of themselves naturally.

Cerney, J.V., D.C., *Acupuncture without Needles,* Parker Publishing, West Nyack, N.Y., 1974. This illustrated book explains how to relieve pains and discomforts with acupressure in an easy-to-follow style.

Chan, Pedro, *Finger Acupressure,* Ballantine Books, N.Y., 1974. A perfect book for nonprofessionals who want to take care of themselves naturally. Thirty-seven specific acupressure treatments are provided.

Coseo, Marc, *The Acupressure Warm-Up for Athletic Preparation and Injury,* Paradigm Books, Brookline, Mass., 1992. This book details meridian stretching exercises, warm-up exercises and finger pressure techniques for athletic preparedness. Illustrations are provided and several 10-minute routines are suggested for pre-event readiness.

Teequarden, Iona Marsaa, M.A., L.M.F.E.C., *Fundamentals of Self-Acupressure,* Jin Shin Do® Foundation, Felton, Calif., 1989. The developer of Jin Shin Do offers easy-to-use techniques for the relief of many common ailments.

acupuncture an ancient, complex diagnostic and healing system that uses needles painlessly inserted in a specific pattern among the 365 points[1] found throughout the energy pathways, called MERIDIANS, to release energy blockages believed to cause disease. It is a major component of CHINESE Medicine, which also includes MOXIBUSTION,[2] or the use of burning herbs placed directly on acupuncture points, Chinese herbal medicine, massage and exercises to balance the body.

Acupuncture has been found to be effective in the treatment of pain, arthritis, gynecological problems, pain-free childbirth, asthma, chronic headaches and migraines, muscle tensions and general stress management. As an integral part of the traditional Chinese approach to healing, acupuncture can treat many illnesses, reduce the side effects of drug withdrawal and maintain optimum energy levels. People of all ages can be treated with acupuncture.

The Chinese may have developed acupuncture and moxibustion as early as the Stone Age when primitive knives and sharp instruments, called *bians,* were used for the treatments. The definition of *bians* dates back to 206 B.C.–A.D. 22 and comes from the *Shuo Wen Jie Zi* (Analytical Dictionary of Characters): ". . . *bian* means using stone to treat disease."[3] These stones were

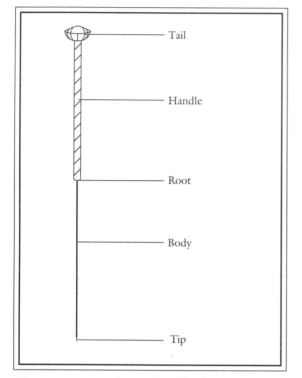

Tail

Handle

Root

Body

Tip

The most commonly used needle for acupuncture treatments is the filiform. Today's needles are disposable, sterilized, stainless steel instruments that consist of five parts: the tip (the part that is inserted into the acupuncture point), body, root, handle and tail.

eventually replaced with needles made of bone or bamboo. It is interesting to note that stones and arrows were the weapons of battle, and it did not go unnoticed when wounded soldiers reported relief from chronic symptoms after injury to certain points on their bodies.[4]

The ancients began to recognize a pattern that stimulation, even by means of injury, to certain parts of the body facilitated healing in other regions. They also observed that similar illnesses had common skin sensitivities, which all patients experienced. They ascertained that a series of points following a particular course affected the health of specific organs and systems. This eventually became the complex, but efficiently organized, system of the meridians, or energy pathways.

The extant *Huangdi Nei Jing* (The Yellow Emperor's Classic of Internal Medicine), c. 300–100 B.C., is the earliest recorded medical text on acupuncture, ACUPRESSURE, the Chinese system of massage, and moxibustion and is still considered to be an important reference source. The *Ling Shi* (Canon of Acupuncture) was part of this tome and described nine different acupuncture instruments called the "nine needles." Indian AYURVEDIC medicine also makes reference to acupuncture in its ancient text, the *Suchi Veda,* written at least 2,500 years ago, as the art of piercing with a needle.[5] This text laid the foundation for Ayurvedic teachings and healing art.

During the Shang dynasty (c. 1766–1122 B.C.), and the advent of bronze casting, metal needles started replacing the more primitive tools. The unique ability of metal to conduct heat, and years of trial and error, led to the discovery of the meridian or channel (*jingluo—jing* means "to go through" and *luo* means "something that attaches") system.

In the middle of the first century A.D., *Zhen Tiu Jia Yi Jing* (A classic of acupuncture and moxibustion) was written and established the names, numbers and locations of each point along the meridians. The characteristics and indications of each acupuncture point were described in great detail. Names were assigned according to their nature, location or benefit. The Imperial Medical College, which dates back to the Tan dynasty (A.D. 618–907), was probably one of the earliest medical schools to promote the use of acupuncture and moxibustion for treating illnesses.

In 1683, German doctor Engelbert Kämpfer introduced acupuncture to Europe. It took another 200 years before *The Medicine of China* was written and published in France in 1863. However, it wasn't until the 1940s, when the French diplomat Soulie de Morant published his stories about the Chinese art of healing, that Western physicians started to take a real interest in acupuncture.

In order to understand how acupuncture works, and the theories behind Chinese medicine, it is important to grasp the intercommunication between the meridians, organs and essence, or substances.

The intricate meridian system is an invisible network that connects organs and essence, or fundamental substances. They transport *qi* energy, blood (*hseuh*) and essence (*jing*) and connect the interior of the body with the exterior and are related to the internal organs. According to the theory of Chinese medicine, there are 12 **regular** channels that are symmetrically paired on the body and 8 **extra** channels. In addition, 15 **collateral** and 12 **subcollateral** channels provide the connecting network of all the channels.

The 12 regular channels, which are set deep in the muscles, are categorized according to the theory of YIN and YANG. This principle, an integral part of Chinese medicine, explains the relationships, patterns and the processes of natural change in the universe. It is based on the construct of polar opposites, which are dependent upon each other for health and balance.

The six yin meridians, LUNG, SPLEEN, HEART, KIDNEY, HEART CONSTRICTOR or PERICARDIUM, and LIVER correspond to the medial side of the body, the yin organs, and the upward flow of energy, while the six yang channels, LARGE INTESTINE, STOMACH, SMALL INTESTINE, BLADDER, TRIPLE HEATER or TRIPLE WARMER, and GALL BLADDER, relate to the lateral side of the body, the yang organs, and the downward flow of energy. The channels flow in a continuous circuit, starting with the lung meridian and ending with the liver.

Each of the channels has a complementary, but opposite, relationship with another meridian, one yin and one yang. This communication explains how they can affect each other when pathologies are present in the body. For instance, pathology or energy blockages within the lung meridian will have an adverse effect on its yang counterpart—the large intestine meridian.

The relationships of the regular meridians are:

Yin	*Yang*
Lung (Lu)	Large Intestine (LI)
Spleen (Sp)	Stomach (St)
Heart (H)	Small Intestine (SI)
Kidney (K)	Bladder (B)
Heart Constrictor (HC)	Triple Heater (TH)
Liver (Lv)	Gall bladder (GB)

These 12 regular channels are named according to three factors: whether the channel runs in the hand or the foot; whether it is a yin or yang meridian; and with which organ it corresponds. Internal organs are either **zang** or **fu,** meaning yin or yang, respectively. The six *zang* (yin) organs are the lung, spleen, heart, kidney, liver, and pericardium, whose physical organ is the parietal pericardium, or pericardial sac. The six *fu* (yang) organs are the large intestine, stomach, small intestine, bladder, gall bladder, and triple warmer, whose physical organ is most often considered to be the CONNECTIVE TISSUE network.

The eight extra channels do not relate to any internal organs, per se, but they do have important functions. These channels serve as reservoirs of *qi,* blood and *jing* for the regular meridians. Two of these extra channels, the GOVERNING VESSEL (GV) and the CONCEPTION VESSEL (CV) are thought of as regular channels because they contain independent acupuncture points not found on the other regular channels. The front midline yin conception vessel, *ren mai,* controls the functioning of all the yin meridians. *Ren* means "fostering and responsibility." The back midline yang governing vessel, *du mai,* controls the functioning of all the yang meridians. *Du* means "governing." These two extra channels are generally combined with the other regular channels to complete the classic meridian system.

The remaining 6 channels, regulate the *qi* of the 12 regular channels and strengthen and connect the internally/externally related meridians.

The remainder of the meridian system consists of various networks of interrelated channels. The 12 **chief branches,** which extend from the regular meridians, run deep in the body. They serve to connect the internal meridians with those that are external and are considered to be a continuation of the regular meridian system. Fifteen **collateral branches,** which also arise from the regular meridians, govern the body surface. Twelve **muscle branches** and twelve **cutaneous branches** are connected with their own regulating regular meridians. The muscle and cutaneous branches are the sites where *qi* and blood nourish the muscles, tendons and skin. The muscle regions are deeply distributed under the skin, and the cutaneous regions are located within the superficial layers of the skin.

When an illness occurs in any part of the body, the channels that pass through the afflicted area may be affected. It is also possible that if a disease affects a particular organ, it may manifest at any point along the respective channels. This helps to explain why an acupuncture treatment on one area of the body can have a beneficial effect elsewhere.

Points along the same channels share common characteristics. If the pathways cross each other, these **crossing points** also have common therapeutic properties.

In Chinese medicine, PULSE READING is considered to be a very effective way to make a diagnosis.[6] In acupuncture, however, pulse reading is used to confirm the diagnosis rather than formulate it. Six pulses are represented on the radial pulse of each arm. Three are superficial, and three are deep, relating to each of the 12 regular meridians. The practitioner feels for the strength or weakness of the beat and its overall rhythm, using six different types of pressure: light, moderately light, medium, moderately heavy, medium heavy and heavy. From this reading, he can determine where and what the problem is within the meridian system of the body.

The pulse found on the right hand corresponds to the yang (superficial) large intestine and yin (deep) lung and are located at the crease of the wrist. One *cun* away,[7] or approximately 1.31 inches, the yang stomach and yin spleen meridian can be palpated. The yang triple heater and yin heart constrictor are two *cun* away from the bend of the wrist. On the left hand, the yang small intestine and yin heart are found at the crease of the wrist, followed by the yang gallbladder and yin liver. Finally, two *cun* from the wrist are the yang bladder and yin kidney meridian pulses.

The acupuncture needles used today are disposable stainless steel. The method of insertion is also considered part of the treatment, and the depth of penetration, which should not draw blood, is generally guided by the anatomy of the body part. The *Ling Shi* (Canon of Acupuncture), part of the *Huangdi Nei Jing* (c. 300–100 B.C.) refers to the nine needles of acupuncture and describes their names, forms and applications.

The *chan* needle is 1.6 *cun* long and is used for external influences that have penetrated the body. The needle tip is arrow shaped and it is inserted at skin level. *Yuan* needle is 1.6 *cun* long, has a rounded tip and is used for superficial massage. *Di* needle is 3.5 *cun* and has a blunt tip, which does not penetrate, and is used on the surface of the skin. *Feng* is 1.6 *cun* and has a sharp edge, which is used for bleeding the acupuncture point. *Pi* is 4 *cun* and .25 *cun* wide. It has a very sharp tip and is used to open the skin and discharge pus. *Yuan li* is 1.6 *cun* and has a sharp, thick, round tip used to treat acute illnesses. *Hao* is 3.6 *cun* and fine. This needle can be left in place on the body and is used primarily to treat joint pain and paralysis. *Chang* is the longest needle, measuring 7 *cun*. It is thin and very sharp and is used in cases of paralysis and obstruction. The ninth needle is *da,* 4 *cun* long with a round, thick, sharp tip. It is used to treat articular swellings and to drain fluids from swollen joints.

The most common needle is *hao,* the filiform

needle, also called the fine or capillary needle. It can be made from gold, silver, alloy, or stainless steel, its most conventional form. When children receive acupuncture, the needle is appreciably smaller, measuring .05 *cun*.[8]

The popular filiform needle is made up of five parts: the tip, body, root, handle and tail. The tip is slightly rounded "like a fir needle, so it moves the blood vessels out of the way."[9] The body should be straight, flexible and consistent in diameter. The root joins the handle to the body. The handle is a tightly wound coil of wire, which should be proportionate to the body. At the end of the needle is the tail, which is a rounded projection.

Acupuncture treats illness by relieving energy blockages and restoring *qi* to an area. The needle can be manipulated to stimulate the arrival of this vital life force. "The most important thing in acupuncture is the arrival of *qi*."[10] The practitioner senses the resurgence of this energy by a gripping around the needle deep within the tissue.

The Chinese have developed very sophisticated techniques to restore *qi* to the ailing patient. The needle is worked in a number of ways to accomplish this goal. **Waiting for *qi*** (*hou qi*) repositions the needle without removing it until the *qi* arrives. A light tapping massage of the channel (*xun an*) is done around the point to bring the *qi* back to the affected area. **Moving *qi*** (*xing qi*) is done by actively manipulating the needle in many directions to stimulate the flow of energy. **Maintaining *qi*** provides the healthy sustenance of *qi* energy.

Electro-acupuncture was developed in Germany in 1934. A current is applied to the needle after insertion. It provides stronger stimulation to a point and affords more control for the practitioner.

Acupuncture can treat, and often cure, a myriad of symptoms. In addition to its therapeutic applications, electro-acupuncture is often used, in conjunction with pharmaceuticals and herbs, as an anesthetic in China, thereby decreasing the dosage of many conventional drugs. In ancient times, the acupuncturist had to constantly turn the needles by hand to produce the anesthetic effect until the medical procedure was completed. Endorphins, pain-controlling compounds, are released into the body when needles are inserted. These chemicals have been found to be almost 1,000 times stronger than morphine in suppressing the pain reflex. Cortisol, a natural anti-inflammatory, is also secreted during acupuncture treatments.

Acupuncture, when used prior and during surgical procedures, has many advantages over Western pharmacology. Since the placement of acupuncture needles in specific points can effectively reduce or eliminate pain, the patient can remain conscious during the surgery. Although pain is suppressed, all biological functions are maintained at normal levels. The patient's immune system is actually stimulated by the treatment, speeding up recovery. There are no harmful side effects of the acupuncture treatment, unlike the use of drugs. Patients who cannot undergo conventional anesthesia for a variety of reasons can tolerate acupuncture treatments. The needles are inserted at least 10 to 20 minutes before the surgery and are left in place throughout the procedure.

Notes

1. Kaptchuk, Ted J., O.M.D., *The Web That Has No Weaver*, Congdon & Weed, N.Y., 1983, p. 80. Classic acupuncture recognizes 365 points on the regular channels of the meridian system. However, miscellaneous points and advance technology have increased this number to at least 2,000.

2. Moxibustion was developed at the same time as acupuncture, but climatic differences made the use of thermal point (heat) stimulation necessary. Ignited herbs, such as mugwort, are placed on or near the acupuncture points, providing deep heat penetration.

3. Xinnong, Cheng, *An Outline of Chinese Acupuncture*, Foreign Languages Press, Beijing, 1975, p. 3.

4. Gach, Michael Reed, *Acupressure Potent Points*, Bantam Books, N.Y., 1990, p. 5.

5. Concon, Archimedes A., M.D., "Principles and Practice of Classical Chinese Acupuncture," *The Best of Health World*, Health Work Magazine, Inc., Burlingame, Calif., 1993, p. 52.

[6] The most respected book about pulse diagnosis is the *Mei Ching* (Classic of the Pulse) written by Wang Shu-ho (c. A.D. 280).

[7] Finding the points is done through a measurement of a *cun,* a proportional unit, which translates to 1.31 inches.

[8] Auterole, B., et al., *Acupuncture and Moxibustion—A Guide to Clinical Practice,* Churchill Livingstone, Edinburgh, 1992.

[9] Ibid., p. 6.

[10] Ibid., p. 2.

Further Reading

Chang, Stephen Thomas, Dr., *The Complete Book of Acupuncture,* Celestial Arts Publishing, Berkeley, Calif., 1976. Provides a concise explanation of the Five Element Theory, energy flow, meridians, procedures and points for treating specific problems.

Kaptchuk, Ted J., O.M.D., *The Web That Has No Weaver,* Congdon & Weed, N.Y., 1983. Considered by many to be a classic explanation and discussion of Chinese medicine. This book is filled with clear illustrations.

Mann, Felix, *Acupuncture,* Vintage Books, N.Y., 1973. Provides an easy-to-understand explanation of the way acupuncture works.

Marcus, Paul, M.D., *Thorson's Introductory Guide to Acupuncture,* Thorson's, HarperCollins, N.Y., 1984. Thorson guides provide simple, concise and instructive information about their subjects. *Introductory Guide to Acupuncture* is no exception.

Shanghai College of Traditional Medicine, *Acupuncture: A Comprehensive Text,* translated by John O'Connor and Dan Bensky, Eastland Press, Seattle, 1981. An extremely clear book in its detailed explanation of the history, applications, procedures and treatments of acupuncture. Illustrations clarify many of the topics.

Xinnong, Cheng, *Chinese Acupuncture and Moxibustion,* Foreign Language Press, Beijing, 1987. This is the revised edition to the classic text. A very detailed explanation of the history of acupuncture and its theories is provided. This book also discusses moxibustion, cupping, ear therapy and tongue diagnosis. Procedures for treating many conditions and anesthetic remedies are provided. Beijing, Foreign Languages Press, 1987.

acu-yoga increases the effectiveness of two ancient healing arts by combining them. ACU-PRESSURE and YOGA share the same holistic philosophy, which recognizes the unity of physical, emotional and spiritual awareness. Together, according to Michael Reed Gach, a massage practitioner who developed this system, their strengths complement and augment each other.

The points used in acupressure manipulate and release energy through the MERIDIANS, while the postures and breathing exercises of yoga purify and revitalize the body. Each posture presses and stretches the acupuncture points against the floor, energizing the meridians and releasing muscular tension.[1]

The breathing techniques of acu-yoga serve many different functions. The basic **breathing technique** is a long and deep breathing pattern used to balance the meridians. *HARA* breathing nourishes the internal organs. According to Eastern healing systems, the *hara,* located one and a half inches below the navel, is the center of the body's strength and energy. The emphasis of this breathing is the visceral organs. **Breath visualizations** encourage the infinite creativity of the mind. The **breath of fire** is used with postures to strengthen the nervous system, cleanse the blood and expand the electromagnetic field surrounding the body. The **holding breath** is a gentle massage of the internal organs.

Meditation is an integral part of acu-yoga. Coupled with the yoga postures, three contracted positions, called **locks,** are performed during the meditations to channel energy through the meridians.[2] The locks increase blood circulation, regulate the endocrine glands and rebalance the reproductive system.

The **root lock,** *mulabandha,* is a tightening of the rectum, sex organs and navel and affects the first (root) and second (sacral) CHAKRAS.[3] The **diaphragm lock,** *uddiyand bandha,* affects the diaphragm and the third (solar plexus) chakra. The **neck lock,** *jalandhara banda,* works on the chest and throat and the upper chakras, the heart, throat, third eye, or the sixth chakra located between the eyebrows, and seventh, crown chakra. The **master lock** is a combination of all three locks performed at once.

Acu-yoga can be performed daily as a way to maintain optimum health and prevent illness. Following the traditional Chinese theory that illnesses are caused by energy blockages along the meridians, acu-yoga can be used to treat specific problems by pressing and stretching the related acupressure points.

Notes

[1] The points used during an acupressure massage are identical to those used in acupuncture.

[2] Gach suggests that these locks be done under the supervision of a qualified yoga instructor.

[3] Chakra is a Sanskrit word, which means "wheel" or "revolving energy." There are seven major chakras, or energy centers, in the body starting at the base of the spine and continuing to the top of the head. Each chakra is linked to a specific organ, color, element, gland, function and sense.

Further Reading

Gach, Michael Reed, with Marco, Carolyn, *Acu-yoga,* Japan Publishing, Tokyo, 1981. This book introduces the philosophy of acu-yoga and provides a section on treating specific conditions. The photographs and illustrations make it an easy-to-follow book. The chapter on the acu-yoga exercises is divided into four parts relating to the spine and flexibility, chakras, regulating channels and organ meridians.

alchemia heart breath was developed by healer Kamala Renner, director of Dovestar Alchemian Institute, Hooksett, New Hampshire, in 1971 as part of the ALCHEMICAL SYNERGY work, a system of universal energy patterns. The physical and emotional changes she observed in her MASSAGE and YOGA clients compelled her to create a breathing system that would continue to develop and deepen personal growth.

Alchemia heart breath is used as an introductory step in discovering energy blockages, which may be held in the body. The system works with the rhythm of the breath directed throughout the body as well as yoga and REBIRTHING breathing exercises. Rebirthing breathing is used to heighten self-awareness and stimulate self-healing. Practitioners will sometimes gently touch the client in areas of tension to help him focus on his breathing.

A light trance state often results, which facilitates a clearer understanding of the causes of the disruptions in an individual's personal growth.

Alchemical Synergy® a system of the universal energy patterns as they were channeled to Kamala Renner, the founder of this system, from a group of spiritual entities. This process focuses on achieving personal transformation by using the **universal four forces: centripetal, centrifugal, gravity** and the **electromagnetic force.**

The centripetal force gives a person an opportunity for introspection, to find what individually designed path is right and natural for him to follow. The centrifugal force controls outward momentum, the interaction of the consciousness and the relationships with others. These two forces represent the classic **yin/yang,** or the duality, polar opposites, of nature.

The third force, gravity, regulates the action of the centripetal and centrifugal energies to provide balance. The electromagnetic force is the life force, which permits the continuing evolution and expansion of the consciousness.

Based on the laws of physics, Alchemical Synergy considers these four forces to be the originating structure of consciousness and are associated with specific characteristics. Balance between the forces ensures a healthy individual. Alchemical Synergy defines every experience in terms of the four forces. When an individual becomes aware of their influences on his life, he can start changing the patterns that are confining and stagnating.

When used as a tool of transformation, this system can help release inappropriate behavior and provide the client with the opportunity to get in touch with life's higher purpose. The ultimate goal of this work, is to help an individual contact his inner master, his center, and achieve maximum potential.

In 1944, when she was 11 years old, Kamala Renner died during surgery for a ruptured appendix. Her inert body was left unattended for at least 15 minutes during which time her spiritual body fought its way back to the physical plane. Years later, this experience resurfaced while she was undergoing HYPNOSIS and was verified by hospital records she subsequently secured.

The next year, she had another near-death experience, this time by drowning. Once again, she left her physical body only to return. At 26, while suffering from polio, she received injections that resulted in a fever of over 106°. For the third time in her life, Renner had a conscious memory of leaving her body.

Since recalling her first near-death experience, Renner has remained in contact with a group of spiritual beings called the White Light Brotherhood. The Brotherhood is composed of 12 male and 12 female spiritual entities. It was through this council's guidance and direction that Renner developed Alchemical Synergy, KRIYA MASSAGE™, REIKI-ALCHEMIA and ALCHEMIA HEART BREATH.

Alchemical Synergy is a composite of several disciplines. Hypnotherapy assists the client to reach his inner child, his spiritual guides, past lives, early childhood memories and to communicate with the different aspects of his personality.

The hands-on aspect of Alchemical Synergy could be any combination of Kriya Massage or Reiki-Alchemia. Kriya Massage was developed by Renner in 1970 and is defined as spontaneous energy movement. The practitioner massages her client while maintaining a dancelike, continuous motion. The practitioner must have a heightened sense of intuition in order to sense what the client requires to enable him to transform his ideas into those that will work for him. The strokes and techniques are taken from ENERGY WORK, SWEDISH MASSAGE, NEUROMUSCULAR THERAPY, and SOMA-EMOTIONAL RELEASE.

Reiki-Alchemia utilizes **keys,** or hand movements above the body, of different geometric shapes to allow healing and vibrational attunements to occur. Each key has its unique effect and practitioners must be properly trained in order to receive the knowledge to use them. Traditional REIKI is combined with the Alchemia model to provide a passive and active blend of healing energies. Etheric (physical), subconscious energy blockages and stored traumas may

be released during this work. The goal of Reiki-Alchemia is to reach a state of unconditional love.

Alchemia Heart Breath was developed in 1971, when Renner noticed changes in her massage and yoga clients' breathing patterns after their treatments. This work is the entrance level to understanding energy blockages. The heart breath works with the client's natural breathing rhythm combined with yoga and REBIRTHING breathing exercises. Rebirthing breathing is used to heighten self-awareness and stimulate the body's ability to heal itself. A light, noninvasive touch is sometimes used to bring attention to the client's breathing. A light trance state sometimes results from this work, which provides an opportunity for the client to retrace and correct obstructions in his personal growth.

Alexander Technique™   an educational process that teaches the client how to use his body properly. Tensions built up from the unbalanced use of the body during common daily activities create inefficient neuromuscular patterning and inhibit free movement, such as the simple activity of bending over and tying a shoe. The Alexander Technique corrects bad postural habits, releases tension and pain and restores joint mobility and optimum health. Alexander Technique provides the client with a greater awareness and control over his movements, which results in more energy and less pain.

Frederick Mathias Alexander (1869–1955) was a Shakespearean actor on the Australian stage. He suffered from frequent bouts of hoarseness and laryngitis, which his doctors and their medicines could not cure. Using a three-way mirror, he examined the way in which he was using his body while on stage and discovered a definite tension pattern between his head, neck and torso. He noticed that whenever he spoke on stage, he would pull his head back and down. When he corrected this posture, after many months, his voice returned. In the 1930s, he began teaching this technique to others and attracted many prominent actors and personages to his system.[1]

Although the technique does not address specific symptoms, Alexander believed that once the head/neck/torso alignment was restored, tensions would be released throughout the rest of the body. He believed that how we use our bodies affects the activity in which we are engaged. His technique provides a way to integrate movements with maximum balance and coordination. Although each session is individually designed, Alexander felt that an elongated spine, with the head balanced on top, would provide the primary focal point for proper body mechanics.

Each session, which is usually private, lasts between 45 and 60 minutes. The client is guided by an Alexander Technique practitioner through a series of individually designed hands-on and verbal instructions to bring awareness to simple movements, such as sitting and standing properly. Clients are asked to practice these instructions daily until they have developed appropriate postural habits.

Chair and massage table work is done in most sessions. The chair is a helpful tool in learning how to sit and stand without straining. The massage table work is completely passive for the client. The hands-on treatment, which elongates the muscles and releases spasms, provides a noninvasive way to lengthen and widen the body, thereby releasing tensions and gaining a new perspective of alignment. A minimum of 10 sessions is required to understand the basic principles of this system.

VISUALIZATION exercises, using mental imagery and thoughts to create a picture of the body, seek to lengthen the torso, freeing it from the pull of gravity, are incorporated into the Alexander Technique.

Modern stresses, emotional factors, possibly genetics and poor habits all contribute to the loss of the kinesthetic sense, the ability to perceive self-movement. The Alexander Technique restores this feeling of movement by providing a means of achieving coordination, fuller and deeper breathing, improved internal organ functioning, stress reduction, improved joint flexibility and fewer joint disorders and a release of psychosomatic and emotional symptoms. Self-confidence and self-esteem are reestablished and physical skills are improved.

Alexander believed that the correct mental outlook was of paramount importance in effecting any physical change. He felt that the client has to be open to new ideas and concepts about himself. Old response patterns, called **inhibitions**, had to be altered before the physical habits could change.

The Alexander Technique has gained international popularity and acceptance and has become a part of the curricula of many prestigious schools around the world.[2]

Notes

[1] Among Alexander's famous clientele are George Bernard Shaw, John Dewey, Aldous Huxley and Lillie Langtry. Kevin Kline, Paul Newman, John Cleese, et al., have all benefited by working with Alexander practitioners.

[2] Julliard School (N.Y.), Boston University, New York University, Los Angeles Philharmonic Institute, London Academy of Music, Royal College of Music (London), etc.

Further Reading

Alexander, F. Mathias, *The Use of Self*, Centerline Press, Long Beach, Calif., 1986. Posthumously published, this book describes the principles and exercises of the Alexander Technique.

Caplan, Deborah, *Back Trouble: A New Approach to Prevention and Recovery Based on the Alexander Technique*, Triad Publishing Co., Gainesville, Fla., 1987. The author asserts that many back problems can be avoided or treated by demonstrating the use of proper body mechanics based on the teachings of F. Mathias Alexander.

Gelb, Michael, *Body Learning: An Introduction to the Alexander Technique*, Henry Holt and Co., N.Y., 1987. This book gives an overview of the history, theory and practice of the Alexander Technique.

Gray, John, *Your Guide to the Alexander Technique*, St. Martin's Press, N.Y., 1990. An easy-to-follow guide about the principles of the Alexander Technique.

Leibowitz, Judith, and Connington, Bill, *The Alexander Technique: The World Famous Method for Enhancing Posture, Stamina, Health and Well-Being and for Relieving Tension and Pain*, Harper & Row, N.Y., 1990. This book details the history, principles, exercises and applications of the Alexander Technique.

Stevens, Chris, *Alternative Health: Alexander Technique,* Mac-Donald Optima, Boston, Mass., 1988. A discussion of the Alexander Technique citing its applications and history.

alignment   defined in *The Random House Dictionary* as "arrangement in a straight line; to bring into line; to ally (oneself) with a group, cause, etc.; to form a line."[1] This term, used by chiropractors, osteopaths and other health care providers, refers to the structural balance and optimum functioning of the spine and corresponding musculature. Although perfect alignment is difficult to achieve and maintain due to daily activity, the spinal vertebrae can be professionally **adjusted,** or moved, to reposition them correctly.

Notes
[1] *The Random House Dictionary,* Ballantine Books, N.Y., 1978, p. 21.

AMMA Therapy®   in Chinese, *amma* means "push-pull." The ancient Chinese believed that rubbing or massaging a painful area would bring relief. This system, which is involved with the balance and movement of life energy (QI), is at least as old as ACUPUNCTURE and MOXIBUSTION. From the time of Huangdi, the Yellow Emperor, 5,000 years ago, the practice of manipulation along energy pathways, or MERIDIANS, was used to treat diseases. AMMA practitioners rely on their hands to work with and balance the life energy force along these channels.

AMMA is a combination of many therapeutic massage techniques: SHIATSU's deep pressure and acupuncture point stimulation, FOOT REFLEXOLOGY, DEEP FASCIAL and CONNECTIVE TISSUE MASSAGE, CHINESE (TUI-NA) and SWEDISH MASSAGE techniques and the skeletal manipulation of *chiropractic.*

The goal of AMMA is to balance and maintain proper energy flow. The **homeodynamic** state, a condition of balance and harmony within an organ system, is sought. The work is done along the 14 regular meridians of acupuncture (lung, large intestine, stomach, spleen, heart, small intestine, bladder, kidney, heart constrictor, triple heat, gall bladder, liver, governing vessel and conception vessel) as well as lesser-known channels, such as the tendino-muscle and connecting channels.

The interest in AMMA has been regenerated by Korean-born Tina Sohn. When she was 12 years old, two intense emotional traumas caused her to fall into a coma for 30 days. After regaining consciousness, she started to have empathic experiences of people, feeling their pain. Following years of intense study and discipline, she developed acute sensitivities and diagnostic skills. These talents are now passed on to her students.

AMMA practitioners must have both physical strength and a deep understanding of anatomy and physiology. They have to develop their own emotional natures in order to understand and be able to help others. Manual sensitivity, which plays a fundamental role in AMMA, must be increased and spiritually heightened.

The precepts of CHINESE MEDICINE, dating back at least 5,000 years, are applied to AMMA: an imbalance in the forces of YIN and YANG may create illness. The ancient Chinese **Eight Principle Theory** of disease classification is used in AMMA. This is a method of categorizing illnesses according to yin or yang, hot or cold, external or internal and excess or deficient.

AMMA shares many, though not all, of the traditional acupuncture points found along the meridians. Those points, which are common to both systems, are called *ah shui* points, which translates to mean "ouch."

The hands of the practitioner are sensors and tools. They can feel and interpret subtle changes and the flow of energy within the channels. The main hand techniques of AMMA are circular pressure, the movement used most often, directly on a point; direct pressure to the point; embracing, where the hand draws a body part up into the palm; and percussion, a type of vibratory tapping.

Each of the strokes can be applied in a variety of ways. Circular pressure may be performed with the thumbs, fingers, palmar surface, ulnar surface (surface of the pinkie finger) or the heel of the palm. Direct pressure may be applied into a point with the thumbs or the fingertips. Stroking may involve thumbs, fingers, palms or loose fists. Embracing is a palmar technique, which draws the body part up in a vertical direction, or a thenar (ball of thumb) technique, which pulls in a horizontal direction. Percussion is performed by cupping in a loose, tentlike hand formation or chopping with the ulnar surface.

The practitioner may sit or stand during a treatment, which generally lasts one hour. The client is lying faceup, clothed, on a massage table. The session usually begins with a massage at the client's head and proceeds down the body. In the prone position, the treatment starts on the back and proceeds down the legs. Points all along the channels are pressed, squeezed or lifted.

Tina Sohn delineates specific principles of AMMA treatment for the practitioners:

1. Physical and emotional health must be maintained by the practitioner to ensure the fluent flow of energy with the client
2. The hands are tools that are guided by the body and the *hara*, which is the center of the body and the source of life's vital energy
3. Appropriate use of the body and proper body alignment is essential for a relaxed treatment
4. The hands should be relaxed at all times
5. Two-handed contact should always be maintained
6. The hand should gather information about the client's physical condition as well as treat
7. The rhythm of the treatment should be maintained throughout the treatment
8. The direction of the treatment follows the lines of the muscle fibers, never across them
9. A clear goal of treatment should be established before beginning each session.

Further Reading

Sohn, Tina, and Finando, Donna, *AMMA: The Ancient Art of Oriental Healing,* Healing Arts Press, Rochester, Vt., 1988. This instructional text offers beginning practitioners the philosophy, principles and practice of AMMA ther-apy. Clear illustrations are provided in the demonstration of the basic, full-body massage technique.

Sohn, Tina, *AMMA Therapy: The Ancient Art of Oriental Healing,* Healing Arts Press, Rochester, Vt., 1988. This book describes the techniques and treatments of AMMA, which combine Oriental medicine theories with Western anatomy and physiology. This is an illustrated guide, which provides specific treatment therapies and nutritional recommendations.

ampaku therapy (see HARA) or ampuku therapy is a diagnostic SHIATSU massage in the abdominal region of the body called the *hara.* The *hara* represents the core and origin of the body's vital energy and strength. In Japanese culture, the *hara* has an inviolability that is echoed throughout the language and the culture. There are specialists who work solely on the *hara* with ampaku therapy. All organs of the body are represented in the *hara,* so work on this limited area has far-reaching effects.

applied kinesiology a physical evaluation system, developed from the chiropractic profession, that uses manual muscle testing to assess the functioning of the body. It was developed in 1964 by Dr. George G. Goodheart, D.C. A patient came to see him with a severe dysfunction of the serratus anterior (anticus) muscle, which caused his scapula (shoulder blade) to "wing" out. Goodheart palpated tender nodules on the insertion[1] of the muscle and proceeded to apply pressure for a few minutes. The pain disappeared and the function of the muscle was restored.

Over a period of time, Goodheart came to recognize that in the absence of obvious pathology, postural distortions manifest themselves with muscles that "fail" muscle testing. Applied kinesiology has advanced beyond using muscle testing as its only assessment tool. Since Dr. Goodheart was skilled in chiropractic as well as MERIDIAN THERAPY, JOINT MOBILIZATION, MYOFASCIAL THERAPIES, reflex procedures, clinical nutrition, CRANIAL TECHNIQUE and other health systems, they all have become incorporated in applied kinesiology.

Applied kinesiology lists the **triad of health** as the three fundamental places where illnesses may manifest: chemical, mental and structural. The chemical aspect of the triangle focuses on illnesses resulting from drugs, allopathic (Western medical practice) medicines, poor nutrition or environmental toxicity. The mental approach is represented by problems, which result in employing psychiatric or psychological therapies, counseling, ministerial intervention or the mind's effect on the body. Structurally, the body is healed by bodyworkers and doctors. The effects of physical traumas or structural anomalies can result in the breakdown of the structural side of the triangle. In applied kinesiology, the triad of health is always evaluated, since it is believed that all health problems stem from one, or several of its parts.

The core of applied kinesiology is its examination procedures. The advantage in using this system is the immediate information that it supplies. The test results will provide instantaneous answers to the location of the problem, which kind of corrections would be most beneficial and if those therapies achieved their goals. As a functional assessment, it is used in conjunction with many other standard diagnostic techniques, including the client's medical history, a physical examination and laboratory tests. After an evaluation has been established, the corrections can include spinal or cranial adjustments, massage, neurolymphatic or neurovascular point work or meridian therapy.

According to applied kinesiology theories, there is a direct relationship between muscles and specific internal organs or glands. This viscerosomatic link explains how applied kinesiology can find the problems: when an organ is weak, dysfunctional or diseased, it may result in its related muscle failing the simple test. There are a number of reasons why this muscle might fail: myofascial dysfunction (injury or trauma to the fibrous membrane covering and separating muscles), peripheral nerve entrapment (pressure on the nerves causing a weakness to its corresponding muscle or organ) or nerve damage,

spinal SUBLUXATIONS, neurological dysfunctions, poor nutrition and eating habits, toxicity in the body, cerebrospinal fluid imbalance, MERIDIAN blockages, or LYMPHATIC sluggishness.[2] Applied kinesiology helps the practitioner ascertain which of these causes is applicable to the client.

The muscle test is a precise indication of a weakness within the body. It evaluates the ability of the nervous system to counter against resistance. The client lifts a particular limb in the position of its function and tries to hold that position against the practitioner's resistance. If the client can maintain the position, the muscle and its related organ or gland are considered to be strong. A muscle that cannot tolerate the minimal pressure will fail, exposing an area of internal weakness.

Accurate testing is of paramount importance. The International College of Applied Kinesiology® provides guidelines for appropriate testing.[3] A practitioner must be knowledgeable in anatomy and physiology and understand functional and synergistic involvement.[4]

1. There must be proper position to the "prime mover," or the muscle being tested
2. The regional anatomy must be stabilized. It is important to avoid recruitment of any other muscles
3. There must be a careful observation of the client's test position
4. There must be a careful observation of the test performance
5. The timing, pressure and position of the test must be consistent
6. It is important to avoid any preconceived ideas of the test outcome, since they can alter the results
7. There should be no pain during the procedure
8. Considerations must be made with respect to the client's physical condition, age, pain level and any other contraindication

The practitioner must also be aware that the test results can be sabotaged by many factors:

1. Transient, unintended directional force to the spine or skeletal system
2. Incorrect stretching of joints, tendons or ligaments
3. If the patient is touching her skin over the area of the dysfunction, called **therapy localization**
4. A repetitive contraction of the muscles
5. Fumes from chemicals
6. Food or nutritional supplements in the mouth
7. A particular phase of breathing
8. Negative mental imagery
9. Any other sensory stimulation that is disruptive[5]

Applied kinesiology has been used to treat many conditions that go undiagnosed by standard medical testing. Very often, a client will complain of "just not feeling well" but not be able to pinpoint anything specific, such as a general malaise. Because of its unique approach to the body, muscle testing directs the practitioner directly to the problem.

Applied kinesiology is also a "functional biomechanics" since it involves an assessment of posture, gait and joint range of motion.

The evaluation procedures of applied kinesiology make it a unique science. In addition to muscle testing, some other examination procedures include reading the client's body language, **challenge, therapy localization,** postural analysis, the **temporal sphenoid line** and the meridian system. Muscle testing can also be used to analyze chemical and nutritional needs. A weak muscle will test strong when the proper amount of supplementation, such as vitamin, mineral or herb, is placed in the client's hand or mouth.

Reading body language is a powerful tool in understanding the client's problems. Structural irregularities can manifest themselves in muscle imbalances or skeletal misalignments. Energy blockages in the meridian system can provide thermal clues. In this instance, regions of the body will feel hot or cool, depending upon the excess or deficiency of energy. The motion and interrelationship of the cranial-sacrum-pelvic structures can be palpated, and the presentation, or posture, of the body itself as a diagnostic tool is understood by the applied kinesiologist.

Challenge is the body's reaction to both positive and negative stimuli.[6] The effect is measured in conjunction with a muscle test. The challenge can be done in many ways. A specific force can be placed into a joint or placed into the joint with specific vectors. These vectors, or directions, will provide information on how to correct the joint's function.

When a client touches an area of dysfunction, it will cause the corresponding muscle to test weak. This is known as **therapy localization.** It indicates that something is wrong but not what it is. It must be further confirmed through other diagnostic techniques.

Postural analysis helps the practitioner recognize which muscles are involved in the client's imbalance. In most cases, the primary cause of postural imbalance is the weak, hypotonic muscle, not the one that is contracted, or hypertonic.

The **temporal sphenoid line** (TS line) is one of the most important diagnostic tools in applied kinesiology. Discovered by Major B. DeJarnette, D.C., and developed by M.L. Rees, D.C., it was originally used to correspond only with organs. But Dr. Goodheart found that it also had a correlation with the muscle/organ/gland/vertebral relationship.[7] Located on both sides of the cranium, the TS line contains diagnostic points that become tender nodules when organs and muscles are dysfunctional. The sensitivity, which is required in this diagnostic technique, is difficult to master, but the TS line is an integral part of the evaluation system of applied kinesiology.

The TS line starts in front of the ear and proceeds to the middle of the temple. From there, it extends upward for about 1 inch, when it returns to the scalp along the temporoparietal suture, the juncture of the temporal and parietal cranium bones of the skull. It ends on that suture, about 1 inch behind the ear.

The MERIDIAN system of Chinese ACUPUNCTURE

is put to diagnostic and therapeutic purposes in applied kinesiology. Vertebral manipulation often affects the meridians through stimulation to the **associated points,** which can correlate with any meridian imbalance. There is also clinical evidence that they are associated with vertebral subluxations.[8] Correcting structural imbalances improves the flow of energy throughout the meridian system.

Neurolymphatic and **neurovascular points** (or **reflexes**) are used to treat weakened muscles. Neurolymphatic points were discovered by Dr. Frank Chapman, D.O., in the 1930s, for stimulation of lymphatic drainage throughout the body. A clinically ''active'' neurolymphatic reflex will have a weak associated muscle strengthened by therapy localizing the point. Neurovascular points affect circulatory function. Discovered by Dr. Terrence J. Bennett, D.C., these reflexes used in applied kinesiology are generally found in the head, unlike those of Chapman's, which are found all over the body. A clinically ''active'' neurovascular point will have a weak associated muscle made strong by therapy localizing the reflex.

Every muscle has an associated organ or gland. A partial list gives a general idea of the interrelationships.

Muscle	Organ/Gland	Meridian
Biceps Brachii	Stomach	Stomach
Triceps Brachii	Pancreas	Spleen
Deltoid	Lung	Lung
Serratus Anterior	Lung	Lung
Latissimus Dorsi	Pancreas	Spleen
Trapezius	Eye/Ear	Kidney
Gastrocnemius	Adrenals	Heart Constrictor
Rectus Abdominus	Small Intestine	Small Intestine
Quadriceps	Small Intestine	Small Intestine
Hamstrings	Rectum	Large Intestine
Gluteus Maximus	Reproductive	Heart Constrictor
Psoas	Kidney	Kidney

Notes

1. The origin and insertion of a muscle are its attachment points. Generally, when a muscle contracts, the insertion of the muscle moves toward the origin.
2. International College of Applied Kinesiology, U.S.A., ''Applied Kinesiology Status Statement,'' International College of Applied Kinesiology, Lawrence, Kans., 1992, p. 1.
3. Ibid., p. 3.
4. A synergist is a muscle that helps the prime mover, or the main muscle, perform its function. An applied kinesiologist must be able to test the prime mover without synergistic involvement.
5. International College of Applied Kinesiology, U.S.A., ''Applied Kinesiology Status Statement,'' International College of Applied Kinesiology, Lawrence, Kans., 1992, p. 2.
6. Walther, David S., *Applied Kinesiology, Vol. I: Basic Procedures and Muscle Testing,* SDC Systems DC, Pueblo, Colo., 1981, p. 25.
7. Ibid., p. 39.
8. Ibid., p. 135.

Further Reading

Biokinesiology Institute, *Muscle Testing,* Biokinesiology Institute, Shady Cove, Oreg., 1982. This easy-to-use guide explains the techniques of self-administered muscle strengthening. The emotional associations, nutritional recommendations, possible causes of disease and massage remedies are listed, with illustrations, for 69 symptoms.

Diamond, John, M.D., *Your Body Doesn't Lie,* Warner Books, N.Y., 1989. An easy-to-follow book on how muscle testing can improve your health and energy.

Kendall, Henry O., P.T., Kendall, Florence P., P.T., and Wadsworth, Gladys E., P.T., *Muscle Testing and Function,* 2d ed., Williams & Wilkins, Baltimore and London, 1971. A comprehensive professional text of muscle-testing techniques. Clear illustrations and photographs elucidate this precision system. The explanations are technical and the book is a wonderful reference text.

La Tourelle, Maggie, and Courtenay, Anthea, *Thorson's Introductory Guide to Kinesiology—Touch For Health,* Thorsons Pub., San Francisco, Calif., 1993. The history of Applied Kinesiology and Touch For Health is clearly detailed. Self-help techniques are listed for many common symptoms.

Walther, David S., *Applied Kinesiology, Vol. 1: Basic Procedures and Muscle Testing,* SDS Systems DC, Pueblo, Colo., 1981. A professional text of the first module of applied kinesiology. Illustrations and photographs clarify the techniques. The history, theories and muscle-testing procedures are technically explained. This is an excellent reference book.

———, *Applied Kinesiology: Synopsis.* SDS Systems DC, Pueblo, Colo., 1988. This professional tome covers postural analysis, applied kinesiology testing, meridian analysis, neurological disorders and provides an in-depth discussion of applied kinesiology.

applied physiology a stress management system that allows the body to express what is out of balance and provides information to restore that balance. It instructs how to detach from unhealthy attitudes, which may contribute to the development of disease.

After being diagnosed with a serious illness for which there was no cure, Richard Utt sought the help of a chiropractor, Dr. Sheldon Deal of Tucson, Arizona, who practiced APPLIED KINESIOLOGY. The treatments assisted Utt in his recovery and interested him enough to study the discipline. In the 1980s, he created a new system, called applied physiology, partially based on his knowledge of applied kinesiology.

Utt felt that conventional healing methods never address powerful, negative dispositions. Applied physiology purports that disease is a sign that certain physical and metaphysical laws have been compromised and need correction in order to ensure health and spiritual growth.

This muscle-monitoring technique combines BIOFEEDBACK with Utt's **seven element theory** and CHINESE MEDICINE'S FIVE ELEMENT THEORY. The Chinese theory classifies everything as either metal, wood, fire, water or earth. To this, Utt added air and ether to create his seven element theory, which provides for the lateral, vertical and horizontal movement of energy. This Figure 8, three-dimensional energy pattern is based on the **holographic super-theory** of reality first discovered in 1794 by Gottfried Wilhelm von Liebniz, who developed integral and differential calculus.

Applied physiology research shows a relationship **between** each muscle and an **object meridian**. This technique, as in applied kinesiology, is done by monitoring a particular muscle, called the **indicator muscle**. This makes it possible to ascertain the energy within its related organ or system. It is used to provide communication between the muscle and the organs and systems of the body. As a muscle is put through its RANGE OF MOTION and monitored, it changes its meridian association. It is monitored at various points to determine where the stresses lie within the body.

Once these areas are identified, the applied physiologist uses ACUPRESSURE techniques, neurolymphatic or neuromuscular stimulation, sound or rhythmic music, color, flower essences such as lavender or rose, or positive affirmations to relax the client. The overall goal of the treatment is to let go of the stress within the holographic body by integrating the physical, mental, emotional and spiritual components of an individual. Applied physiology has been used successfully to increase the muscle coordination in muscular dystrophy and polio victims and control allergic reactions.

Further Reading The following books have been written by Richard Utt and published by Applied Physiology Publishers, Tuscon, Ariz.
Muscle Monitoring Workbook, 1993.
Attitude with Essence Workbook, 1993.
Seven-Element Figure 8's Workbook, 1992.
Can-Opener Workbook, 1994.
Seven-Element Anatomy and Physiology Holographic Workbook, 1988.

appropriate touch a bodywork treatment for survivors of sexual and physical abuse created by massage therapist Bob Yoder in 1989. Yoder recognized that many aspects of traditional massage therapy were inappropriate for abuse survivors due to their associations with "bad touch."

Appropriate touch respects the client's needs and wants, while honoring her personal boundaries and past experiences. This system is concerned with more than the hands-on aspects of treatment. The practitioner must keep in mind his client's reticence to touch and make the working environment as safe and as comfortable as necessary.

For example, a well-lit room shows no hidden corners but is not too bright to appear antiseptic or foreboding. Dimmer switches can adjust the lighting level, so the client feels comfortable. Keeping the door of the treatment room closed may provoke anxiety in a survivor. Here too, the practitioner must sensitize himself to the client's wishes. Incense and candles could provide a sense of security to some clients. They may also be a terrifying reminder of ritual abuse to others.

The practitioners of appropriate touch are aware that their manner and proper attire are important in creating a safe feeling. They learn how to stay focused on the client's needs, so that recovery is not hindered by the therapist's own touch issues and personal history. The gender of the practitioner ought not make a difference, since this is a professional service and setting. A physical history should be medical in scope, permitting the client to explain, if and when she is ready, the origin of the pain or injury.

The practitioner does not probe into the client's life but lets it unfold at her own pace. Since most massage treatments require the client to be nude, although draped and covered at all times, the appropriate touch practitioners are proficient in fully clothed techniques as well. It is important to let the client dictate how much clothing she feels safe removing.

Although appropriate touch is not used to learn about past abuse, it is not uncommon for the nature of touch therapy to induce flashbacks. Practitioners of appropriate touch recognize this phenomena and can bring the client back to the present moment without embarrassment or shame, which is so often associated with abuse.

An important distinction makes this system different from most other healing systems: appropriate touch is not linear. Setbacks are common and expected. It is important to continue honoring the bravery of the survivor to confront her demons and to provide a safe haven to feel whatever she needs.

This system can be combined with many forms of touch therapy. Regardless of the form that is used, appropriate touch offers a healthy and nurturing way for survivors to relearn the pleasures of touch.

aromatherapy the use of essential plant and vegetable oils is most commonly associated with **massage,** although they are properly added to bath waters, used in herbal wraps, constitute primary ingredients in perfumes and cosmetics, are burned as incense or are taken internally as medicines. The aromatherapy massage employs a combination of SWEDISH MASSAGE and SHIATSU techniques. The goals of the practitioner are to provide a deeply relaxing treatment (or a stimulating one, depending on the oils used in the lubricant) and to work on problem areas, which the client may have.

The therapeutic action of the essential oils take place either through skin absorption or through the respiratory tract as inhaled vapors. The aroma of the herbs also contributes to their healing effect. In order for the essences to penetrate during a massage, the skin must be clean and free of toxins and dirt. Heating the skin, either with rapid rubbing (friction) or by applying a moist, heated cloth before the treatment, opens the pores and allows the oils to be absorbed.

Fragrance molecules reach the brain through inhalation. The cells of the olfactory **membranes** in the nasal cavity are bring cells. In fact, this **membrane** is the only place in the body where the central nervous system is in direct contact with the external environment. With each breath, we smell.

There are several theories explaining the olfactory sense, or the sense of smell. One theory maintains that substances emit gaseous particles, which dissolve in the mucus of the nasal membrane. This fluid chemically acts upon the nasal hairs to create a nerve impulse. Another theory suggests that radiant energy, given off by the stimulating substance, is the actual stimulant, rather than smell molecules. A final belief holds that smell molecules are fat soluble and are dissolved directly into the nasal membrane where a nerve impulse is created.

Pheromones, hormonelike substances secreted by each person, influence physical attraction. Memories and emotions can be recalled or stimulated from odors. Within the limbic system, the oldest part of the brain, neurotransmitters are released that create specific responses. Fragrances govern the functioning of sexuality, attraction and aversion, moods, memory and creativity, etc., within this system.

The first recorded use of aromatherapy can be traced back to ancient Egypt, where priests were the first practitioners. They made incense, religious unctions and perfumes from aromatics. Physicians soon followed by incorporating essential oils and herbs in medicinal formulas. Papyrus records exist, dating from 2800 B.C., that describe herbal remedies. Oils were even used in their mummification process.

Essential botanical and vegetable oils have been used in a variety of ways throughout history. In 1660, the famous herbologist, astrologer and physician, Nicholas Culpeper, wrote *Arts Master-Piece, or the Beautifying Part of Physick,* which contained herbal recipes for health and beauty. Many of his formulas are still being prepared commercially today.

The oils come from all parts of the plant: leaves, flowers, barks, roots, resins and fruit rinds. The chemical composition of the essences can change according to which part of the plant they come from and the soil and climatic conditions. The essences are usually clear, although slight coloration can be found in some oils.

Essences are extracted through a variety of methods. Distillation is the most common procedure. The plant matter is placed in a vat and steamed. The essences evaporate and are then cooled. Since they are not water soluble, the oils separate from the water and are collected. The plant material is washed in an appropriate solvent until it dissolves. Separation takes place by heating the solution, which condenses the oil. A third technique is squeezing, most often used for citrus fruits. The fruit peel is removed and hand squeezed over a bucket.

Aromatics are highly volatile, meaning that they can evaporate easily in the open air. In order to ensure potency, they should be stored in airtight, dark glass containers and kept in a cool, dry environment.

The medicinal and therapeutic properties of herbs have been recognized since ancient times. Many of today's pharmaceuticals are adapted from herbal sources. As such, the dosage and combination of essential oils are determined by a client's constitution and illness. The appropriate mixture can alter a client's physical condition as well as her state of mind. In most cases, when treating with herbs, the treatments should not exceed four weeks.

The medicinal action of herbs has been classified as follows:

Abortive—causing abortion in high doses

Adrenal Cortex Stimulants

Analgesic—pain relieving (e.g., eucalyptus)

Anaphrodisiac—lessening sexual desire

Anodyne—pain relieving

Anthelmintic—expelling intestinal worms

Antibilious—relieving bile

Anticonvulsive—inhibiting convulsions and seizures

Antidepressive—uplifting (e.g., bergamot)

Antiemetic—controlling vomiting

Antiphlogistic—reducing vascular inflammation

Antiseptic—inhibiting bacterial growth (e.g., chamomile)

Antispasmodic—controlling muscle spasms (e.g., hissop)

Antisudorific—inhibiting perspiration

Antitoxic—defeating poisons

Aphrodisiac—stimulating sexual desire (e.g., cardamon)

Astringent—contracting tissues

Carminative—promoting expulsion of intestinal gas and easing gripping pains (e.g., frankincense)

Cephalic—stimulating to the mind

Cholagogue—stimulating the flow of bile from the gallbladder

Choletic—increasing secretion of bile

Cicatrizant—promoting the formation of scar tissue

Cordial—toning for the heart (e.g., benzoin)

Cytophyletic—regenerating cells

Demulcent—relieving inflammation

Deodorant—inhibiting body odor (e.g., clary sage)

Depurative—purifying the blood

Digestive—aiding digestion (e.g., peppermint)

Diuretic—increasing urine production

Emetic—promoting vomiting

Emmenagogue—pertaining to the female reproductive system (e.g., myrrh)

Emollient—softening and soothing inflammations

Expectorant—promoting the expulsion of respiratory catarrh (e.g., cedarwood)

Febrifuge—reducing fever (e.g., camphor)

Galactagogue—increasing flow of milk (e.g., fennel)

Hemostatic—stopping blood flow

Hepatic—pertaining to the liver

Hypertensor—raising blood pressure

Hypoglycemiant—lowering blood sugar

Hypotensor—lowering blood pressure

Laxative—promoting bowel movement (e.g., fennel)

Mucilaginous—a substance of thickness soothing to inflamed areas

Nervine—promoting nerve relaxation

Ophthalmicum—remedy for eye diseases

Parturient—easing labor pains

Rubefacient—stimulating circulation (e.g., black pepper)

Sedative—calming to the nervous system (e.g., marjoram)

Splenetic—tonic for the spleen

Stimulant—exciting systems of the body (e.g., ylang-ylang)

Stomachic—a tonic for the stomach (e.g., chamomile)

Tonic—providing tone to particular systems of the body

Uterine—a tonic for the uterus (i.e., clary sage)

Vasoconstrictor—constricting capillaries (e.g., cypress)

Vermifuge—eliminating intestinal worms (e.g., bergamot)

Vulnerary—an external, topical agent for healing wounds and sores (e.g., benzoin)

The use of herbs, in appropriate dosages, has been used to treat many symptoms. The following is a brief list of common ailments and a partial inventory of the herbs used to treat them:

Allergies—chamomile, balm

Anxiety—angelica, neroli orange, ylang-ylang

Coughs—myrtle, hyssop, fennel

Digestive problems—angelica, mint, tarragon

Headaches—lavender, balm, rose

Insomnia—rose, lavender, marjoram

Muscle pains—rosemary, Swiss pine, ginger

Nervousness—angelica, balm, galbanum

Stress—bergamot, clary, lavender

Throat soreness—bergamot, cajeput, slippery elm

Further Reading

Culpeper, Nicholas, *Culpeper's Complete Herbal and English Physician,* W. Foulsham, London, England, 1994. Updated version of the classic text written by England's foremost aromatherapist/physician. Some of the recipes he provides are still being used today.

Gattéfosse, René Maurice, *Gattéfosse's Aromatherapy,* Atrium Pub., Santa Rosa, Calif., 1995. Gattéfosse is considered by many to be the father of aromatherapy. This book, translated from French, details his research into the use of essential oils.

Rose, Jeanne, *Aromatherapy Book,* North Atlantic Pub., Berkeley, Calif., 1992. This popular aromatherapist lists hundreds of ailments and the herbs that treat them.

Tisserand, Maggie, *Aromatherapy for Women,* Thorson's Publications, N.Y., 1985. Gynecological remedies for everyday stress, menstruation, pregnancy, postpartum, skin and hair skin and childhood diseases are listed in this easy-to-use book.

Tisserand, Robert, *The Art of Aromatherapy,* Destiny Books, N.Y., 1977. Written by one of America's leading authorities, this book offers a concise and detailed description of the history of aromatherapy, herbal recipes and lists the medicinal properties and applications of the essential oils.

Worwood, Valerie, *The Complete Book of Essential Oils and Aromatherapy,* New World Library, Los Altos, Calif., 1991. Over 600 homemade recipes and beauty products are described in this comprehensive book.

Aston-Patterning® unlike many bodywork systems that seek to restore physical symmetry to a client's posture, Judith Aston's paradigm, the core of her work, is that "all human movement occurs in asymmetrical and three-dimensional spirals."[1] Symmetry is illogical since each half of the body is different: there are different internal organs, there is usually a predominant side where strength and dexterity is greater, and each hemisphere of the brain controls different physiological functions. "People look the same in tension and different in ease"[2] or holding patterns of tension are common, while relaxation is an individualized posture.

Aston-Patterning is a holistic and integrated system of movement education, soft tissue bodywork, fitness training and environmental design custom-tailored to suit each client. Aston's innate ability to recognize, analyze and absorb what most untrained eyes could not sense, led her to develop a system of modifying body patterns, which can lessen pain, provide stability and grace and enhance physical performance.

Judith Aston received her master's degree in dance and fine arts in 1965. Two car accidents, in 1967 and 1968, left her with severe back and neck problems. When her doctors proposed a spinal fusion, she sought alternative care. She contacted Dr. Ida Rolf at the Esalen Institute in Big Sur, California. The ROLFING® treatments she received gave her an almost immediate decrease in back pain. She became a student of Rolf's and was invited by Dr. Rolf to develop a series of movements that would help maintain the corrections gained by the Rolfing treatments.

In 1971, this curriculum, which became the Rolf-Aston Structural Patterning™, became an integral part of Rolfing. She taught bodyworkers to recognize the proportions, dimensions and interrelationships in their clients' bodies; to impart this physical data to the clients so they could use it in their movements; and to use their own bodies correctly and efficiently when working. Environmental modification, or the proper use of everyday items and furnishings, such as chairs, tables, etc., were added to the program later.

In 1977, as a result of differences in philosophy and biomechanical models, Judith Aston left to form her own organization.

Each Aston-Patterning session contains all or some of the current forms of the system: **Aston-massage, neuro-kinetics, arthro-kinetics, myo-kinetics, Aston fitness training,** and **ergonomic modification.** There is also a facial toning form. A detailed personal history of the client is taken at the first session. Pretesting provides information about how the client uses his body while doing basic movements and tasks, such as sitting and walking, as well as an evaluation by palpation of the hyper- and hypotonicity of the tissue and the hyper- and hypomobility of the joints. Activities that are specific to the client's lifestyle, such as sports, are videotaped and analyzed.

Movement education, also called **neuro-kinetics** is the core of Aston-Patterning. It provides efficient ways of adapting movement principles to daily life. The movements are divided into basic "units of work," such as an arm unit or a walking unit. All of the units are eventually utilized for total body integration.

The most basic unit is called **arcing,** where the pelvis, chest and head are raised into a full extension from a flexed position. Arcing teaches weight transfer, eye tracking, breath release and finding **neutral,** which is the halfway point between flexion (bending) and extension (standing erect).

The bodywork is composed of **Aston-massage, myo-kinetics** and **arthro-kinetics.** The strokes of the massage match the direction of the tissues in a three-dimensional path, called **spiraling.** The client is comfortably propped with pillows and towels in the most natural position, which offers the least amount of stress.[3] At first glance, the strokes appear to be similar to the EFFLEURAGE strokes of Swedish massage, but, instead, it is performed with both hands in three-dimensional contour to each other, following the grain of the muscles.[4] This massage does not use unnecessary compression in the strokes, which Aston believes violates the structural integrity of a muscle.

Myo-kinetics is used by a certified Aston practitioner and concentrates on specific muscles and fascia. It is also a two-handed technique, although the firm fingertip pressure can stretch and release tight muscles. Deep tissues are painlessly reached as the overlying layers are gently moved into slack.

Arthro-kinetics is the deepest and most powerful massage technique, since it addresses the joints that move in spiral patterns, matching the action of the attached muscles.[5] This work has a profound physical effect, since it can affect the deepest level of the body.

After the movement education and bodywork is performed, posttesting and often an ergonomic consultation complete the session. The posttesting is a repeat of the pretested activities to offer the client a recognition of the changes that have taken place. The ergonomic consultation considers the everyday objects that the client uses and makes appropriate adjustments for more beneficial use. The Aston-Line® offers a line of ergonomic products, which support this paradigm for greater ease in daily living. A fitness program to loosen, tone, stretch and improve cardiovascular health is also a part of Aston-Patterning.

Every treatment session sets out with the same goals for the clients: to have an experience of physical change; to learn how to facilitate these changes on their own; and to apply these changes to their lifestyles.

Notes

Aston-Patterning also concerns itself with the practitioners' use of correct body mechanics in order to avoid strain and injury and to increase the effectiveness of the treatments.

[1] Low, Jeffrey, "The Modern Body Therapies: Aston-Patterning," *Massage Magazine,* October/November 1988, p. 49.

[2] Ibid., p. 49.

[3] This is contrary to Ida Rolf's theory that the client should be placed in a position that exposes physical blockages and stresses.

[4] One hand might massage up a flexor muscle in one direction while the other hand massages down the opposing extensor.

[5] Arthro-kinetics is taught in an advanced class after certification has been granted. Not all Aston practitioners are trained in this form of the work.

aura therapy   or the treatment of the HUMAN ENERGY BIO-FIELD, is made up of radiant, luminous emanations, which create a halo of colors around the body. All of nature generates an aura; even inanimate objects radiate this energy. The aura can be perceived by clairvoyants, psychic healers and those especially trained to see the emanations. Kirlian photography utilizes special film, which can photograph the energy bio-field.

Auras are outward manifestations of a person's physical, emotional, psychological and spiritual health. Any mood changes, physical illnesses or heightened emotions will alter the color and strength of the aura.

Scientific research has proved the existence of auras. As early as 1939, Drs. H. Burr and F. Northrop of Yale University, were able to measure the energy fields surrounding a plant seed, the eggs of frogs and human ovulation. Dr. Viktor Inyushin, from the Kazakh University in Russia, started his experiments with the human energy bio-field during the 1950s. He recognized that a bioplasmic energy field made up of living matter, some of which is emitted into space, enveloped the body. In 1979, Dr. Robert Becker of Upstate Medical School in Syracuse, New York, charted an electrical field, which was shaped like the body and the central nervous system. He called it the direct current control system, which changed shapes according to physical and psychological alterations.[1]

In more recent times, the Superconducting Quantum Interference Device, SQUID, developed by research scientists, can measure the electromagnetic field that surrounds the body.

Religious recognition of the aura dates back over 5,000 years to the ancient Indians who spoke of *prana,* or universal energy. Yogis practicing meditation and breathing exercises learned to control and use this energy to expand their consciousness and rise to more enlightened lev-

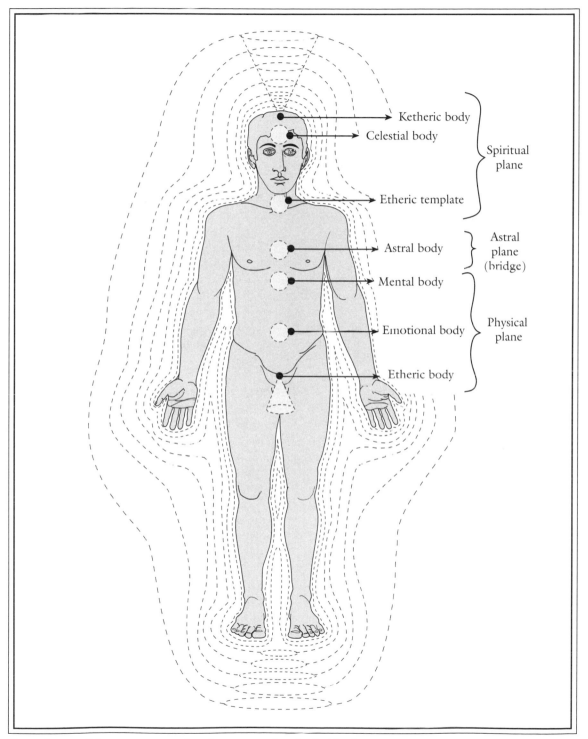

Ketheric body

Celestial body

Spiritual plane

Etheric template

Astral body

Astral plane (bridge)

Mental body

Physical plane

Emotional body

Etheric body

Seven layers of the aura surround and penetrate the physical body. Each layer represents a different aspect of the individual and emanates an energetic field of varying colors.

els. The ancient Chinese believed that all matter is made up of QI, or CHI, energy and that any disruption to its natural flow will result in illness. Most occult and esoteric philosophies recognize and speak of the human aura.[2] Paintings often depict spiritual masters and religious adepts with a golden halo at the crown CHAKRA.

Occultists recognize humans as septenary beings—we are made of seven main auric levels (also called bodies, planes, layers, templates, etc.) of being or consciousness. Each of these seven auric levels has its own function and is closely associated with a chakra. In optimum health, the energies of each plane supports and balances the others. The densest, most mundane levels are the **physical** (functioning—at the lowest), **etheric** (physical sensations), **lower mental plane** or **emotional,** and the **higher mental plane.** On the spiritual level, the fifth level is the **spiritual causal plane** also known as the **etheric template,** the sixth is the **intuitional plane** also known as the **celestial body,** and the seventh level is the **divine, absolute** or **ketheric template body.**

These auric levels are overlapping and interrelated currents, which encircle the body in an oval-shaped design. The strength and extent of the emanations depend upon the health and spiritual evolution of the individual.

The first aura emanates from the physical body and surrounds it in a cloud-shaped configuration composed of physical and etheric forces. Its color is a bluish white, and health is manifested as straight lines extending in all directions from the edge of the body, approximately ¼ to 2 inches beyond the body. The physical auric level is related to physical functioning, pleasure and pain, and autonomic functioning. In illness, the lines appear to bend or droop at the source of the problem. "Being run down" is the experience of weak radiations on the physical level.

The second auric level, the etheric level, stems from the emotional center in the spleen and circles the astral body from a distance of 12 to 18 inches. Although this level contains all the colors of the rainbow, the color and strength of this level depend upon the health of the individual. The aura changes with mood swings, thoughts and emotions. In health, it is luminous and in illness, dark spots and patches appear within the aura.

The lower mental plane, or the emotional level, is the center of action based on knowledge and intelligence. Linear thinking and mental organization are controlled on this level. Its shape is oval and its rays are shiny, bright or pale yellow. In cases of perversities or evil consciousness, dark spots appear on the aura and the emanation is deformed.

The fourth level, the higher mental plane, is a partner to the third level. This is the level of the higher mind, or the soul. It relates to the heart chakra and its color is rose. Inspiration and intuition make the aura grow. Dormant thoughts or negative mental activity will manifest in a dim aura.

Entering into the higher spiritual plane, the fifth aura, or the spiritual or etheric template, is where the essence of the spirit dwells. It is the soul's "life history." According to occult science, all conditions of the lower four planes are results of the forces within the spiritual, or causal, body and are directly affected by its state. The fifth plane, which controls divine will, is the meeting juncture between the cosmic and the physical levels. Its colors, which are barely perceptible in most people, are delicate subtones, often represented in ethereal shades of blue. The rays emanate 1½ to 2 feet from the body.

The celestial body, or the intuitional plane, which is the sixth level, and the divine, or seventh level, are parts of the cosmic aspects of the individual and blend together at the periphery of the aura. Highly spiritually developed people manifest this aura as a white light, which is transmitted to them from a supreme cosmic source. The light is absorbed into the seven chakras.

The sixth level is made up of opalesque gold-silver colors and radiates 2 to 2¾ feet from the body. Celestial love or spiritual ecstasy, the higher mind and the integration of the body and spirit stem from this level.

The seventh level is egg-shaped and is made up of a gold-silver shimmering light. It can reach 2½ to 3½ feet from the body. This divine white light can produce a condition of health and harmony. The inability of the light to penetrate the body may indicate the presence of illness. These **blocks** will affect a specific auric level and all those below it, ending in the physical level.

Barbara Brennan describes six types of energy blocks.[3] The **blah** block is caused by suppressed feelings, which causes the energy to stagnate. In this instance, the body tends to bloat or accumulate fluids in the blocked area. The **compaction** block holds unexpressed feelings of rage, which become buried under layers of fat from overeating or excessive muscular development. **Mesh armor** prohibits feelings, especially fear, by moving them around the body when the individual is challenged. Although this block does not normally result in illness, the individual carries the sense that something is missing. **Plate armor** contains feelings by freezing them with high tension. Life for this person is unfulfilled and lacking in deep personal connections. **Energy depletion** is a decrease of energy as it flows down the legs, producing a sensation of not being able to stand on one's own feet. The **energy leak** diverts energy out of the joints rather than letting it flow through the limbs. People like this lose the strength and ability to respond to experiences and tend to have cold limbs. Arthritis and other joint problems may result from this block.

Auric healing commences with an analysis of the client's energy system. An observation of his physical condition, his movement capabilities, a CRYSTAL reading of the chakras, and FOOT REFLEXOLOGY may be used to evaluate the general condition of the energy field.

The practitioner (healer) will then align the three energy systems vital to the healing: her own, the client's and those of the **guides,** and the universal energy bio-field. Guides are used to help channel and direct the healing energy.

The lower four levels (bodies) are healed first, using **chelation,** which is charging and clearing the aura, spinal cleaning and addressing specific auric needs. The fifth layer is treated through spiritual surgery, then the sixth and the seventh. Cosmic healing of the eight and ninth layers concludes the healing. The latter two levels are the levels of reincarnation.

There are two approaches to the healing journey: the inner and the outer. The inner healing establishes balance and health on all levels by focusing on the physical, emotional, mental and spiritual aspects of an individual. The outer healing helps reestablish balance in the layers of the aura by applying energy from the universal energy bio-field. The length of the healing process depends upon the condition of the individual.

The process of inner healing, also called full spectrum healing, treats each level differently. The physical plane receives massage, exercises, postures and sound (voice) vibrations to release any of the physical blocks. The second level is healed by LAYING ON OF HANDS, which repairs and restructures this body so the energy flow is released. For the third level, the healer challenges imbalanced thought processes and seeks to discover new ways for the client to solve his problems. Emotional healing takes place when emotional traumas have been removed. The astral body, the fourth level, is healed as the practitioner channels the love of humanity to the client, so that defense mechanisms can be dropped safely.

In the spiritual levels, the fifth level is healed through spiritual surgery, which realigns the client's will with the divine will. The celestial body, or the sixth level, is healed as the practitioner is enveloped in universal love and channels it to the client. The ketheric template, or the seventh level, is healed by challenging a faulty belief system.[4]

Outer healing is done in conjunction with inner healing to eradicate physical symptoms generated by a faulty belief system. It is accomplished by the use of traditional or alternative

health care practices, such as MASSAGE, CHIROPRAC-
TIC, ACUPUNCTURE, homeopathy, etc. Inner and
outer healing are best achieved when people start
taking responsibility for their own health.

Notes
[1] Brennan, Barbara Ann, *Hands of Light: A Guide to Healing
through the Human Energy Field,* Bantam Books, N.Y.,
1988, p. 20.
[2] Ibid., p. 29.
[3] Ibid., p. 101–104.
[4] Ibid., p. 148–149.

Further Reading
Brennan, Barbara Ann, *Hands of Light: A Guide to Healing
through the Human Energy Field,* Bantam Books, N.Y.,
1988. A comprehensive book that clearly explains the
human energy bio-field, the chakras and the auric layers.
Black-and-white and color illustrations help describe and
elucidate the information.
Bruyere, Rosalyn, *Wheels of Light,* Healing Light Center,
Glendale, Calif., 1987. Considered to be a classic on the
subject of chakras and the human energy bio-field. A
comprehensive easy-to-use book.
Burks, A.J., *The Aura,* CSA Printers & Publications, Lakemont, Ga., 1962. An informative guide to the aura.
Butler, W.E., *How to Read the Aura,* Samuel Weiser, Inc.,
N.Y., 1971. This book describes the levels of the human
aura and provides exercises and techniques to perceive the
emanations.
Cayce, Edgar, *Aura,* ARE Press, Virginia Beach, Va., 1945.
Cayce explains how health and illness can be evaluated by
reading the auras.
Powell, A.E., *The Astral Body,* Theosophical House, London, 1972. This book describes the aura that surrounds all
animate and inanimate objects.

autogenic training (autogenics) "self-gener-
ated" training, a system of meditative and self-
hypnosis exercises used for profound relaxation
and self-awareness. It was developed by Dr.
Johannes H. Schultz, a psychiatrist/neurologist
in Germany, during the 1920s. He was a student
of Dr. Oskar Vogt from whose work Schultz
derived his theories. During the late 19th century, Vogt observed that his psychiatric patients
were often able to hypnotize themselves or
entrance themselves, resulting in appreciable
levels of stress reduction.

Schultz recognized that autohypnosis produced two noticeable physical responses: there
was a heaviness and warmth in the limbs and

throughout the body.[1] He felt that if he could
teach people to make suggestions to themselves
as these changes occurred, he could introduce
them to a state of "passive concentration,"[2]
where control over the autonomic nervous
system could be brought about.[3]

Most people are dominated by the sympathetic, or stress-induced, arousal state. Autogenic training teaches clients how to switch this
to a physiological state where relaxation dominates.

There are three principles of autogenic training. First, there is a mental repetition of six
verbal formulas while the client is "contacting"
each body part. There are suggestions of sensations of heaviness, warmth, a calm and controlled heartbeat, easy respiration, abdominal
warmth and finally a cool forehead accompanied
by a sense of peace. These six physiologically
oriented directions make up the core of the
autogenic training, called the **autogenic standard exercises.** As each step is repeated over and
over again, the client has an easier time lapsing
into a relaxed state.

The second principle of autogenic training is
called **passive concentration,** where all activities
of the autonomic nervous system are influenced
by learning to let go and release during the
process.

The third principle is the use of specific
training postures to avoid distractions by reducing sensory input. This provides an undis-
turbed atmosphere in which to practice the
process.

Under the supervision of medical personnel
or an autogenic training practitioner, individuals, or small groups, are lead through the relaxation techniques. The course lasts 8 to 10 weeks,
and each session is one hour per person or one
and a half hours for the group. Ideally, the client
will learn the system and be able to perform the
relaxation exercises on his own, at any time, in
any place. The recommended practice is three
times a day, for 10 to 15 minutes per session.
The client can be seated, lounging or lying
down. Once the system is learned, it is always

available to the client. Mini sessions serve as quick "pick-me-ups" to dispel pent-up tensions throughout the day.

Autogenic training is thought to be a westernized version of Eastern meditation practices. There are, however, no religious or philosophical overtones. It is all directed, very specifically, to physical release and functioning.

Autogenic training can benefit most people, regardless of their physical condition. According to Wolfgang Luthe, Schultz's successor and leading authority, autogenic training can help cure asthma, hypertension, lower back pain, migraine headaches, endocrine and metabolic dysfunction such as diabetes, epilepsy and cerebral palsy, sexual dysfunction, cardiac arrhythmias, and ulcers.[4] It has also been used to break destructive habits and addictions and to improve athletic and academic performances.

There are some situations where autogenic training is contraindicated. Patients with severe mental illnesses, personality disorders, acute psychoses and people with no or very low motivation should abstain from using this system.

In order to bring a session to an end, the client cancels the training by clenching his fists and bringing them to his shoulders. He takes a deep breath and stretches. Although he returns to normal consciousness, a sense of deep relaxation and alertness is maintained sometimes up to several days.

Notes

[1] Vasodilation of the peripheral arteries produces the sensation of warmth. Deep muscular relaxation allows for the feeling of heaviness. "Hanging Loose," *Harper & Queens,* May 1980, p. 1.

[2] Ibid., p. 1.

[3] The autonomic nervous system is made up of two opposing but mutually functioning branches: the sympathetic and parasympathetic nervous systems. Together, they govern functions such as endocrine gland secretions, constriction and dilation of blood vessels, respiration and other involuntary actions of the body. The sympathetic branch is concerned with arousal associated with stress and movement. The parasympathetic branch is concerned with the return to normalcy after the stress reaction. In other words, relaxation, recuperation and normal internal organ functioning are controlled by the parasympathetic branch.

The branches should work together for optimum health and homeostasis (balance).

[4] "Hanging Loose," *Harper & Queens,* May 1980, p. 2.

Further Reading

Linden, Wolfgang, M.D., *Introduction to the Methods of Autogenic Therapy,* Association for Applied Psychophysiology and Biofeedback, Wheat Ridge, Colo., 1977. This text is considered to be a classic in its field. It includes information about the techniques of autogenic training (therapy), rules for the clients and practitioners, contraindications, practice patterns and autogenic formula phrases.

Linden, Wolfgang, M.D., and Schultz, Johannes, *Autogenic Training: A Psychophysiologic Approach to Psychotherapy,* 1959.

Linden, Wolfgang, M.D., *Autogenic Training: A Clinical Guide,* Guilford Press, N.Y., 1990.

Avatar® an avatar is a Hindu deity who assumes physical form in order to participate in the ongoing process of creation. In 1987, Harry Palmer, an educational psychologist, developed a personal transformation system based on the concept that people's beliefs, prejudices and preconceived ideas are mirrored in their lives. One attracts what one believes. The purpose of Avatar training is to create an ideal life by shedding negative attitudes and replacing them with positive, healthy ones.

The system teaches the client to quiet her mind and remove the clutter in order to create desired results. **Dis-creation,** or the ability to dissolve unwanted situations, includes getting rid of bad habits and addictions and changing illness to health.

The Avatar course is divided into three sections. Section I is called **Creativism.** It explains the philosophical principles of the system and teaches exercises, which produce insights into higher levels of consciousness. Section II, **The Exercises,** explains the principles of creation and experience. Exercises in awareness are done to heighten perception and to enable the client to create her own reality. **The Rundowns,** Section III, teaches the principles of dis-creation.

All three sections take seven to nine days to complete. Avatar Master courses and Avatar Wizard courses are available for advanced students.

Further Reading

Palmer, Harry, *Living Deliberately: The Discovery and Development of Avatar,* Star's Edge International, Altamonte Springs, 1994. This book, available from Star's Edge International, describes how the author develops this system, what belief systems are and how to create your own reality.

_____ , *Resurfacing,* Star's Edge International, Altamonte Springs, 1994. This book describes the relationship between belief and experience and supplies techniques for exploring consciousness.

Ayurvedic medicine an Indian folk medicine and one of the oldest organized techniques of treatment and prevention to embrace the principle that illnesses relate to disharmony within the body. The word Ayurvedic is made up of two Sanskrit words *ayur* and *veda,* which translate to ''life's knowledge'' or ''life's science.''[1] Practiced in Nepal and Sri Lanka, dating back at least 3,000 years, the teachings spread to China, where many of the traditions of Chinese medicine, such as CUPPING, PULSE READING and the theory of balanced energy, were adopted. Ancient texts report the use of Ayurvedic surgical techniques for major and minor procedures as well as the use of herbal remedies.[2]

The type of cure the client will receive is determined after an analysis of his *doshas,* or three fundamental life forces. The *tridosha* doctrine of Ayurveda is the theory of these three basic elements. Although each person is a combination of all *doshas,* one will predominate in his constitution and provide the key to treatment.

Vata, air, is the *dosha* of movement. People with excess *vata* will have restless and nervous personalities. *Kapha,* earth, is a stabilizing force, which is responsible for physical structure. An excess of *kapha* will produce a strong, even-tempered person prone to gaining weight. *Pitta,* fire, is the connection between air and earth and is allied with heat, digestion and dehydration. An excess of *pitta* will produce fiery individuals who are passionate, quick to anger and subject to rashes and ulcers.

Each *dosha* is ruled by one or two of the five senses and responds to different aromas and tastes. *Vata* types rule hearing and touch and are prescribed warm, sweet and sour essences such as orange or rose geranium. *Kapha* governs taste and smell and responds to spicier, warm essences such as eucalyptus. *Pitta* controls sight and is benefitted by sweet and cool aromas, such as rose or mint.

According to Charak Samhita, a noted doctor who, along with Susruta Samhita, a famous surgeon, wrote massive encyclopedias about Ayurveda 3,000 years ago, there are four types of life. *Hita* is a useful life; *ahita* is harmful; *sukha* is happy; and *dukha* is an unhappy existence. He believed that there are four primary objects in life: *dharma* is performing religious rites; *artha* is acquiring wealth; *kama* is satisfying sybaritic, sensual pleasures; and *moksa* is attaining salvation. Ayurveda tries to balance more than just the body; the holistic human experience is cared for.

A further determination of body type is achieved through the investigation of skin and hair color, body size, weight, eye size, muscle strength, food preferences, voice pitch, sex drive and even dream analysis. Tissues of the body and elimination pathways are examined for additional physical typing.

Ayurvedic doctors seek to find a balance between the basic *doshas* by prescribing a number of techniques including herbal remedies, element-specific diets,[3] meditation and yoga exercises. *Panchakarma,* a detoxification process, is an important component of Ayurveda. Herbal steam baths, enemas, laxatives and nasal cleansing are some of the ways the purification process is accomplished.

Primordial sounding, or the use of sound and toning for healing purposes, is also employed. Pulse diagnosis helps the doctor determine the client's *dosha* so the proper treatment can be prescribed. A *kapha* pulse is slow and gliding and is considered to be swanlike. A *pitta* pulse is quicker and throbbing, like a frog, while the *vata* pulse is the fastest of all and is thought to be snakelike.

Marma therapy, the use of 107 **junction** (or acupuncture) **points,** is an Ayurvedic treatment for the relief of disease. Three important *marma* points, which can be self-stimulated on a daily basis for revitalization, are found between the eyebrows, at the top of the diaphragm (the xiphoid process) and at the *hara,* (conception vessel—CV 6) 1½ inches below the navel on the midline of the body.

The **bliss** technique is used to recapture joy, or ***ananda*** in Sanskrit. A special sound is intoned whose purpose is to restore the vibration of bliss to the client.

Gandharva music, a form of music therapy, is used in Ayurvedic healing to bring balance and harmony to the client.

Notes
1 Pati, Kumar Dr., ''Ayurvedic for Health,'' *The Best of Health World,* Health World Magazine, Inc., Burlingame, Calif., 1993, p. 1.
2 Reader's Digest, *Family Guide to Natural Medicine,* The Reader's Digest Association, Pleasantville, N.Y., 1993, p. 54.
3 The *doshas* are also characteristic in foods, seasons and the time of day. Food is particularly emphasized when designing a diet to fit the person's *dosha* and physical condition.

Further Reading
Chopra, Deepak, Dr., *Ageless Body, Timeless Mind,* Crow Pub. Co., N.Y., 1993. A best-seller featuring Ayurvedic philosophies to stay healthy and maintain a youthful vigor.
——— , *Quantum Healing: Exploring the Frontiers of Mind/Body Medicine,* Bantam Books, N.Y., 1989. This best-selling book explains the philosophies of Ayurvedic medicine and the connection between the mind and the body.
Frawley, David, *Ayurvedic Healing,* Passage Press, Sandy, Utah, 1989. Three divisions of the book explain the theory of Ayurvedic medicine, principles and therapies and treatments of disease and Ayurvedic remedial, preventative steps.
Lad, Vasant, *Ayurveda: The Science of Healing,* Lotus Press, Santa Fe, N.Mex., 1985. The author explains the principles and theories of Ayurvedic medicine. Diagrams and charts are included.
Svoboda, Robert E., *Prakruti: Your Ayurvedic Constitution,* Geocom Ltd., Albuquerque, N. Mex., 1988. This book explains the Ayurvedic analysis of physical types. Specially designed diets and lifestyles are recommended to maintain balance.
Tiwari, Maya, *Ayurvedic: Life of Balance,* Inner Traditions, Rochester, Vt., 1994. A description of the history and theory of Ayurvedics.

B

barefoot shiatsu was developed by SHIATSU expert Shizuko Yamamoto. It is a system of Japanese shiatsu bodywork, which employs the fingers, palms and feet of the practitioner. Barefoot shiatsu is a component of MACROBIOTIC SHIATSU.

Bartenieff Fundamentals[SM]**,** developed by Irmgard Bartenieff (1900–1981), is a system that increases ease, efficiency and expression in movement. It is a type of body reeducation used to minimize daily tensions and enhance movement for dancers and athletes. The system incorporates basic principles of movement and exercise, which can be performed on the floor, seated or standing.

Bartenieff was a student of Rudolf LABAN (1879–1958) who had created an innovative system of movement structure and intent. She applied her knowledge of Laban's work to physical therapy and dance therapy and created Bartenieff Fundamentals.

Her work explores movement initiation and sequencing, weight shift, spatial tension and breath support. It helps to develop dynamic alignment, strength, flexibility, coordination, kinesthetic awareness and physical expression.

This system balances the deep and superficial muscles by using simple movements in an aware, relaxed manner. The individual experiences the entire body moving fluidly in all spatial directions, reducing injury and stress.

Bartenieff opened the Laban/Bartenieff Institute of Movement Studies in New York City in 1979.

Bates method of vision training a system of eye exercises and relaxation techniques created by ophthalmologist Dr. William Horatio Bates (1881–1931) to improve vision.

Dr. Bates was a pioneer in his time. He questioned conventional medical treatments for vision problems and the accepted prescription of corrective lenses to fix them. He set up a laboratory at Columbia University and studied tens of thousands of eyes before developing his theory. Poor vision, he believed, was caused by weak eye muscles and that tension in the mind and body (eyes) interferred with correct functioning. He considered the mental aspect of vision to be equally as important as the physical exercises. He created a system that resembled MEDITATION, BIOFEEDBACK (still in its infancy) and stress-reduction training.

His experiments also included the discovery of the functions of the six sets of muscles that control the eyes. Vision is normal when all the muscles work together. However, if one muscle, or any combination of them becomes tense, the eye cannot focus properly. The recti muscles are found at the top, bottom and sides, while the two oblique muscles go around the middle of each eye. For the most part, they are striated, voluntary muscles, except at their attachment point on the sclera (white of the eye), where they become smooth muscle.[1] The smooth portion focuses the eye while the recti muscles flatten the eye to accommodate for distances. The obliques squeeze the eye, lengthening it for close vision.

In 1920, Dr. Bates developed his method of vision training designed to strengthen the muscles and improve vision without the aid of glasses. As an extra benefit, his relaxation techniques often resulted in the relief of many stress-related physical ailments. His method, however, will not work on eye problems that are organic in nature, such as glaucoma or cataracts.

His vision training has helped thousands of people improve their sight and possibly prevent vision problems from developing. It has benefited people with myopia (nearsightedness), hyperopia (farsightedness), poor peripheral vision, strabismus (crossed eyes) and amblyopia (lazy eye). Athletes have found improved eye-hand coordination, and airline pilots claim to sharpen their focus and depth perception with Bates's exercises. In 1939, Aldous Huxley credited this vision system with helping him recover from near blindness.

Some of Bates's exercises for eye relaxation are focusing, blinking, palming and shifting. To improve focus, hold one extended finger 3 inches from the face and the other finger at arm's length. Focus on the closest finger with both eyes, blink, then focus on the farthest finger. Repeat several times.

Blinking once or twice every 10 seconds keeps the eyes lubricated. Palming helps relax the eye muscles. While sitting comfortably, cover the eyes with cupped hands (which may be briskly rubbed together to produce heat). Palm twice daily for 10-minute periods. Bates also suggests to avoid staring at objects and to shift eye focus constantly.

Note
[1] Striated muscle tissue provides controllable, voluntary action, while smooth muscle action is considered to be involuntary.

Further Reading

Bates, William H., M.D., *Better Eyesight without Glasses,* Henry Holt & Co., N.Y., 1981. This revolutionary book provides a detailed explanation of Bates's vision training system complete with exercises and an eye chart to measure vision improvement.

Chancy, Earlyne, *The Eyes Have It,* Samuel Weiser, York Beach, Me., 1987. Natural treatments to strengthen vision including the Bates method, yoga, massage, herbal and folk remedies are explained. Conventional methods of treatment are also listed.

Goodrich, Janet, *Natural Vision Improvement,* Celestial Arts, Berkeley, Calif., 1986. Based on the Bates method, this book's theme is one of choice: choosing to improve vision and see without glasses.

Leviton, Richard, *Seven Steps to Better Vision,* Eastwest Natural Health Books, Brookline, Mass., 1992. Practical, hands-on information about vision improvement is offered in a seven-step plan.

Rosanes-Benett, Marilyn, Dr., *Do You Really Need Glasses?* Station Hill Press, Barrytown, N.Y., 1990. This book provides a thorough discussion of eye anatomy and physiology, dysfunctions and an eye exam and vision improvement exercises based on the Bates Method.

Benjamin system of muscular therapy a

deep muscle therapy, which combines individu-ally designed treatment and education to reduce chronic tension and promote health.

In 1958, at the age of 14, a serious back injury sent dancer Ben Benjamin to the doctor. He was told that he would never dance again. Unsatisfied with that dismal prognosis, Benjamin sought treatment from the French massage therapist, Alfred Kagan, dubbed "Doctor" Kagan by the dance community. After only three massages, Benjamin was able to dance again without pain.

He was so inspired by the healing effects of the deep massage, that he studied with Kagan and eventually developed his own system, which uses over 700 muscle manipulations. The Benjamin system of muscular therapy incorporates exercises for warmup, stretching and strength training with massage, employing area-specific strokes, pressures and rhythms to control pain and tension. Body awareness exercises minimize and control the build-up of tension, and a conscious awareness of the causes and effects of tensions provides the client with alternative choices to poor postural habits.

"We assist people in healing themselves."[1] The Benjamin system is so precise that practitioners can ascertain whether the cause of the tension comes from injury, MISALIGNMENT or emotional stress. The treatment is then designed to meet the client's individual needs.

Benjamin was profoundly influenced by the pioneering works of F.M. ALEXANDER (Technique), Dr. Wilhelm Reich and DR. JAMES CYRIAX. The Alexander Technique provided Benjamin with the insight of appropriate movement habits and body mechanics. His practitioners, as well as their clients, benefit by learning to use their bodies more effectively. Reich's work details the emotional life within muscle tension. **Armoring,** or the physical tension within the body, is the result of stored emotional traumas and inhibited expression. Benjamin recognized that by understanding the emotional-physical connection, his practitioners would be able to determine the best course of treatment. Dr. Cyriax's ideas provided Benjamin with injury evaluation skills and deep friction massages, which reduces adhesive scar tissue.

In 1974, Ben Benjamin founded the Muscular Therapy Institute in Cambridge, Massachusetts. In addition to training in the muscular therapy technique, a strict code of professional ethics is emphasized along with training in compassion and self-awareness. Students of the two-year program are also required to fulfill 35 hours of an outreach program, which brings the work into the community of people who need it.

Benjamin categorizes muscle tension as either mechanical or emotional. Mechanical tension, which responds well to his system of treatment, can be brought on by several factors including physical trauma, surgery, poor posture and body mechanics, environment, injury or misalignment. Emotional tension, which results in chronic muscular tightening—or armoring—may require psychological intervention rather than muscular therapy.

Tension may also be examined from the perspective of time, whether it is a current tension or residual one. Current tension usually lies in the superficial muscles and has been present for a short amount of time. Conversely, residual tension is present in the body over a long period of time and is often located in deeper tissue. Either of these tensions can be mechanical or emotional in origin.

The system is divided into four parts: deep massage, tension-release exercises, body-care techniques and postural realignment.

Deep massage reaches into those muscles that store residual tension and pain. Complex hand and finger techniques can penetrate muscles or muscle groups, relieving the tension and enhancing local circulation. Benjamin's system uses two basic types of deep massage: **stroking/kneading,** which increases general circulation, particularly venous flow, and **pressure,** which breaks down the tension.

The stroking/kneading stroke begins with a light pressure that gradually deepens. The movement follows the direction of the muscle fibers.

Pressure strokes are applied across the muscle fibers and help treat spasms, injuries and problems from long-term tension.

The practitioner initially identifies tension through observation and then by touch. Correct pressure is necessary for effective treatment. The touch should be pleasantly deep, without eliciting pain or discomfort. Excessive pressure would be counterproductive, since the client would tense up.

Lubrication is used to reduce friction. Deep massage is contraindicated in cases of: bone, muscle or skin diseases; skin infections; pain from an unhealed fracture; cancerous tumor; severe arthritis affecting brittle bones; on recently injured or ruptured soft tissues; and in cases of general poor health.[2]

The tension-release exercises help dissolve the tightness found in specific muscles. They can be performed alone and are considered to be as important as the deep massage. Ideally, they should be done between treatments to encourage relaxation. The exercises used in the Benjamin system of muscular therapy were created to release mechanical tension.

Body care techniques provide a means to maintain lower levels of tension and help reduce their build-up in a gentle way. They are more passive than the tension-release exercises and can easily be done at home. These simple techniques include baths, showers, saunas and steam baths, deep breathing exercises, proper diet and nutrition, adequate sleep and rest.

Postural alignment plays an integral part in maintaining a body that is relaxed and free of tension. Until the underlying postural anomalies are corrected, the pattern of stress will be repeated.

Clients of muscular therapy receive many beneficial effects from the work: they are more aware of their bodies, have better circulation, heal faster from injury, display more energy, are more flexible, have better sleep although they require less, have reduced pain, lose weight faster and generally feel better.[3]

Notes

[1] Brown, Lonny J., Ph.D., "Training Good Hands with Heart at Cambridge's Muscular Therapy Institute," *Whole Health Network*, no date, p. 10.

[2] Benjamin, Ben E., Ph.D., *Are You Tense? The Benjamin System of Muscular Therapy*, Pantheon Books, N.Y., 1978, p. 53.

[3] Ibid., p. 9.

Further Reading

Benjamin, Ben E., Ph.D., *Are You Tense? The Benjamin System of Muscular Therapy*, Pantheon Books, N.Y., 1978. This illustrated and photographed book describes the Benjamin system of muscular therapy and provides instructions for a full-body massage.

_____ , *Exercise without Pain* (formerly) *Sports without Pain*, Summit Books, N.Y., 1979. Preparation, postevent and prevention of sports injuries are illustrated in this book.

_____ , and Gordon, Gale, M.D., *Listen to Your Pain: The Active Person's Guide to Understanding, Identifying, and Treating Pain and Injury*, The Viking Press, N.Y., 1984. This book describes how to assess and treat pain and injury problems.

Bindegewebsmassage a massage technique to the CONNECTIVE TISSUE. In 1929, Elisabeth Dicke of Germany suffered from an untreated tooth abscess, which eventually resulted in general toxemia (blood poisoning) and an infection that spread to her right leg. Due to the severe circulation problems she was having, her doctors were considering amputation to save her life.

The night preceding the surgery, she began to massage her back, noticing a thickness and tightness in the musculature. After hours of self-administered treatments, she noticed an appreciable reduction of her back pain accompanied by an increase in circulation to the afflicted limb.[1] Dicke discovered that the inelastic, insensible and rigid tissues on the painful side of her back were loosened by these pulling strokes, and the skin's tension was sufficiently lowered to equal that of the uninvolved side.[2] The idea that reflexes on the body could directly affect internal organs was discovered.

Studies made by Dr. Henry Head[3] and Dr. J. Mackenzie[4] corroborated Dicke's findings of the reflex relationships between skin zones and internal organs.

The connective tissue layer between the skin and the muscle is the most abundant tissue in the body and functions to protect, support and hold together various organs. It is present throughout the body, mucous membranes and around blood vessels and nerves. It protects individual organs and forms the subcutaneous layer, which attaches the skin to underlying tissues and organs.[5] *Bindegewebsmassage* works primarily within the loose connective tissue network.

A detailed system of reflex zones was established on the body to treat various illnesses. The treatment should not be painful and the pressure of the strokes is determined by the client's tolerance.

The treatment begins with a diagnostic stroke, which determines visceral pathologies. The tissues are gripped between the thumbs and fingers and are lifted on each side of the spine, from the fifth lumbar vertebra (L5, the lowest vertebra) to the first cervical vertebra (C1, also called the atlas) just under the cranium. Tissues that cannot be lifted, are too tight or painful or produce a redness or raised wheal along the spine may indicate a problem in the reflected organ. Treatment is then applied to the affected area.

The massage technique is "a pull on the skin" as the fingers create tension on the connective and subcutaneous tissues.[6] The distinctions in angle and rhythm of the movement can affect the degree of tension on the massaged area. The client and practitioner are usually seated during the treatment, although the practitioner may stand if that is more comfortable. The strokes follow a particular sequence.

Bindegewebsmassage to the back is done in three sections. The **basic section** (called *grund auf bau*), extends upward from the coccyx to the first lumbar vertebra in the lower back. The **thoracic section** includes the thoracic vertebra of the middle back (T12–T1, from the bottom upward). The **cervical section** starts at the seventh cervical vertebra and proceeds up the neck to C1. All treatments, regardless of the pathology, include the basic section.

Strokes using the flat of the middle finger are performed three times without lubricant. The direction of the pressure on the back follows the **dermatomes,** or skin reflexes of *Bindegewebsmassage.* On the extremities, pressure can be in the direction of the muscle fibers, fascia, tendons or at right angles to fascial borders. **Balancing strokes** are performed at the end of each treatment to calm stimulated nerve endings.

Effects may occur during the treatments as well as some time after. Circulation is increased, histamine-like substances are secreted by the skin, and Dicke, along with other proponents of CONNECTIVE TISSUE MASSAGE state that there is an influence on internal organs, which directly improved pathologies.[7]

Notes

[1] Kisner, Carolyn Dieball, M.S., and Taslitz, Norman, Ph.D., "Connective Tissue Massage: Influence of the Introductory Treatment on Autonomic Functions," *Physical Therapy,* Vol. 48, No. 2, p. 108.

[2] Ibid., p. 108.

[3] Bischof, I., and Elmiger, G., Licht, Sydney, ed., "Connective Tissue Massage," In *Massage, Manipulation and Traction,* 1960, pp. 57–85 (cited, p. 119). Kisner, Carolyn Dieball, M.S., and Taslitz, Norman, Ph.D., "Connective Tissue Massage: Influence of the Introductory Treatment on Autonomic Functions," *Physical Therapy,* Vol. 48, No. 2.

[4] Mackenzie, J., *Krankheitszeichen und ihre Auslegung,* Wurzburg, Germany, 1917. (cited Ibid., p. 119).

[5] Tortora, Gerald J., and Anagnostakos, Nicholas P., *Principles of Anatomy and Physiology,* 3d ed., Harper & Row, N.Y., 1981.

[6] Kisner, Carolyn Dieball, M.S., and Taslitz, Norman, Ph.D., "Connective Tissue Massage: Influence of the Introductory Treatment on Autonomic Functions," *Physical Therapy,* Vol. 48, No. 2, p. 108.

[7] Langen, D., "Study on the Mechanism of Action of Massage of Reflex Zones in Connective Tissue," *Psychotherapy,* Medical Psychology, 1959, (cited Kisher p. 119).

Further Reading

Ebner, Marie, *Connective Tissue Massage,* The Williams & Wilkins Co., Baltimore, 1962. This is a definitive text on connective tissue massage complete with illustrations and photographs of the massage techniques.

Tappan, Frances M., *Healing Massage Techniques,* Reston Publishing Co., Inc., Reston, Va., 1980. This book is very thorough in describing some of the most common forms of hands-on bodyworks, including *Bindegewebsmassage.* Illustrations and photographs clarify the explanations of the systems, which include Eastern and Western techniques.

bioenergetics a therapeutic process that studies the personality in terms of the energetic processes of the body. According to its originator, Alexander Lowen, M.D., it is "a therapeutic technique to help a person get back together with his body and to help him enjoy to the fullest degree possible the life of the body."[1] The therapy is a combination of deep breathing, talk therapy, bioenergetic exercises and positions and hands-on work to ease tensions and release blocked feelings.

The work is an offspring of REICHIAN THERAPY, which was one of the first body-oriented psychotherapies. Dr. Wilhelm Reich (1879–1957) created a system that maintained that we are our bodies. Reich purported that repressed emotions were stored as muscular contractions he called **armoring.**

Dr. Lowen met Reich at the New School for Social Research in New York City and studied with him from 1940 to 1952. He helped popularize Reich's work during the 1950s. In 1953, Lowen met Dr. John C. Pierrakos (see CORE ENERGY THERAPY) and his classmate Dr. William B. Walling, all neo-Reichians. They founded the Institute for Bioenergetic Analysis in New York in 1956 with the idea of modifying or expanding Reich's technical procedures.

Bioenergetic analysis strives to achieve three goals: to enable the patient to understand his personality in terms of his body; to improve all functions of the personality by releasing the energy that is blocked by muscle contractions; and to increase the patient's experience of pleasure by resolving the **characterological** (body) **attitudes,** which have cut him off from his feelings.

Bioenergetics makes no distinction between mental and physical illness or pain. Every disturbance is believed to affect the whole person. Most people, however, need to understand the correlation between their problems and how these manifest in their bodies. Once they realize this, patients can begin the bioenergetic work.

In a typical session, the patient relates his history and something of importance he wishes to discuss with his therapist. The therapist studies the patient's body, movements and the sound of his voice in order to ascertain where and how the emotion is held. Having the patient assume a variety of bioenergetic positions indicates the tension spots. All distortions and denials of reality are compensated by **body attitudes**. Once these energy blocks are located, any combination of breathing exercises, stretching or expressive exercises may be used to release the tension.

There are two important principles to keep in mind when working with the body: any limitation of movement is both a cause and effect of emotional problems, and any restrictions of natural respiration are both a cause and effect of anxiety.

The integration and coordination of physical responses depend upon the unity of respiration and movement. In bioenergetics, the physical tension is released concomitantly with the psychological. Special movements and positions enable the patient to regain body awareness and release repressed emotions.

Note
1 Lowen, Alexander, M.D., *Bioenergetics,* Penguin Books, N.Y., 1976, introduction.

Further Reading
Baker, Elsworth, M.D., *Man in the Trap,* Macmillan & Company, N.Y., 1967. This book describes the history of Reichian therapy.

Lowen, Alexander, M.D., *Bioenergetics,* Penguin Books, N.Y., 1976. Written by the originator of this body/mind approach to personality, it details the history and application of bioenergetics. Case histories are cited throughout the text.

———, *The Betrayal of the Body,* Simon & Schuster, N.Y., 1969. Dr. Lowen describes how the body can mask repressed feelings.

biofeedback a term coined in 1969, is a system that relays information about the physical condition of the body, which is measured on sensitive instruments. Feedback, a term taken from the electronics field, is data that is recorded and then sent back into the system where the information helps make appropriate adjustments, such as a timer, which can "read" a clock and turn on a light.

Used as a primary therapy, or in conjunction with others, the goal of biofeedback is to provide deep relaxation and stress management skills to prevent stress-related disorders or illnesses. It is a powerful teaching tool, with immediate reinforcement, which offers self-regulation and control over mental, emotional and physical processes for improved function and health.

Biofeedback principles can be traced back as far as the 18th century, where Indian yogis demonstrated the ability to control functions of the body previously considered to be involuntary such as heartbeat.[1] It was believed that strong meditative powers gave them this ability.

During the 1950s, scientists learned that clients were able to control certain physiological functions by responding to data from specialized medical apparatus. The research continued into the 1960s, when rats were taught to regulate their blood flow even after muscle paralyzing drugs were administered. The developer of the present biofeedback system is Norbert Wiener, a mathematician who referred to it as "a method of controlling a system by reinserting into it the results of its past performance."[2]

The biofeedback instruments are sensitive electronic devices, which monitor physiological processes. Sensors are placed on the body that can measure muscle tension, skin temperature, etc. The information is amplified and converted into visual responses or tones (sometimes both), meter readings or computer displays. The client uses the information as a guide and practices certain relaxation procedures to change the readout and reduce physical stress.

Deep breathing, relaxation techniques and GUIDED IMAGERY are used as part of the biofeedback system. These procedures must be practiced in order to bring about a physical change. Eventually, the client may be able to achieve her goals, without the use of the biofeedback machinery, on a self-regulatory basis.

The practitioner guides the client by helping her to interpret the information, leading the VISUALIZATION and facilitating the treatment. The result is greater control over autonomic body functions, such as blood pressure, heart rate, digestion, perspiration, etc.

There are a few variations in biofeedback instrumentation. The **electromyograph** (EMG) is a commonly used machine. This instrument measures the electrical activity of the muscles by applying sensors on the skin. EMG feedback is the primary system for general relaxation training, muscle rehabilitation after trauma or injury, tension related conditions such as headaches, TEMPOROMANDIBULAR JOINT conditions and bruxism (grinding of the teeth), chronic pain, acne vulgaris,[3] muscle spasm and muscular dysfunction due to stroke. Asthma and ulcers, also illnesses often brought on or exacerbated by stress, can be relieved.

Thermal, or **blood flow feedback,** measures skin temperature. An increase in blood flow will produce a higher temperature, while a decrease in circulation will lower skin temperature. Finger blood vessels are particularly sensitive to stress, which explains why hands feel cold when we are anxious. The thermal feedback device is used on the fingers to monitor blood flow and relaxation. This machine is useful for vascular disorders, such as migraine headaches, Raynaud's disease,[4] hypertension and the vascular complications of other diseases.

Electrodermal feedback (EDR) measures skin conductivity from fingers and palms, which is associated with the sweat glands. It is sometimes referred to as **galvanic skin response** (GSR). It can sense emotional changes in some people and is used, in conjunction with other methods, in lie detector tests for that reason. EDR is used to treat performance anxiety in athletes, excessive sweating and for relaxation and desensitization training.

Brain wave feedback, or the electroencephalograph (EEG), monitors brain wave activities. Sensors are placed on the scalp and brain wave emission is measured. Alpha waves are present during relaxation, so the client learns how to enhance this particular brain activity. Epilepsy, insomnia, hyperactivity, attention deficit disorder in children, alcohol and chemical dependencies and traumatic brain injury can be treated using the EEG.

Additional biofeedback machines, even handheld devices for home use, have been developed to treat many conditions. Self-regulation in stress-related disorders such as heart arrhythmias, incontinence and irritable bowel syndrome may all be controlled.

The length of therapy depends upon the severity of the symptoms and the motivation of the client. The stress reduction and relaxation skills must be practiced on a regular basis to ensure success.

There are few contraindications to biofeedback. Medical consultation is necessary for any serious diseases and people suffering from endocrine imbalance, such as diabetes, should inform their doctors about their decision to use biofeedback, since medication doses might be affected.

Notes
[1] Kastner, Mark, L.Ac., Dipl. Ac., and Burroughs, Hugh, *Alternative Healing,* Halcyon Publications, La Mesa, Calif., 1993, p. 37.
[2] Ibid., p. 37.
[3] Hughes, H., Brown, B.W., Lawlis, G. Frank, and Fulton, J.E., Jr., "Treatment of Acne Vulgaris by Biofeedback Relaxation and Cognitive Imagery," *Journal of Psychosomatic Research,* Vol. 27, No. 3, Pergamon Press, Ltd., 1983, p. 186. This study showed a relationship between acne and psychological stress. During periods of duress, there is an increase in the secretion of hormones that causes acne. By reducing the participants' anxiety level through biofeedback and guided imagery, there was a significant improvement in their skin condition.
[4] Raynaud's disease is a condition that causes blood vessels in the fingers or toes to constrict upon exposure to cold or excessive stress.

Further Reading
AAPB Applications Standards and Guidelines Committee, *Biofeedback Applications: Standards and Guidelines for Biofeed-*

back *Applications in Psychophysiological Self-Regulation,* AAPB, Wheat Ridge, Colo., 1992. This small book provides information about the indications of clinical use, how the service is provided, the process of assessment, instrumentation and safety and the ethics of biofeedback.

AAPB, *Biofeedback: A Client's Information Paper,* AAPB, Wheat Ridge, Colo., 1993. An informative pamphlet about biofeedback and how it works for the clients' use.

biomagnetics See MAGNETIC THERAPY.

bladder meridian in oriental bodywork, a YANG meridian with 67 ACUPUNCTURE points, whose element is water, relates to the midbrain, which cooperates with the kidney hormone system and pituitary gland. It also relates to the autonomic nervous system as it corresponds to the reproductive and urinary organs.

It helps with the elimination of urine, the final product of the body's liquid purification process. It combines with the SMALL INTESTINE meridian and is used to treat all the major symptomatology of the tendino-musculor-skeletal systems, such as neck and back pain, sciatica, arthritis, scoliosis, headaches, tennis elbow, etc.

The bladder meridian flows downward bilaterally from the corner of the eyes, down the back of the head, where it separates into two channels on each side of the spine. It converges again behind the knees and ends outside the little toes.

body-centered transformation created by Gay and Kathlyn Hendricks, psychologists in Colorado, allows people to reconnect with their fundamental nature, called **essence.** They purport that in early childhood, mixed messages from parents about appropriate behavior, traumas and suppressed feelings are finally expressed through unhealthy means, such as physical tightness, pain, in dreams and fantasies and through faulty communication. People learn early in life to control their feelings and deny the experiences of their bodies. This **integrity dilemma** tells us that who and what we have become is unacceptable.

The goal of body-centered transformation is to peel back the layers of suppression and dis-

cover the essence within. Essence is the part that is connected to the self, others and the Divine, at the same time.

According to this system, people lose their essences in two possible ways: through rapid learning, such as trauma or shock, or through slow learning. The latter is experienced most of the time, and people find themselves assuming roles and postures in order to adapt to situations.

Recapturing **integrity,** or the **integrity tripod,** is the heart of the work. The trinity is composed of: recognizing and expressing one's nature—one's truth—; being aware of feelings; and holding to agreements. Integrity is "operating in a state of wholeness."[1]

There are nine strategies, combinations of principles and techniques, which the Hendrickses have found to be effective in achieving their goals.

Breathing patterns, which can be inhibited by early childhood traumas, are used as a diagnostic tool. People's feelings are reflected in their breathing. For example shallow chest breathing might indicate a need to remove oneself from experiencing feelings or sensations. The Hendrickses urge their clients to breath with, rather than against, the feeling to amplify sensation. Correct breathing is deep belly breathing complimented with spinal movement.

Movement strategy is an authentic representation of a person's essence. The movement component is the expression of full creativity.

The **communication principle** concerns itself with a truthful awareness of what is going on at the moment. The ability to communicate allows a shifting from rigidity and argument to a flow of harmony. Clients are advised to have their feelings, speak the truth about them and keep the agreements that were made about them.

Presencing is actively being in the experience.

Magnification is making something larger, so it can surface and be addressed.

The **responsibility principle** does not seek blame or find fault, but rather provides the client with the ability to respond to a situation and make the appropriate corrections and adjustments. There are three levels of learning responsibility. The entry level is taking responsibility for having acted as a victim in the past. The midlevel concerns itself with actively assuming responsibility for one's actions. On the senior level, a person may inspire other people to behave in a similar manner. "Responsibility is the act of claiming that you are the source for whatever is occurring."[2]

The **love strategy** is the ability to love and accept all aspects of self, even those elements that have been difficult to embrace. Body-centered transformation suggests that people should think of someone or something that they love and then use that feeling to diffuse any problems.

Grounding deals with having feet planted firmly on the ground to deal with reality.

Manifestation asks the client how he would like to be and what his desires are. This serves to open the arena for people to design their own realities.

Body-centered transformation does not follow the conventions of traditional talk therapies. The work is sometimes done on a mattress or seated directly on the floor. The emphasis is on being present with feelings and not focusing on the past. The client's breathing, body movements and sounds are monitored as an indicator of feelings. Many deeply buried sensations are released once the client gets in touch with those feelings. With essence in their lives, clients of this system report more vitality, humor and the ability to examine different perspectives objectively, without losing themselves.

Notes
[1] Nurrie Stearns, Mary, "Rediscover Your Essence," *Lotus,* Spring, 1994, p. 95.
[2] Ibid., p. 95.

Further Reading
Hendricks, Gay and Kathlyn, *At the Speed of Life,* Bantam Books, N.Y., 1993. The history, development and philosophy of body-centered transformation is discussed in this book.

Body-Enlightenment® a path toward enlightenment where the physical body is used for transformation and self-realization. The body, heart and mind are recognized as an inseparable unit that is designed to guide human beings toward healing and wholeness.

The Body-Enlightenment process uses letting-go bodywork and emotional release combined with CHAKRA work, breathing and belief-shifting techniques to reprogram the body/heart/mind connection. The session also combines soft rocking and joint release to relieve muscular tightness and physical pain and to free blocked energy. Once the physical and emotional traumas or blocks are healed, and old beliefs are identified and released, then new positive life-affirming beliefs will be implanted and anchored in the body on a cellular level. As a result, the body becomes lighter, the heart is free to love and joy, and the mind changes from an enemy into an ally. Finally, the body/heart/mind can begin to express its highest purpose in life and can truly act as a divine guide, showing one the way toward enlightenment.

Body-Enlightenment is a synthesis of bodywork derived from TRAGER, BREEMA and body awareness methods. It also includes breathing, HYPNOTHERAPY, EMOTIONAL RELEASE and MEDITATION techniques. It was developed in the mid 1980s by Ranjita Koubenec, Ph.D., and first taught in 1988 under the name rebalancing. Body-Enlightenment is a registered trademark since 1992 and taught at the Somantra Institute of Body-Enlightenment at Harbin Hot Springs, California.

Body-Mind Centering® an approach to physical, emotional and spiritual change using movement and touch. Body-Mind Centering recognizes that the mind expresses itself through the body and the body through the mind.

Experiential anatomy is the foundation of the work. Participants and practitioners learn the structure and function of the body as well as experiencing each tissue "from the inside."[1] This sensitive awareness holds the key to the therapeutic potential of the system. The participant learns to identify, differentiate and finally integrate the tissues of the body. Changes occur not only on a physical level, as energy and movement are transmitted to specific tissues, but also in a conscious awareness of self and others.

Body-Mind Centering explores how to "embody" the tissues. The flow of fluids within the body, bones, ligaments, muscles, fascia, fat, skin, organ systems, nervous system and endocrine system are experienced through their movement and touch. The practitioners of this system can work directly with the tissues of the participants because they are consciously aware of their own.

Bonnie Bainbridge Cohen, the developer of Body-Mind Centering, grew up in a circus family. Her mother was a performer and her father sold tickets for the Ringling Bros. and Barnum & Bailey Circus. Bainbridge Cohen began to study dance at the age of three and received a B.S. in OCCUPATIONAL THERAPY and dance from Ohio State University in 1963. She came to New York City and studied modern dance with Erick Hawkins, who was instrumental in teaching her graceful, effortless movement.

Effortless movement, according to Body-Mind Centering, is established when the brain responds to information rather than controlling the body. This may lead to new experiences, sensations and patterns of moving.

Bainbridge Cohen moved to Amsterdam, the Netherlands, in 1968. Her work with injured dancers in a language she hadn't mastered led her to develop her hands-on work. Back in America, she established the School for Body-Mind Centering in Amherst, Massachusetts, in 1973.

The development of the work was slow and methodical. "It took me two years to figure out how to get into my blood, to differentiate it from lymph."[2] It takes four years to complete the school's course of study.

Within Body-Mind Centering is the common idea she shares with the Chinese FIVE ELEMENT THEORY: the organ relation with emotion and character. The correlation is repeatedly revealed as memories and emotions surface when renewed movement takes place within a particular organ. In Body-Mind Centering, for example, the skeletal system provides a physical framework as well as support for thoughts and ideas; the muscles, in addition to moving the body, represent and express vitality, power, resistance and resolve.[3]

The work includes developmental movement, touch and repatterning, breathing and vocalization and perception. Developmental movement underlies movement through the body system. Inner cellular awareness and movement, along with outer awareness and movement through space, help to alleviate developmental problems.

Touch and repatterning provide transference of energy between people. The hands-on work brings an awareness of the force, space and rhythm of the body. Repatterning is facilitated when a mutual resonance is established between the same tissues of the practitioner and participant. Expanded choices and consciousness become available to the participant through repatterning.

Breathing and vocalization provide insight into the relationship between self and the environment. Breathing may help relieve emotional or physical blocks, while vocalization reflects the integration of the body's systems by providing an avenue of expression between the conscious and unconscious mind, self and others.

Body-Mind Centering includes work with infants and young children. Early intervention can prevent unhealthy perceptual-motor development patterns of movement from becoming the norm for a child. With young children, much of the work is done with touch and play.

Notes
[1] Golden, Stephanie, "Body-Mind Centering," *Yoga Journal,* September/October 1993, p. 86.
[2] Ibid., pp. 89–90.
[3] School for Body-Mind Centering, Certificate Program in Body-Mind Centering, School for Body-Mind Centering, Amherst, Mass., 1990, p. 2.

Further Reading
Cohen, Bonnie Bainbridge, *Sensing, Feeling, and Action: The Experiential Anatomy of Body-Mind Centering,* Contact Editions, Northampton, Mass., 1993. The originator of the system discusses the theory and application of Body-Mind Centering. Specific applications for dancers are detailed.

Bodymind Integration the philosophy that all aspects of a person, the physical, emotional and mental, must be connected and balanced in order to maximize well-being and the fulfillment of human potential. This system combines DEEP TISSUE bodywork, GESTALT and REICHIAN techniques to encourage emotional release and balance.

Movement reeducation and methods of personal maintenance retain and expand upon what the client has learned.

Techniques of MYOFASCIAL manipulation are included in each session.

Bodymind Integration simultaneously helps individuals to achieve natural physical balance, reduce tension and expel emotional blocks. It is a short-term bodywork system, generally 10 to 15 sessions, with an overall goal of attaining real personal growth emerging from a total, harmonized "bodymind."

Body Mind Integrative Therapy™ a therapeutic process that works on the physical body to achieve integration of the total self—mind, emotions and spirit. It seeks to free characterological holding patterns found in the body, reinstate natural healing and align the physical with the spiritual self.

It is based on the tradition of Elsa Gindler (see SENSORY AWARENESS) and MARION ROSEN. Body Mind Integrative Therapy is a gentle but powerful form of touching and energy work with the purpose of providing the foundation for safety and ease in the expression with one's body and feelings. Facilitators touch from the heart, nonjudgmentally, and follow somatic cues. The work is intuitive in nature and respectful of the participant.

Body Mind Integrative Therapy has four main components: the physical (muscular), spiritual (energetic), emotional and mental. The work provides a safe environment for validation and the unfolding of the self.

This system has been found helpful in healing gaps in personal development when there has not been a healthy bond with the primary parent. It frees up physical and emotional holding patterns, providing for more spontaneous expression. Deeply held traumas and stored memories are released in a secure environment. Physical, emotional and sexual abuse issues may be resolved gently through Body Mind Integrative Therapy as the participant learns to respond to "good touching."

This system also cultivates unconditional self-love by helping the client to build ego strength to consciously reconnect with the self.

Bodywork for the Childbearing Year^{SM} was created specifically to address the dynamic changes in a pregnant woman's body throughout her pregnancy, labor and postpartum period. Women with low risk, normal pregnancies can reap many benefits from this sensitive work. High risk pregnancies, or women with special needs, are requested to consult with their doctors or midwives before beginning any massage (or exercise) program.

Bodywork for the Childbearing Year was developed in 1984 by Kate Jordan and Carole Osborne-Sheets, both registered massage therapists and mothers. Osborne-Sheets studied DEEP TISSUE MASSAGE and structural MYOFASCIAL work, while Jordan brought her training in SWEDISH MASSAGE, FOOT ZONE THERAPY, NEUROMUSCULAR THERAPY, CROSS-FIBER MASSAGE, the ALEXANDER TECHNIQUE and VISUALIZATION to their system. Their diverse backgrounds contribute to the eclectic techniques and modalities blended in their work.

The treatment consists of specific features of deep tissue sculpting, SWEDISH MASSAGE, JOINT MOBILIZATION, foot zone therapy, CONNECTIVE TISSUE MASSAGE, and TRIGGER POINT THERAPY designed to alleviate many of the physiological, musculoskeletal and emotional stresses that may

accompany pregnancy. Pregnancy massage allows women to approach labor with more confidence and less anxiety.

The client lies on her side, or in a semireclining position, with pillows or support devices surrounding her to help maintain her position comfortably. She is draped throughout the session.

Massage during pregnancy increases blood and lymph circulation, thereby relieving edema, or swelling, in the legs and hands and can relieve pain from varicosities.[1] Pregnancy bodywork can alleviate strain on weight-bearing joints and myofascial structures and provide relief from muscle spasms and cramps. It prepares the pelvic musculature for childbirth, aids in the development of the kinesthetic awareness necessary to give birth and models the nurturant touch that enables a woman to successfully mother her newborn. Pregnancy massage also provides stress reduction, which has a profound impact on pregnancy outcome.

The postpartum bodywork relieves many of the discomforts experienced immediately after birth and helps to return the client's body to its prepregnancy state by restoring the abdomen, repositioning her pelvis and reorganizing her body use to reflect the postpregnancy change in weight distribution.

The professional course, which began in 1984, includes INFANT MASSAGE training. The beneficial effects of infant massage are numerous to both baby and parent, and studies have shown that the physical, emotional and intellectual development of the child is stimulated and bonding is enhanced through touch.[2]

Notes

[1] Pressure directly on varicose veins must be avoided.
[2] Stillerman, Elaine, L.M.T., *MotherMassage: A Handbook for Relieving the Discomforts of Pregnancy,* Delta Books/ Delacorte Press, N.Y., 1992. A study at the Rainbow Babies' and Children's Hospital in Cleveland, Ohio, showed that intellectual development, reading scores, IQs and language skills were raised by infant massage.

body wraps are relaxing, often therapeutic treatments of heated herbs, clay, mud or paraffin. They can help relieve chronic muscle pains, detoxify the body, beautify and smooth the skin and may be beneficial in treating joint disorders such as arthritis and rheumatism. There is still much debate on whether cellulite, weight or inch loss is permanent through the use of body wraps. Most practitioners agree that water loss through perspiration is responsible for any weight loss. Still others claim that inch loss can be permanent.

The herbal body wrap is a 20-minute treatment, which uses a mixture of dried herbs in one of three basic formulas: stimulating, relaxing or cleansing.

Sheets, towels and a cheesecloth bag of the herbal mixture are placed into a vat of steaming water until they are infused with the herbal properties. A massage therapist pulls the sheets and towels out, drains them of excess liquid and drapes a sheet over a massage table.

The client lies nude on the table and the warm sheet is folded over her, topped with a steaming wool blanket and a plastic blanket to retain the heat. Cool cloths are placed on her forehead to prevent overheating. It is not uncommon for the body wrap to be accompanied by a foot massage, or REFLEXOLOGY, treatment.

The healing properties of clay have been known since ancient time. Heated mud is deeply penetrating and therefore beneficial to muscle relaxation, increased circulation and perspiration, lymph drainage and stimulating to the release of toxins. The mud bath is a large tub filled with mud kept at a constant temperature of 103°F. The client submerges herself up to her neck and remains for 15 minutes. After a shower, she enters a whirlpool, and showers again. She may then opt for a full-body massage or just relax in a darkened room, draped with a light blanket.

In a mud wrap, the client's body is coated with a layer of mineralized mud and covered with a plastic wrap and blanket. The treatment can last for half an hour.

A more localized treatment is the mud pack, which is an application of a mud-soaked cloth

pack to a specific body part. The pack is held in place with a plastic wrap and covered with a blanket for half an hour. The mud pack is beneficial in the treatment of joint pain and muscle spasms.

The parafango, or fango pack, is another localized treatment. Common in European spas, this combination of muddy volcanic ash and paraffin is heated and placed on a particular area and covered with a cloth. The paraffin hardens, sealing in the hot mud. It is kept in place for 20 minutes.

There are a few contraindications for these wraps and packs. Pregnant and lactating women should avoid them. People with high blood pressure are cautioned about the excessive heat they may experience. Treatments seem to work best on contaminated or sluggish systems, which require intensity to eliminate the stagnation.

Clients are advised to drink plenty of water, to avoid eating before the treatment and to avoid alcohol for 72 hours after the wrap.

Bowen body balancing   See FASCIAL KINETICS.

breath therapy   the use of respiratory exercises, such as yoga breathing, called *pranayama,* to open lung passages, oxygenate the blood and cleanse the body by eliminating gaseous toxins. Deep breathing can ease anxieties and reduce stress. Historically, air therapy, or fresh air breathing, has been used for centuries. The ancient Incas used to put sick people on mountain tops to expose them to sunlight and pure air.

Individuals with nervous ailments, stomach acidity and some neurotic conditions such as hyperactivity, can benefit from deep breathing exercises. They are also particularly advantageous to individuals with lung and respiratory problems, such as asthma (spasmodic muscles of the bronchioles, which limit breathing and cause wheezing), emphysema (lost elasticity in lung walls, which remain filled with air on exhalation) and bronchial infections (inflammation of bronchi and bronchioles). Deep breathing increases lung capacity, minimizing the effects of those illnesses that restrict the breathing mechanism.

One calming breathing exercise is to inhale deeply through the nose for a count of 10. Hold the breath for a count of 10 and exhale to a count of 10. Eventually, the count can be built up throughout the entire breath cycle. Repeat this exercise for five minutes.

In addition to the physical ailments, which breath therapy can treat, many physical tensions that are primarily emotional or psychological in origin, may also be treated with breath work (see EMOTIONAL RELEASE). This approach believes that unexpressed emotions are stored in the body and constricted breath further inhibits their expression. Participants in breath work are encouraged to breathe deeply into the chest or abdomen while the therapist gently works on those muscles that are being held to numb the feelings. Although emotions can be stored in any part of the body, especially areas of injury or trauma, working the sensitive areas of the chest and abdomen provide an opportunity for emotional release. Deep breathing allows the feelings to flow freely throughout the body. The participant is urged to permit the spontaneous expression of these feelings to surface.

This type of bodywork can be used to deal with current stress but is especially useful in dealing with chronic holding patterns originating from childhood. Participants often report increased energy, a deep sense of release from the past and a greater sense of aliveness from breath work.

breema   a hands-on or self-administered system that uses gentle, yet firm, rhythmic brushes, stretches and holds to create a profound and fluid balance with the physiological and structural systems of the body, the MERIDIANS (energy pathways), and the CHAKRA systems. Self-healing forces are activated, increasing physical vitality, mental clarity and emotional balance.

The mountain villagers of Breemava, a Kurdish region that separates Iran from Afghan-

istan, have been practicing breema for centuries. These farmers and shepherds have developed a unique relationship with nature that rewards them with abundance in a land that would normally be barren and uninhabitable. This fact is not unusual in these remote, mountainous villages. What sets the people of Breemava apart, however, is the development of the system of bodywork they practice, which is based on movements and exercises passed down for centuries. This system was eventually incorporated into daily life as a way to sustain physical and mental health and happiness.

Breema was brought from this distant land in the 1950s by a native who traveled all over the world studying healing methods and finally settled in California, where he opened the Institute for Health Improvement in Oakland.

The participant lies clothed on a soft mat on the floor. The breema touch helps one become more centered, energized and harmonious in mind and emotions. The body is used as a unit, integrating the attention of the mind with the activity of the body.

People who practice breema say that they treat "from the HARA, returning to the *hara*," which is considered to be the most important area of the body.[1] Breema bodywork concentrates on opening the *hara*. "For someone who has *hara*, events of life can be nourishing and supportive. Someone without *hara* is drained by the events of life."[2]

In breema, illness is thought of as an imbalance between the body, mind and spirit. In order to correct this, breema chooses an activity in which all of these aspects will support each other. Emphasis is placed on experiencing one's body, weight and breath, encouraging the mind to recognize the body and inviting the feelings to be balanced.

Breema may also be self-administered. **Brushing**, which has a nurturing effect, is an important segment of the exercises. It allows the preceding section of an exercise to penetrate deeper into the body. **Leaning** on parts of the body is done with an open hand that conforms to the shape of that part. The "leans" easily and comfortably transmit body weight from one area to another. **Holding** with both hands over the *hara*, heart or eyes for three breaths is done to understand the effects of the exercises on the body.

Self-breema begins with three breaths. The first one is an experience of the upper body. The second breath brings the experience of the whole body into focus. The third breath is one of joy accompanying the intake of life energy.

The exercises of breema developed from the people's daily activities and are named to represent these movements. "Grinding the wheat," or "gushing spring" are names used to describe the exercises.

When the body is viewed as an energy system, strengthening exercises can heal certain illnesses and conditions. Breema exercises can be used to treat many ailments such as headaches, asthma, depression and fatigue.

Notes
[1] The Institute for Health Improvement, "The Breema Touch," Oakland, Calif., 1992, p. 1. The Kurdish for *hara* is *del-aka*.
[2] Ibid., p. 2.

Further Reading
Schreiber, Jon, Dr., *Touching the Mountain: The Self-Breema Handbook*, California Health Publications, Oakland, Calif., 1989. This book provides a clear and concise guide to the history and philosophy of breema. Illustrations of the self-breema exercises are easy to follow.
_____, *Walking into the Sun: Stories My Grandfather Told*, California Health Publications, Oakland, Calif., 1991. This book is a collection of stories. Each story is a celebration of the mystery of life.
_____, *Flame of the Unchartered Heart: Essential Poetry*, California Health Publications, Oakland, Calif., 1992. This inspirational collection of poetry is accompanied by 40 illustrations.

Barbara Brennan Healing Science supports the idea that an imbalance in the HUMAN ENERGY FIELD (human AURA) may result in illness. The energy field is composed of seven overlapping and interrelated levels, from the physical levels at the bottom to the spiritual levels at the top. Levels 1, 3, 5 and 7 are structured patterns of lines of light that form a vessel to hold and direct the fluid, flowing bioplasmic levels 2, 4 and 6. Each level corresponds to a particular CHAKRA and vibrates at a unique color and sound frequency. The purpose of Brennan's work is to balance and heal the energy field to prevent or treat disease.

Distortions at any level of the energy field will cause an imbalance in the body, possibly resulting in disease. Brennan believes that by balancing and healing the human energy field, disease can be arrested before it affects the physical body or be more effectively treated if it has already reached the physical body.

Brennan's work includes using **High Sense Perception** to examine the energy field and the interior of the physical body. High Sense Perception employs the five senses and expands them. Brennan uses clairvoyance (seeing beyond the visible light spectrum), clairaudience (hearing beyond normally audible sounds) and clairsentience (the ability to sense someone's emotions and feelings) as part of her diagnostic skills.

She uses touch to help release any energy blocks, which may be caused by either current life conditions or situations in the past, as well as past lives. Brennan believes that all people are capable of learning how to heal on this level, and has a four-year program to train people to do so.

Each level in the human energy field has its unique function. The first level, the **etheric body,** relates to physical functions and sensations and the autonomic functioning of the body. It is associated with the root chakra, found at the base of the spine. The etheric body is made up of scintillating light lines in the pattern of the physical body. These lines of light wrap every cell in the body. This "pattern of health" also extends out from the body for about half an inch. The color varies from light blue to gray.

The second level, the **emotional body,** is associated with emotions and feelings and the sacral chakra. If this energy field is weak, the person may be "out of touch" with his feelings

about himself. In such a case, by focusing in that area, especially working on self-acceptance and self-love, the second level will become charged. This level is associated with immunity, so a good charge is needed for health. It contains all the seven colors of the rainbow.

The third level, the **mental body,** is associated with the solar plexus chakra and controls our mental awareness and linear thought processes. Yellow is the color that emanates from this level. This is also a structured level and is composed of many fine yellow lines of light.

The **astral level** is the fourth level, associated with the heart chakra. This is the level of love where we are able to relate with others. A person with a strong fourth level will have many deep, heart-connected relationships with others, while a person with a weak field will tend to be more of a loner and more interested in other things than people. A vibrant rose color is present on this level, as well as all colors.

The fifth level of the human energy field, the **etheric template body,** is associated with divine will, the power of the word, speaking, and taking responsibility for one's behavior and actions. The related chakra is the throat. A powerful fifth level will provide purpose and attentiveness to work, while a weak field often results in the inability to complete tasks. Cobalt blue is the background for this level.

The sixth level, the **celestial body,** is related to the brow, or third eye chakra, and is associated with divine love. Spiritual pursuits, such as MEDITATION and chanting will stimulate this field. Opalescent pastel colors radiate out in great light streams from this level.

The seventh level, the **ketheric template** or **causal body,** and crown chakra are associated with the higher mind. This level produces a protective shield around the entire field. Creative ideas and the integration of difficult concepts into one's life are stimulated with a powerful seventh level. A weak field will produce a weak person with limited ability to integrate creative ideas into his life. Very powerful and strong gold shimmering lines of light are perceived at this level. These lines, which form an egg-shaped boundary, hold the whole system together.

Brennan says that she was aware of auras and energies in her childhood in Wisconsin and thought everyone was. When she turned to academic pursuits, she forgot about the life energy fields. She earned her undergraduate degree in physics and her graduate degree in upper atmospheric physics from the University of Wisconsin. She spent the next six years at NASA's (National Aeronautics and Space Administration) Goddard Space Flight Center as a research scientist and atmospheric physicist. In 1971, she left NASA and traveled to Mexico for a while, where she renewed her interest in spirituality, meditation and life energy fields.

She then went to the Pathwork Center in Phoenicia, New York, and studied the lectures of Eva Pierrakos, a channel. For nine years, she studied, meditated and developed her unique psychic abilities. Brennan claims that we all have "guides" who communicate with us and help us in our lives. It was during this time that she began to integrate her scientific training and experience with the information she accumulated about the human energy field through High Sense Perception and working as a healer. Out of this, she developed accurate ways to train others to work with the human energy field very precisely to bring about health.

Brennan practiced as a professional healer in New York City for 15 years and founded the Barbara Brennan School of Healing (East Hampton, N.Y.) in 1982 to instruct others in the art of Healing Science. The school offers a four-year program designed for people all over the world. An International Directory of Healers containing the names of people who have graduated from the school is available.

Brennan's work has captured the attention of many doctors and scientists. The National Institutes of Health in Washington, D.C., asked her to cochair an ad hoc committee on Structural and Energetic Therapies. She has also participated with the Russek Foundation, in Boca Raton, Fla., in researching the mind/body connection in health, on a panel on cardiovascular disease with eminent cardiologists and psychologists.

Further Reading

Brennan, Barbara, *Hands of Light: A Guide to Healing Through the Human Energy Field*, Bantam, N.Y., 1987. This best-selling, illustrated book instructs healers how to use High Sense Perception to treat the chakras and energy levels. Brennan offers us a comprehensive explanation, which is a must for all students of metaphysical healing.

_____ , *Light Emerging: The Journey of Personal Healing*, Bantam, N.Y., 1993. Written to help people understand the healing process and heal themselves, this clearly illustrated book offers insights focusing on self-care. Many case histories are described.

C

Cayce/Reilly massage a preventive and curative massage treatment based on Cayce's psychic readings and Dr. Reilly's massage and manipulation methods.

Edgar Cayce (1877–1945) was born in Kentucky. At a very young age, it became apparent that he could "see" and "talk" to nonphysical being or spirit entities, some of whom he recognized as deceased relatives. He related once that, as a school child, he slept for a few moments on a spelling book and was able to remember every word in the book. This did not last, however, and the ability soon faded.

Cayce completed his formal education and took his first job at Hopper's Bookstore in Hopkinsville, Kentucky. In March 1900, he became ill and lost his voice. No longer able to talk with customers, he studied photography where conversation was unnecessary. While employed at the studio of W.R. Bowles in Hopkinsville, he had his first experience with a hypnotist called "Hart, the Laugh Man." Under hypnosis, he was able to speak normally. By experimenting with a friend, Al C. Layne, later known as Dr. Layne, an osteopathic physician, Cayce discovered that he could put himself into a state of altered consciousness that seemed to resemble the hypnotic state. Layne asked Cayce how to correct the problem and from this altered state, Cayce directed Layne to make the suggestion to increase the circulation to his throat. When this was done, Cayce was able to speak normally again, but the loss of his voice was to recur throughout his life.

Cayce, called the "Sleeping Prophet" after the publication of Jess Steran's book *Edgar Cayce Sleeping Prophet* in 1967, was able to tune into the subconscious mind of others by being given their names and addresses. At the time of his death in 1945, he had given over 14,306 readings in the categories of health, business, mental/spiritual/dreams and life readings for 5,787 people.[1] These readings comprise the largest body of psychically derived information in the world.

Dr. Harold J. Reilly (1895–1987) was a noted chiropractor, physiotherapist and proponent of natural therapies. The Reilly Health Institute in Rockefeller Center in New York City was a health mecca for over 30 years. Reilly's association with Cayce began in May 1931, when the sleeping Cayce started sending patients to "Reilly's in New York." While the two men did not meet for two years after this relationship was established, a fast friendship formed and Reilly remained a staunch supporter of Cayce's work until his death in 1987.

Upon closing his office in Rockefeller Center in 1966, Dr. Reilly established a therapy department at the Association for Research and Enlightenment (A.R.E.) in Virginia Beach, Virginia, offering the health services recommended in the readings to the members of the A.R.E. In 1985, Dr. Reilly worked closely with Gladys Davis Turner, Jeanette Thomas and Dr. James C. Windsor in establishing the Harold J. Reilly School of Massotherapy. Reilly was quite explicit in the creation of the term **massotherapy.** He defined massotherapy as a new healing art form, which is a unique combination of suggestions and therapies offered in the Cayce readings.

Some of those therapies included: physiotherapy applications such as packs applied to the body; hydrotherapies included various baths, steam with fume additives and colonic irrigations.

The Cayce/Reilly pattern combines many different massage techniques with passive joint manipulation and mobilization. A synthesis of many disciplines, the Cayce/Reilly pattern incorporates elements of REFLEXOLOGY, LYMPHATIC DRAINAGE, ACUPRESSURE and SWEDISH MASSAGE.

Reilly defines massage as a "systemic therapeutic friction, stroking and kneading of the body."[2] Manipulations, hydrotherapies, including colonic irrigations and massage, were considered to be an integral part of Cayce's drugless therapy. He suggested self-massage as well as professional care.

The strokes of the Cayce/Reilly massage are touching, stroking (effleurage), kneading (petrissage), friction, rolling, wringing, nerve compression, percussion and manipulation.

The massage always begins on the left with a long, slow stroke from the wrist to the shoulder to lubricate and begin contact with the body. Stroking is always performed in the direction of the heart and away from the head, with all circular motions being up and out. The therapist must learn to use both right and left hands equally when changing sides of the body. Stroking prepares the body for deeper work by inducing relaxation and improving venous circulation.

Kneading is the most important therapeutic stroke since it affects the nerves, blood vessels, glands, equalizes blood and lymph flow, increases cellular exchange and speeds up waste and elimination removal.

Friction is often applied without lubrication to the surface of the skin. The underlying tissue is not manipulated.

Rolling moves a limb back and forth with the hands in alternate directions. Wringing is occasionally used on the side of the waist, on excess fat. It is a squeezing movement, drawing back and forth in opposite directions.

Nerve compression normalizes circulation, speeding waste product removal through increased blood and lymph circulation.

Percussion can be performed in a variety of ways. As in Swedish massage, cupping is a tentlike hand position, beating is a relaxed fist with the contact on the ulnar surface, hacking is done with the sides of the open hands, and slapping is performed with open palms. The stroke is rapid, one hand following the other.

Cayce's readings provided many formulas for massage oils as one of many modalities in the treatment of specific ailments or for general use. He frequently suggested the use of peanut oil, alone or in combination, to treat arthritis. Olive oil was said to stimulate muscular or mucous membrane activity. A general tonic calls for:

6 oz. peanut oil
2 oz. olive oil
1 Tb. dissolved lanolin
2 oz. rosewater. Shake well before each use.[3]

Atlantic University, chartered in 1930, is the oldest Cayce organization. Originally conceived as a four-year liberal arts program, the university today offers a master's degree in transpersonal studies. Under the direction of its own board of directors, President Jerry Caldwell administers a program, which offers courses through the mail and in residence. The school received accreditation from the National Home Study Council in June 1994.

The Association for Research and Enlightenment was chartered in 1931. Over 100,000 people from all over the world are involved in the activities of the A.R.E., which has one of the largest parapsychological libraries in the world with over 60,000 volumes. The A.R.E. Press, established in 1992, publishes Edgar Cayce material.

The Edgar Cayce Foundation, chartered in 1948, is the legal owner and physical custodian of Edgar Cayce's and related records. The foundation maintains the Edgar Cayce readings as original transcripts, in microfiches and master database.

The Harold J. Reilly School of Massotherapy was established in 1985 and is a 600-hour credit program in the unique healing modalities of Cayce readings combined with Reilly's massage.

Notes
[1] The Association for Research and Enlightenment.
[2] Reilly, Harold J., Dr., and Brod, Ruth Hagy, *The Edgar Cayce Handbook for Health through Drugless Therapy,* Jove Publications, N.Y., 1975, p. 247.
[3] Ibid., p. 278.

Further Reading
Duggan, Joseph, Ms. T., and Duggan, Sandra R.N., *Edgar Cayce's Massage, Hydrotherapy and Healing Oils,* Home Health Products, Virginia Beach, Va., 1989. Cayce's preventive care and healing recipes are detailed in this book.

Reilly, Harold J., Dr., and Brod, Ruth Hagy, *The Edgar Cayce Handbook for Health through Drugless Therapy,* Jove Publications, N.Y., 1975. Cowritten by Cayce's associate, this how-to book details treatments recommended by Cayce while in trance. Chapters include preventive care, home health and a beauty handbook and longevity guide.

chair massage   a way to provide massage, usually ACUPRESSURE, to clients who are in a seated position. Because it is done through the clothing, this massage requires no lubrication. These 5- to 20-minute massages leave clients feeling revitalized, relaxed and alert.

Practitioners often use specially designed chairs, which allow access to the client's neck, shoulders, back, arms, hands and scalp. Many of these chairs are portable, which makes massage readily available to clients at the workplace, at conventions, in airports, in shopping malls, at street fairs or in many other public venues.

The concept of chair massage was popularized by David Palmer who began working with seated clients in 1983 as a way of providing job opportunities for graduates from his massage school. In 1986, he developed the first massage chair and began a national program to teach table practitioners the techniques and marketing strategies of chair massage. By 1995, there were 15 different massage chairs being manufactured by Palmer's seminar film, *Skilled Touch Institute of Chair Massage,* had trained over 5,000 chair massage practitioners.

Skilled Touch Institute currently offers national certification in chair massage and referral service for practitioners in the United States and Canada.

Further Reading
Palmer, David, *The Chair Massage Handbook,* Skilled Touch Institute of Chair Massage, San Francisco, Calif., 1992. This manual contains over 200 pages of information to help practitioners define and develop their chair massage business.

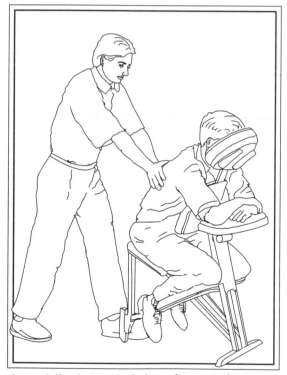

A specially designed chair makes seated massage comfortable and readily available. Massage therapists can carry this portable, lightweight table to offices, convention sites, hotels and practically any place a clothed, short, invigorating massage is requested.

chakra balancing   a system that equalizes the energy vortices of the body. Chakra is a Sanskrit word, which means "wheel" or "revolving energy." The seven major chakras are energy centers of life's vital force, which start at the base of the spine and continue up the body to the top of the head in a vertical power current. In occult anatomy, two currents of energy, + and −, flow on the right and left sides of the body. These currents cross at points between the chakras.

Each chakra is linked to a specific organ, color, element, gland, function, sense, etc. Clairvoyants and highly perceptive individuals contend that chakras are located in the front of the body, relating to feelings, and the back of the body, relating to will, and are funnel-shaped. The openings are wider on the outside of the

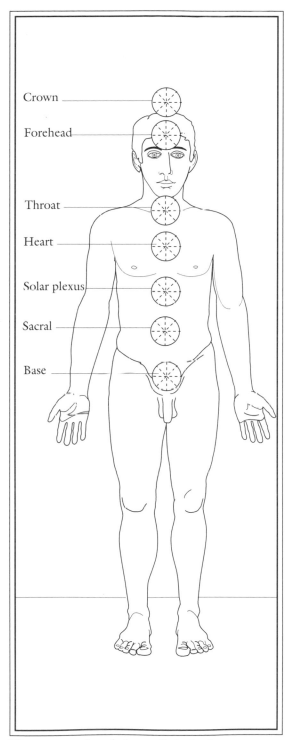

Crown

Forehead

Throat

Heart

Solar plexus

Sacral

Base

The seven major chakras of the body are energy centers of life's vital force. They start at the base of the spine and continue up the body to the crown of the head.

body where they appear to be 6 inches in diameter and are 1 inch away from the body. The small tips are internal, close to the spine.[1]

There are also 21 minor chakras found on the body: one behind each eye, one in front of each ear, one on the sternum (breastbone) where the clavicles (collarbones) meet, one above each breast, one near the liver, one connected to the stomach, two connected to the spleen, one near the thymus gland, one near the solar plexus, one in the palm of each hand, one related to each gonad, one on the sole of each foot and one behind each knee. These chakras are smaller than the seven major ones. They are about 3 inches in diameter and 1 inch from the body.[2] There are also lesser chakras, which are believed to correspond to ACUPUNCTURE points.[3]

The seven major chakras have three functions: to vitalize and energize each AURIC and physical body, to develop the different aspects of self-realization and to transmit energy between auric levels.

The seven major chakras are located on the body along the midline. The first chakra, the **root** or **base** chakra, is located at the base of the spine, between the legs. It is associated with kinesthetics, the sense of body position, proprioception, the sense of physical movement and tactile senses. The first chakra provides the will to live and supplies vitality to the body. The element of the root chakra is the quality of solidarity, or the earth. This chakra governs all that is solid in the body, such as bones, spinal column, teeth and nails. The kidneys are also ruled by the first chakra. The endocrine glands that are associated with the first chakra are the adrenals. The root chakra is often symbolized with the color red and by the vibration of the musical note G, below middle C.

The second chakra is the **sacral** chakra, located above the pubic bone in the front and back of the body. This is where the experience of internal fluidity is derived, therefore its element is water. Emotions, sensuality and sexuality are based at this point. The color of the sacral chakra is orange and it vibrates at the same level as the musical note D. The sacral chakra rules the reproductive organs.

The third chakra, called the **solar plexus** chakra, is found directly under the tip of the sternum in the front and back of the body. At this level, expansiveness and warmth are experienced, so the chakra is associated with the element of fire. The solar plexus chakra provides the visceral organs with energy and relates to intuition and linear thinking. The endocrine gland governed by this chakra is the pancreas. Its color is yellow and its musical note is F.

The fourth chakra, the **heart** chakra, relates to love in the front and will in the back of the body. The element is air and the sense of touch is derived from this element. Energy is provided to the heart, circulatory system, thymus, vagus nerve and upper back from the fourth chakra. The thymus is the endocrine gland at this level. Its color is green and the musical note is G.

The fifth chakra, the **throat** chakra, is found on the front and the back of the body. Its element is ether, which gives the sense of sound. Energy at the throat chakra is supplied to the thyroid gland, bronchi, lungs and alimentary tract. The thyroid is the endocrine gland of the throat chakra. Articulating truth, giving and receiving come from the center, whose color is blue and musical note A.

The sixth chakra, the **brow** or **third eye** chakra, is located on the forehead between the eyebrows and at the back of the head. It supplies energy to the pituitary gland, the corresponding endocrine gland, the lower brain, left eye, ears, nose and nervous system. The front of this chakra rules the power of thought or conceptual comprehension, while the back is related to the ability of actualizing tasks. Sight is the sense of the sixth chakra. Its color is indigo and musical note is D.

The seventh chakra, the **crown** chakra, is located at the top of the head and has the highest frequency of energy vibration. It supplies energy to the brain and right eye. It is associated with

spirituality and knowing. Religions depict the seventh chakra in various ways: halos were painted around the heads of holy or highly evolved people; the tonsure of monks has its origins in the crown chakra; statues of Buddha usually show the crown chakra at the top of his head; and Jewish men and women cover the top of their heads in deference to the Lord and to contain power energy. The pineal gland is the endocrine gland of the crown chakra. Its color is violet, or sometimes white, and the musical note is G above middle C.

Ancient texts have acknowledged the presence and function of chakras. In AYURVEDA, in addition to their organ, element, sense, color, etc., association, each chakra is represented by a deity. The first chakra is pictured as a four-petal lotus (these petals are rapidly rotating vortices, vibrating at different frequencies) represented by Muladhara and the element of earth. It governs waste, elimination and the skeletal system. The second chakra is the element of water, represented by Swadisthan and controlling reproduction, the LYMPHATIC system and body fluids.

The third chakra has Manipura as its deity, the element of fire and rules digestion and metabolism. Air is the element for the fourth chakra, the god is Anahata, and it controls respiration, circulation and the nervous system. The fifth chakra is represented by Visuddha, the element of ether, and controls voice production, hearing and the joints.

The sixth chakra is represented by the god Agyan. The seventh, located at the crown of the head, is represented by an inverted lotus of 1,000 petals.[4]

HATHA YOGA prepares the lower energies to be raised to the higher levels. Kundalini yoga draws energy up from the spine to the crown of the head to achieve enlightenment. The chakras are considered to be subtle force centers, which energize and control the physical body.

Metaphysically, there are seven layers of consciousness that are represented in the chakras. At the top of the head is the spirit and at the base of the spine is matter in its densest form. In between, the energy gets denser in a descending order. The accompanying vibrations also become lower in a descending order. If there are any imbalances or blocks in these vital centers, physical, emotional or mental dysfunction could result.

There are many forms of treatment to clear, or balance, the chakras. COLOR THERAPY reflecting each chakra's color is often employed. CRYSTAL HEALING, or the use of stones and gems placed directly on the chakras, can alter the frequency of vibrations. VISUALIZATION techniques, SOUNDING (or toning) to vibrate at a specific chakra pitch, breathing, exercises and ACUPUNCTURE are all used to balance the chakras.

Psychics report that at the time of death, there is an opening of all the chakras. The three lower chakras dissolve as cords of energy are emitted and the four upper chakras form holes into another dimension.

Notes
1 Brennan, Barbara Ann, *Light Emerging,* Bantam Books, N.Y., 1993, p. 28. Chakras and auras, or the emanation of the human energy field, cannot be discerned by the naked eye. People with highly developed intuitive skills and psychic abilities can "read" auras and "see" chakras. Kirlian photography proves the presence of the human energy field, which surrounds each of us.
2 Ibid., p. 28.
3 Ibid., p. 28. Dr. David Tansely, a RADIONICS expert, proposes this theory in his book, *Radionics and the Subtle Anatomy of Man,* Health Science Press, Devon, England, 1972.
4 Reader's Digest, *Family Guide to Natural Medicine,* Reader's Digest Association, Inc., Pleasantville, N.Y., 1993, pp. 53–54.

Further Reading
Brennan, Barbara Ann, *Hands of Light,* Bantam Books, N.Y., 1988. This text is full of beautiful illustrations, some in color, depicting the human energy field, chakras and auras. Her text is detailed and carefully annotated.
———, *Light Emerging: The Journey of Personal Healing,* Bantam Books, N.Y., 1993. A beautifully illustrated, detailed text about the author's gift of healing. This book is a personal account of her experiences as a healer, citing many cases.
Bruyere, Rosalyn, *Wheels of Light,* Healing Light Center, Glendale, Calif., 1987. A comprehensive book describing the nature of each chakra, the chakra system, energy flow to the chakras, spin direction, diseases and dysfunctions and a balanced energy field. A popular book for healers and their clients.
Leadbeater, C. W., *The Chakras,* Theosophical Publishing House, London, 1974. An easy-to-follow explanation of the functions of the chakras.
Rendel, Peter, *Introduction to the Chakras,* Samuel Weiser Inc., N.Y., 1974. This small paperback provides detailed information about the chakras, how to clear them, the chakra zodiac and includes a few illustrations to clarify the author's theories.
Tansely, David, Dr., *Radionics and the Subtle Anatomy of Man,* Health Science Press, Devon, England, 1972. This is an innovative scientific study of the human energy field.

chi, also called *qi* in Chinese, *ki* in Japanese, and *prana* in Hindi, is the fundamental energy force that powers all life. The concept of *chi* is deeply rooted in the Chinese philosophy, religion and culture. It is the life force in which the body/mind/spirit are inseparable.

Chi is the source of strength and vitality, which flows within the body in a network of energy pathways called MERIDIANS. It is believed that if there is a block anywhere along the meridians, energy becomes stopped up and disease will result.

Chi, blood and body fluids are basic substances, which keep the body in a state of HOMEOSTASIS, or normal functioning. They are the materials that promote healthy activities of internal organs, tissues and meridians.

CHINESE MEDICINE believes that *chi* is the basic substance of the universe and all phenomena were caused by the movement of *chi.* The word denotes both essential substances that maintain the body's vital activities and the functional activities of the organs and tissues.

The body derives *chi* energy from a variety of sources, which are dependent on each other for production and nurishment. *Chi* that is inherited from the parents is called **congenital chi.** *Chi* that comes from food and water (almost 50 percent of *chi* comes from the transformation of the food we eat), air (almost 50 percent of *chi* comes from breathing) or light is called **acquired chi.**

Chi works in different ways throughout the

body. It promotes growth and development of the body; it acts as a warmth regulator, keeping the body at a normal temperature; it defends the body against external pathogens; it checks, controls and regulates metabolism and body substances; it transforms the essences (*chi,* blood and body fluids) into food essences to permit healthy growth; it assists in organ functions; and it helps extract nourishment from food substances that circulate throughout the body.

Physical exercise, ACUPUNCTURE, MOXIBUSTION, MASSAGE, MEDIATION, etc., may be used to stimulate the flow of *chi* and release any blocks for optimum health.

Further Reading

Chia, Mantak, *Chi Self Massage: The Taoist Way of Rejuvenation,* Healing Tao Books, Huntington, N.Y., 1986. Exercises and massage techniques to stimulate *chi* energy.

Olson, Stuart A., *Cultivating the Chi,* Dragon Door Publications, St. Paul, Minn., 1993. Photographed book providing exercises for strength, breathing, Tai Chi, meditation and *qi gong.*

Reed, William, *Ki: Practical Guide for Westerners,* Japan Publications, N.Y., 1986. This book defines *chi (ki)* in basic terms and shows how to develop it as a practical force for everyday life.

Tohei, Koichi, *Ki in Daily Life,* Japan Publications, N.Y., 1978.

———— , *Book of Ki: Co-ordinating Mind and Body in Daily Life,* Japan Publications, N.Y., 1976. Exercises and explanations of how *ki* energy is created and used.

chi nei tsang,　or internal organ massage, is a massage technique, which was developed to relieve obstructions of CHI energy in the internal organs and restore health. Taoist sages of ancient China believed that blocks in the flow of *chi* led to knots, stoppages and diseases. Negative emotions, invasive traumas, such as surgery or drug abuse, and stress can contribute to internal problems.

This system was created to relieve congestion in the internal organs and optimize health. The organs are allied with the five forces of nature[1] (see FIVE ELEMENT THEORY), the related emotions and energy pathways (see MERIDIANS).

The energy channels of *chi nei tsang* consist of the 12 traditional meridians[2] plus the GOVERNING VESSEL MERIDIAN and the CONCEPTION VESSEL ME-

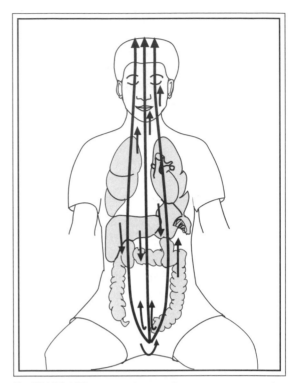

In Chi Nei Tsang, or internal organ massage, the three thrusting channels create a central energy route. *Chi* energy can flow up or down.

RIDIAN, three **thrusting channels,** and the **belt channel,** which make up the body's energy grid.

The thrusting channels are vertical pathways, 1 to $1\frac{1}{2}$ inches wide, which connect with the universal and earth's energy axis. They are connected to all channels and are thought to be a part of the "sea of twelve channels," feeding energy throughout the entire body. The left thrusting channel begins in the left testicle or ovary and ends in the left hemisphere of the brain. The middle thrusting channel, *chong mai* (sea of blood), begins at the scrotum or cervix and ends at the crown of the head. This channel breaks up congestion of *chi* and blood in the abdomen and chest. The right thrusting channel starts at the right testicle or ovary and ends in the right hemisphere of the brain.

The belt channel encircles the entire body with energy, protecting the *chi* and inhibiting negative external energy from physical penetration.

A negative energy cycle is created when blocked energies build up within the organs or move into the abdomen. The diseases that follow can be treated once the toxins and negative influences are removed. *Chi nei tsang* is a direct massage to the viscera and the energy pathways to assist in the release of these obstructions.

The facilitator first observes the general health of the organs by examining the skin, shape and musculature of the abdomen, the breathing pattern, the musculature of the back (as it compensates for a weaker or unhealthy abdomen) and general posture. The Taoists believed that all the energy channels enter and exit from the navel center, called *tan tien* (*tan den*—see HARA).[3] It is the portal between the physical body and the pervasive energy. The massage stimulates and directly affects this vital center.

The shape of the navel is also an indicator of internal organ health. Distortions, or pulls, to any side reflect specific internal problems. The navel is divided into eight sections. Upper pulls toward the sternum (breastbone) indicate problems in the intestines, with the menstrual cycle, prostate, breathing and coughing. Pulls to the upper left indicate problems in the right hip, right leg, stomach, spleen and digestive system. Left pulls indicate right side problems of the kidneys and intestines. Lower left pulls indicate upper right side problems including liver, gallbladder, duodenum and right kidney.

A navel pull downward indicates intestinal trouble, mental confusion, menstrual and bladder problems. Pulls to the lower right indicate upper left abnormalities in the pancreas, stomach, spleen and left kidney. Pulls to the right indicate left side involvement of kidneys and intestines. Pulls to the upper right affect the left hip, left leg, liver, gallbladder and the intestines.

A hands-on examination of the abdomen is part of the diagnosis. The facilitator feels for heat and energy emanations from each organ. Other diagnostic techniques include face reading, TONGUE DIAGNOSIS and PULSE READING.

The Taoists recognized **winds** that circulate within the body, affecting health and spirit. Evil winds are trapped as toxins and blocked energy. These winds must be cleared at the beginning of each session by pressing and holding points on the abdomen where the block is felt.

The session is conducted with the recipient lying clothed on his back with pillows or cushions under his knees to relax the abdomen. The facilitator will use his thumbs, fingers, open palms and the sides of his hands to press, squeeze, shake, push and pull, rock, pat, scoop and/or spiral on the abdomen, generally in a clockwise direction. Elbows are used on large or muscular abdomens.

Chi nei tsang may also be self-administered.

Notes
[1] The traditional Chinese Five Element Theory classifies nature as being made up of fire, water, earth, metal and wood.
[2] The twelve regular channels, or meridians, are bladder, kidney, small intestine, heart, heart constrictor, triple warmer, large intestine, lung, gall bladder, liver, stomach and spleen.
[3] The actual acupuncture point of *tan tien* is located on the midline of the body, along the conception vessel meridian, $1\frac{1}{2}$ inches below the navel. The point is numbered CV 6.

Further Reading
Chia, Mantak and Maneewan, *Chi Nei Tsang: Internal Organs Chi Massage,* Healing Tao Books, Huntington, N.Y., 1990. This illustrated book is written in an easy-to-use style. Preparation for internal organ massage as well as the techniques are clearly explained.

Chinese massage See TUI-NA.

Chinese medicine an ancient and complex art and science, which describes the physiology, pathology, diagnosis and treatment of the human body in intricate and mutually related terms. The theories of YIN/YANG, FIVE ELEMENTS, *zang-fu* (internal organs), MERIDIANS, *qi* (CHI), blood and fluids, which are diagnostic filters for herbal and ACUPUNCTURE treatments, are all part of Chinese medicine.

All of the ancient bodywork systems from China, such as Acupuncture, MOXIBUSTION, ACUPRESSURE, etc., can trace their roots and philosophies to Chinese medicine. Many of the related Oriental healing arts also follow the theories of this sophisticated healing art and science.

The *zang-fu,* the internal organs, are the core of the human body and are interconnected by an intricate network of meridians (energy pathways), which carry the vital life force, *qi,* blood and fluids. Chinese medicine treats the individual holistically, as well as prescribing specifically for particular symptom-complexes.

Any pathology to the *zang-fu* could be manifested in many ways. It may be superficially reflected in the channels and their collaterals. Or the tissues of the involved organ may show signs of disease. The affected *zang* or *fu* organs might also influence each other internally. One way Chinese medicine seeks to regulate the functions of the internal organs is through the use of acupuncture. The treatments will take into consideration the environmental influences of the seasons and temperature.

Syndromes are differentiated in order to find the appropriate treatment. They are analyzed in order to define its essentials, the cause of the problem, its location and its nature. Chinese medicine stresses the difference of syndromes, not of diseases, so it is not uncommon to have varying treatments for the same disease.[1]

The concept of yin/yang and the Five Element Theory were developed by the Chinese by observing the cycles of nature. They recognized the dynamic movement of yin and yang forces and that the physical world was made up of wood, fire, earth, water and metal. When applied to medicine, these theories helped explain the physiological activities and pathological changes a body may undergo. Treatments are also based on these principles.

Yin and yang represent the two complementary opposites of every object, their interdependence and contrast, which are involved in a constantly transforming relationship. Medically,

it is understood that an organic connection exists between all structures and tissues, which can be divided into the polar aspects of yin/yang.

The yang portion of the body is the upper torso, from the waist up, while the yin portion of the body is located in the lower half, from the waist down. The exterior is considered to be yang, while the interior of the body is yin. The back is yang, the front is yin. The lateral aspect of the body is yang, medial is yin. The *zang-fu* organs also have yin/yang relationships. The six *fu* organs are yang and the five *zang* organs are yin. Health is considered to be a state of balanced yin/yang. Disease can also be a result of body resistance, **zheng qi,** or pathogenic factors, **xie qi.** Each of these factors are divided into yin or yang in order to ascertain its nature.

The Five Element Theory postulates that all of nature is made up of wood, fire, earth, metal and water, which are in constant motion and change and deeply interrelated. This theory was used to study the physiological and pathological connections between the *zang-fu* organs and tissues with the environment. Each element is classified with specific characteristics and functions.

This theory asserts that between the elements are connections of varying support or destruction. In Chinese medicine, these relationships help guide the diagnosis and treatment of disease. The *zang-fu* theory explains the physiological functions, changes and relationships of each *zang* and *fu* organ. The six *zang* organs are the heart (pericardium), lung, spleen, liver and kidney. The six *fu* organs are the gall bladder, large intestine, stomach, small intestine, urinary bladder and **san jiao** (three areas of the body cavity, including the connective tissue).[2] The classification is determined by their functions. For instance, the *zang* organs manufacture and store fluids, blood and *qi,* while the *fu* organs digest food, assimilate nutrients and excrete waste.

Another category, called the **extraordinary** *fu* organs, includes the brain, marrow, bone, vessels, gall bladder and uterus.[3]

Qi, blood and body fluids are essential substances, which keep the *zang-fu* organs and tissues healthy. According to Chinese medicine, there are four types of *qi,* classified by their origin and function. **Primary *qi*** (*yuan qi*) is the most important *qi,* developing in utero. It is called the ***qi* of the kidney. Aggregative *qi*** (*zong qi*) is a combination of inhaled *qi* and nutritionally assimilated *qi.* It promotes respiration and blood circulation. **Nutrient *qi*** (*ying qi*) originates from the food transformed by the spleen and the stomach. **Defensive *qi*** (*wei qi*) is derived from food and water. It circulates outside the vessels and helps defend against external pathogenic factors.

The blood is the creation of food catabolism in the spleen and stomach. ". . . when the *qi* and blood are abundant, there can be high spirits and clear minds."[4] Body fluids include all other liquids, such as saliva, tears, nasal discharges, sweat, urine, etc. These fluids are a result of food and drink digestion and absorption by the spleen and stomach.

The meridian system is vital to Chinese medicine. There are 12 regular (6 yin/6 yang) channels, 8 extra channels, 15 collaterals, 12 divergent channels and the musculotendinous and cutaneous regions of the 12 regular channels. These are the energy pathways where *qi* flows.

Chinese medicine diagnoses diseases using four basic methods: looking, hearing and smelling, asking and feeling. Looking, or inspection, provides information about a client through observation of his expressions, demeanor, color, spirit, facial organs and channels. The colors of the facial complexion are very revealing: white is a sign of *qi* and blood deficiency; yellow skin reveals a spleen deficiency; red indicates excessive heat and full blood vessels; green indicates a liver dysfunction and deficiency; blue indicates coldness, pain, blood stasis; and black indicates blood stasis and kidney deficiency. The face and eyes are of particular importance in diagnosis because the organs of the body are reflected in certain parts of them. The tongue is carefully examined (see tongue diagnosis), along with the teeth, gums and throat. Colors in the ears and nose also reveal the presence of certain pathologies.

Hearing (auscultation) and smelling (olfaction) are an integral part of the diagnostic process. The practitioners will listen to the voice, respiration and cough. In addition, body smell, breath and excretions may be examined.

Asking questions reveals not only what personal medical history is stated, but also what is overlooked. Questions are generally asked about overall health, chills and fevers, sweating, thirst, pain, gynecological problems, sleep, excretion habits, etc. The characteristics of each description will help in diagnosing and treating the problem.

The fourth diagnostic method is feeling, or palpation. This includes pulse reading and general body palpation. The best time for taking the pulse is in the early morning, but it is not always possible to do so. The practitioner uses her first three fingers on each of the client's radial pulses while she regulates her breathing to match her client's. The normal pulse is described as having stomach *qi,* spirit and root.[5]

After the diagnosis, the symptoms are differentiated according to the **Eight Principles of Differentiation:** exterior/interior, hot/cold, deficiency (*zu*)/excess (*shi*) and yin/yang. They are further analyzed according to the zang-fu organs and channels.

The therapies prescribed are guided by the principles of treatment, which include **root** (*ben*) and **branch** (*biao*), In other words, according to the principles of cause and effect. Considerations are also made on the strength of the client's *qi* energy, pathogenic factors, the need to tonify or reduce and/or the client's constitution.

The treatments of Chinese medicine may include, but are not limited to, acupuncture, moxibustion, herbs and medicines.

Notes
1. Junying, Geng and Zhihong, Su, *Practical Traditional Chinese Medicine: Basic Theories and Principles,* New World Press, Beijing, 1990, p. 5.

2 Ibid., p. 24.
3 Ibid., p. 25.
4 Ibid., p. 46.
5 Macicocia, Giovanni, *The Foundation of Chinese Medicine: A Comprehensive Text for Acupuncturists and Herbalists,* Churchill Livingstone, Edinburgh, 1989, p. 166. Stomach *qi* is a gentle pulse, four beats per respiratory cycle. A pulse with spirit is soft, but strong and regular. A pulse is said to have root in two different senses when it is healthy. In one instance, it is a sign of good health, and secondly, it is representative of the kidneys.

Further Reading

Chang, Chung-Ching, *Chin Kuei Yao Lueh—Prescriptions from the Golden Chamber,* trans. Wang Su-yen and Hong-yen Hsu. Oriental Healing Arts Institute, Taiwan, 1983. This is a Chinese and English text of Chinese medicine herbal remedies.

Hong-Yen, Hsu Dr., and Peacher, William G. Dr., *Chen's History of Chinese Medical Science,* Oriental Healing Arts Institute, Taiwan, 1977. Photographs and illustrations depict the history and the great physicians and contributors to this complex theory.

Junying, Geng and Zhihong, Su, *Practical Traditional Chinese Medicine and Pharmacology—Basic Theories and Principles, Vol. I.* New World Press, Beijing, 1990. This is an illustrated guide to the theories of Chinese medicine. Yin/yang and the Five Element Theory are described in detail as the basic philosophical elements of Chinese medicine. The meridians and *zang-fu* organs are discussed.

Macicocia, Giovanni, *The Foundation of Chinese Medicine: A Comprehensive Text for Acupuncturists and Herbalists,* Churchill Livingstone, Edinburgh, 1989. This is a detailed text of Chinese medicine with specific analyses of each meridian.

Shang, Han Lun, *The Great Classic of Chinese Medicine,* trans. and edited by Hong-yen, Ph.D., and Dr. William G. Preacher, Oriental Healing Arts Institute, Taiwan, 1981. This text, in Chinese and English, studies the herbal remedies of Chinese medicine.

Yan, Wu and Fischer, Warren, *Practical Therapeutics of Traditional Chinese Medicine,* Paradigm Books, Brookline, Mass., 1995. This clinically specific text is based on Chinese medicine practices in the medical centers of the People's Republic of China. Over 100 conditions are differentiated according to their patterns and related biomedical pathologies.

chiropractic a preventive and therapeutic hands-on health care system that realigns the spine (and extremities) to help restore normal functioning of the nervous system, which controls most body functions. It is a natural approach that addresses the relationship between the spinal column, nervous system and disease.

The term comes from two Greek words: *cheiro* and *praktos,* which translates to mean "done by hand." Doctors of chiropractic manually remove interference to the nervous system (without drugs or surgery), permitting innate energy to flow unimpeded throughout the body, thus promoting the body's inborn ability to heal itself.

Chiropractic is the largest alternative health care system in the Western world. It is estimated that over 15 million patients go to the chiropractor as their primary care practitioners. It is the second largest health care system after traditional allopathic medicine. There are over 40,000 chiropractors in the United States, 16 percent of whom are women, with 2,500 getting licensed each year.[1]

Although chiropractic was not formerly introduced to the United States until the late 19th century, spinal manipulation has been practiced since ancient times. Healers in India, Europe and the Orient practiced a form of chiropractic. Hippocrates advised doctors to observe the spine for "dislocations" when treating disease. Native Americans and Mexicans manipulated the spine to treat back pain and disease.

During the Renaissance, "bone setters" were considered to be gifted healers, and spinal manipulation became a widespread practice in Europe.

Chiropractic came to the United States almost accidently. Daniel David Palmer (1845–1913) was born in Ontario, Canada, in a small town called Port Perry. As a young child, he would often treat injured animals by splinting their broken bones. He left Canada in 1865 and came to the United States where he became a student of Paul Caster, a MAGNETIC HEALER from Burlington, Iowa.

For nine years, Palmer practiced as a magnetic healer, studying and researching the anatomy and physiology of the spine. These studies convinced him that spinal MISALIGNMENT could be responsible for disease.

One day in 1895, Harvey Lillard, a janitor in Palmer's building, told Palmer of his 17-year deafness, which occurred when he was exerting himself from a stooped position. Palmer palpated Lillard's spine and repositioned one of his vertebrae, which seemed to be out of ALIGNMENT. Lillard soon regained his hearing. The science of chiropractic was born.

His second success came when he treated a heart patient using spinal manipulation. This convinced Palmer that spinal misalignments had far-reaching effects, which might account for discomforts and diseases. (Palmer also has the dubious distinction of being the first chiropractor jailed for practicing medicine without a license.)

He opened the first chiropractic school in the United States, Palmer College of Chiropractic, in Davenport, Iowa, in 1897.

Chiropractic has been used to treat neuro-musculo-skeletal disorders, neck stiffness and pain, whiplash, paraesthesia, back sprain, sciatica (inflammation of the sciatic nerve, which runs down the back of the leg), arthritis, headaches and migraines, pregnancy and postpartum structural changes and nervous disorders. Chiropractic has helped patients with many diseases, but chiropractors claim to improve the overall health of the patient, which may in turn affect a specific disorder.

A chiropractic session usually lasts less than 30 minutes. On the first visit, a complete physical examination and medical history are taken, reflexes are tested, muscle testing may be included (see APPLIED KINESIOLOGY), flexibility is measured, and X rays may be taken to check spinal **alignment** and to look for any preexisting pathologies.

The vertebrae of the spine fit together so that nerve impulses from the brain may filter down the spinal cord and out through the nerves, and to promote physical flexibility. These neural messages communicate information all over the body in order that growth, repair and healing may occur. When vertebrae are out of their natural position, or alignment, the potential for nerve interference, or **spinal nerve stress,** is great. Chiropractors call this a **subluxation.**

When there is nerve interference, which is commonly known as a "pinched nerve," the critical communication between the brain and the spinal column with the body is impeded.

Subluxations may be the cause (or result) of abnormal posture, placing tension on the vertebrae, muscles, ligaments and tendons. Blood flow to internal organs is hindered. This may result in organ dysfunction or disease. Rather than treating a patient symptomatically, chiropractors treat subluxations to restore normal function.

Chiropractors place their hands on the back and gently realign the vertebrae with quick thrusts called **adjustments** or manipulations. The frequency of the healing process can be weeks or months, depending upon the condition of the patient and the extent and duration of misalignment. Periodic treatments maintain the adjustments and prevent injuries, while specific problems are treated more often.

There are many kinds of chiropractic adjustments. Two common types are the high velocity, low force **recoil** thrust and the **rotational** thrust. With the recoil thrust, the patient lies face down on a specially designed, sectional table. The doctor presses against the skin of the spine and quickly thrusts.

The rotational thrust is performed with the patient lying on her side. The upper body is twisted counter to the pelvis, rotating the spine to its limit of movement. A short, fast thrust adjusts the spine.

Once the spine becomes aligned, nerve impulses flow more effectively and healing takes place as symptoms minimize and finally disappear.

Spinal movement was described by a theory coined by the Lovett brothers, both chiropractors. The spine functions with a specific harmony. The top three cervical verbebrae, C1–C3, move synchronously with the bottom three lumbar, L5–3.[2] This means that if the first cervical vertebra (called the atlas) rotates to the right, the fifth lumbar also rotates to the right. The potential of movement changes at the fourth cervical (C4) vertebra down to the second lumbar (L2), when movement compensates in opposite directions. At this level, and all vertebrae below (to L3), rotate in opposite directions (i.e., C4 rotates right as L2 rotates left).[3]

An interesting phenomena of the healing process is something that chiropractic refers to as **retracing.** Basically, it is a reexperiencing or reawakening of old pains and symptoms, including emotions, which may surface, as part of the healing process. Patients may complain about feeling worse after several treatments and are dissuaded by this reaction from continuing the care. However, further treatment will clear these reactive symptoms as overall health improves.

The chiropractic explanation of retracing is that all body tissues, especially CONNECTIVE TISSUE, store the memories of all traumas, shocks and injuries. The emotional component, which may accompany the injury, will also be expressed and finally dissolved as healing proceeds.[4]

Retracing can happen in many other types of bodywork as well. In psychotherapy, it is called "progressive abreactive regression" (PAR). It is considered to be a phase the patient passes through on the way toward healing and wholeness and normal in human growth at all levels.[5] It is, however, uncommon in allopathic medicine because prescribed drugs tend to suppress the disease and mask its symptoms.

The medical community has often frowned upon chiropractic, often calling it quackery. However, in the 1970s, a number of scientific studies brought respect and recognition to the healing powers of chiropractic. The Oregon Workmen's Compensation Board found that chiropractors restored the health to patients with back injuries twice as effectively as conventional medicine.[6]

Those practitioners who use traditional chiropractic care as the primary treatment are called "straight" doctors. These doctors exclusively perform spinal adjustments to restore nerve function. "Mixers," however, use chiropractic in conjunction with other therapies, such as MASSAGE, nutritional advice, traction, ULTRASOUND electric stimulation and other systems to provide comprehensive health care. Currently, there are about 150 different techniques, some of which do not involve any manual (osseous) adjusting.

People of all ages can benefit from chiropractic care. Athletes, both professional and amateur, perform better when the spine is aligned. Those activities, which are one-sided, such as tennis, golf, baseball, racquet sports, etc. create a situation where the spinal column loses its natural balance and stress is always placed on one side. Microtraumas, caused by repeated movement, can still cause damage to the body.

Professional athletes, dancers, especially involved in contact sports, absorb a great deal of shock to the spine and corresponding nerves. Chiropractic care can realign the spine, strengthen the muscles, enhance recuperation and prevent injuries.

Doctors of chiropractic must be licensed to practice throughout the United States and Canada.

Notes

1. *Prevention Magazine,* "Hands on Healing," Rodale Press, Emmaus, Pa., 1989, p. 58.
2. The spine is made up of 7 cervical vertebrae in the neck (C1–7), 12 thoracic (or dorsal) vertebrae in the middle of the back (T1–12), 5 lumbar vertebrae in the lower back (L1–5), the sacrum and the coccyx, totaling 24 vertebrae.
3. Spinal movement, however, does not always follow the Lovett brothers' pattern of subluxation. Any variation on this structure may indicate a neurological disorganization called **switching.**
4. Upledger, John E., Dr., and Vredevoogd, J. D., *Craniosacral Therapy,* Eastland Press, Seattle, 1983, p. 251.
5. Stein, A., " Comprehensive Family Therapy,' *The Psychotherapy Handbook,* R. Herink, ed., New American Library, N.Y., 1980, p. 204–07.
6. Prevention Magazine, *Hands on Healing,* Rodale Press, Emmaus, Pa., 1989, p. 61.

Chua Ka[SM] a bodywork system that is either self-administered or used by Arica practitioners in sessions with their clients. It was created by Oscar Ichazo, the founder of the Arica School headquartered in New Rochelle, New York. Ichazo brought Chua Ka to America in 1971 to support internal development. This system refines the body to its highest level of vitality, awareness and strength and restores balance to the mind.

The words *chua ka* mean "cleaning stick" since the *ka,* a tool made from wood, bone or plastic, is often used in the treatments.

Ichazo says that everything that happens to the body is reflected in the mind, and vice versa. Unreleased tensions, which remain within the muscles and CONNECTIVE TISSUE, cause the body to lose its suppleness and energy. Joint RANGE OF MOTION is diminished and the aging process is accelerated.

Chua Ka identifies 27 areas, called **zones of karma,** which are worked in ascending order from feet to head and face. Each zone holds tensions of specific experiences and their related emotional/psychological components.

The Chua Ka method uses three techniques. The hands and the *ka* stick are used like sculpting tools, in precise positions on the body. The connective tissue and the muscles, particularly the tendons,[1] are worked deeply with the fingertips. Heat and vital energy are consciously directed and transmitted to the area. The *ka* stick is used to smooth or separate the muscles.

Skin rolling lifts or pinches the skin between the fingers and thumbs. It stimulates the ACUPUNCTURE MERIDIANS. It increases the flow of blood and LYMPH, stimulates nerve transmissions to the brain and increases skin elasticity by freeing it from underlying muscles to which it had adhered.

There are 72 **vortex points** in Chua Ka. Pressing these points increases the vitality of various muscle groups, relaxes muscle spasms and speeds the elimination of toxins from the body.

Chua Ka acts like a tonic on the body and the mind. Immediate effects can produce increased energy and awareness, while the long-term result is a stronger, more vital body with restored youth and elasticity to the skin.

Note
[1] Tendons are connective tissue, which attach muscle to bone.

Further Reading
Ichazo, Oscar, *Arica Theory and Practice,* Arica Institute, New Rochelle, N.Y., 1972. This clearly written book describes the theory and philosophy of Arica and the massage technique of Chua Ka.

Bonnie Bainbridge Cohen system See BODY-MIND CENTERING®.

color therapy, or chromotherapy, is an ancient system that uses specific color rays to treat diseases of the body and the mind. Color therapy is based on the idea that all organs and body systems vibrate at certain frequencies. Colors are made of specific vibratory energies. By applying a particular color ray on an area, which is deficient or diseased, the correct vibration, and therefore health, will be restored.

The ancient Egyptians were practitioners of color healing. They used healing bowls and jars that were filled with fruit and vegetable juices and left out in the sun to "collect the energy of Ra."[1] The sick patients then drank the irradiated potion. Jewels of the same color were sometimes added to the bowls to increase the potency of the brew.

Sunlight transmits seven major colors through the atmosphere. When sunlight is passed through a prism, the **spectrum,** or rainbow, of colors are visible: red, orange, yellow, green, blue, indigo and violet (purple). These colors match the colors of the CHAKRAS and the AURA. The three primary colors, red, yellow and blue combine to create the secondary colors or orange, green and violet.

Exactly how the healing color energy penetrates the body is hypothetical. One theory purports that permeation of the cells is accomplished through osmosis. The most popular theory maintains that light and color affect the body through synchronized vibrations within the organism. Others hold that the rays enter through the chakras.

There are several ways to use color for healing purposes. Lamps are employed and fitted with one of seven color gels. The treatment can be a general diffusion of color where the whole body is exposed to the rays, or it can be a local concentration of color on a diseased body part. Treatments should last no longer than 30 minutes.

Color breathing incorporates deep BREATHING exercises with VISUALIZATIONS of absorbing the specific ray from the atmosphere. Since the air is full of light and color, the recipient imagines inhaling a color into his body.

Food and water may be imbued with color without affecting their taste. When exposed to color radiation for at least five minutes, the healing powers of the rays are absorbed into the food or water before being consumed.

Recipients may MEDITATE that they are surrounded by a particular color or that this ray is directly affecting a diseased area. Wearing colored clothing or gemstones may have similar effects.

Color massages, which last only 10 to 15 minutes and are localized treatments, are performed by "bathing" the facilitator's hands under colored rays for 5 minutes. The hands are then vigorously rubbed together to produce heat before the massage starts.

Color therapy may be either contact or absent healing. In contact healing, the recipient sits passively with his eyes closed. The facilitator makes a mental affirmation of the color and its properties and then passes clenched hands above the recipient's head. Her hands pass down and open at his forehead. She spreads her fingers slightly and continues down his body with a sweeping motion. It takes 30 seconds to spread the color over his entire body.

Absent healing is done when the two cannot be in the same room. The facilitator mentally transmits the healing rays to the recipient while he places a dampened swatch of colored cloth between his palms for two minutes and concentrates on absorbing the rays.

The exact color ray that is to be used in the treatment is determined in a number of ways. The physical ailment is considered as well as the general condition of the recipient. In some instances, the facilitator may "read" auric vibrations to determine the deficiency. Care must be taken when using colors, since negative effects may result by treating with the incorrect ray. For healing purposes, a main color is often followed by another for balance.

Occultists recognize that all **cosmic rays** emanate from the **divine white light** and that each ray is made up of seven intrinsic elements: physical or material, life-giving or vital, psychological, unifying, specifically healing, inspirational and spiritual.

Red, the ray of universal love, rules every life form. It heats, energizes, stimulates and governs physical vitality and activity. It is used for blood deficient diseases, such as anemia, and is the color of the adrenal glands. Plants grown under red glass grow four times faster than in ordinary sunlight (and slower under green or blue light).[2] An excess of red is dangerous and can produce fiery conditions, aggressiveness and rage.

Orange, the ray of etheric vitality and energy, is warm, positive and stimulating. It enhances assimilation, circulation and mental wisdom. It increases the immune system, sexual potency and regulates food intake. It is the color of the reproductive organs and the spleen.

Yellow, the cosmic sun and the Christos, is a nervine. It relates to the higher mind and soul. It inspires, stimulates, cleanses, purifies, clears a "foggy" head and is the color of the pancreas.

Green, the ray of balance, harmony and abundance, provides the vibration of harmony and balance within the soul and spirit. It is in the middle of the spectrum, a nervine, soothing, is sympathetic, controls blood and circulation and is related to the thymus gland. Green is a master tonic for restoring frazzled nerves.

Blue, the cosmic ray, controls pain, is a healing color, is antiseptic, anti-inflammatory, astringent, sleep inducing, calmative, peaceful, treats fevers, is the spirit ray and is the color of the thyroid gland.

Indigo, the cosmic ray of inner knowledge and wisdom, rules the eyes, ears, nose and the pituitary gland. It is used to treat nervousness, mental disorders, to expel negativity, promote introspection and induce higher consciousness.

Violet (purple), the ray of mysticism, rules the brain and the pineal gland. It is mental and spiritual in nature and assists in transmutation to higher consciousness by affecting the CROWN CHAKRA.

The zodiac and planetary system, gemstones and music all share vibratory frequencies with specific colors.[3] Black and white also take their place in healing and significance. They are opposites of each other. Black is the feminine, passive, negative, and concealing color. White embodies the masculine, active, positive, and revealing. Blackness is interpreted as the background for the cosmos and the absence of light, while white embraces man's highest concepts.

The seven colors of the spectrum are further combined to produce a myriad of other colors. They too produce emotional and/or psychological responses:

Blue with lavender—high spirituality
Blue with dark reddish brown—selfish religiosity
Blue with grey—religiosity tinged with fear
Blue with black—religiosity with superstition
Lavender—high spirituality
Violet—complete spiritual dedication
Orchid—clairvoyance
Lilac—altruism
Yellow—spiritualized intellect
Orange—intellect
Orange with brick red—mental cunning
Light green—sympathy, a magic color

Medium green—adaptability
Medium green with reddish brown or reddish black—jealousy
Green with grey—deceit
Carmine—affection
Scarlet—pride or strong will
Brick red—anger
Deep red with brown—sensuality
Pure rose—affection
Old rose with reddish brown—selfish affection
Brown—acquisitiveness
Red brown—greed
Green with red brown—selfishness
Dark grey with brown red—depression
Pale grey—fear
Black—occult, secretive.[4]

Notes
[1] Ouseley, S.G.J., *The Power of the Rays: The Science of Colour Healing*, L.N. Fowler & Co., Ltd., Essex, England, 1951. Ra was the sun god worshipped by the ancient Egyptians.
[2] Ibid., p. 11.
[3] Heline, Corinne, *Healing and Regeneration through Color*, J.F. Rowny Press, Santa Barbara, Calif., 1943, p. 18.
[4] Ibid., p. 55–56.

Further Reading
Birren, Faber, *Color Psychology and Color Therapy*, Carol Publishing Group, N.Y., 1984. This is a comprehensive study of the effects of color in everyday life by an authority on color and color healing.
Brennan, Barbara A., *Hands of Light: A Guide to Healing through the Human Energy Field*, Bantam Books, N.Y., 1988. An illustrated text about the human energy field, auras, chakras, and colors. This is an important reference book for all people interested in energetic healing.
Hunt, Roland, *Seven Keys to Color Healing*, Harper & Row, San Francisco, Calif., 1991. This book describes how color can be an effective, drugless way to heal. Color breathing techniques are explained.
Wills, Pauline, *Reflexology and Colour Therapy Workbook*, Element Books, Rockport, Mass., 1992. This book combines the use of color healing with reflexology. Color visualizations are sent into zones of the feet to help those who are too sensitive for normal reflexology treatments.

conception vessel (Meridian) **yin** meridian, which regulates all other yin meridians and yin energy. It is called "the sea of yin." It flows unilaterally up the midline of the body, starting from the perineum (the space between vagina and anus, or the scrotum and anus) to the edge of the lower lip. There are 24 ACUPUNCTURE points along the conception vessel.

connective tissue the most widely distributed tissue in the human body. It is rich in blood and LYMPH and is therefore considered to be **vascular.** Connective tissue binds muscles to bones as tendons, bones to bones as ligaments, tissues to each other, forms cartilage and bones, stores fat, helps in the production of blood cells by producing anticoagulants and provides immunity to disease by ingesting bacteria.

There are two classifications of connective tissue, which differ in their cellular material: **loose** connective tissue, with a soft, gelatinous intercellular structure and **dense,** with a rigid intercellular structure.

Loose connective tissue is composed of three different fibers: **collagenous** or **white,** which are strong, resistant to stretching and flexible; **elastic** or **yellow,** which can stretch up to 50 percent of their length; and **reticular** loose connective tissue, which provides strength and support.

Dense connective tissue contains all of these fibers, but collagenous fibers are the most abundant.

Adult connective tissue is further classified as **connective tissue proper,** made up of **loose connective tissue** (areolar), **adipose** tissue, dense (collagenous), **elastic,** and **reticular. Cartilage,** another form of connective tissue, is made up of **hyaline, fibro-,** and **elastic** cartilage. **Bone** (osseous) **tissue,** is also a form of adult connective tissue, in addition to **vascular** (blood) tissue.

Loose connective tissue (areolar) is the most abundant type of connective tissue found in the body. It is continuous within the body and found in mucous membranes, around all blood vessels, nerves and organs. The subcutaneous (under the skin) layer, made up of areolar and adipose tissues, is also called the **superficial** FASCIA.

Adipose tissue stores fat cells and energy and protects the organs.

Dense (collagenous) connective tissue makes up tendons, ligaments and aponeurosis (sheaths of connective tissue). It also makes up the deep fascia, which wraps around each muscle.

Elastic connective tissue is very flexible and makes up the lungs, intervertebral ligaments, true vocal cords, cartilage of the larynx, elastic arterial walls, the trachea and bronchial tubes.

Reticular connective tissue forms the frameworks of internal organs, such as the liver, spleen and lymph nodes. It also binds smooth muscle cells.

Hyaline cartilage, also called gristle, is the most common cartilage in the body. It is found at the ends of long bones at the site of joints, at the juncture of the ribs, in the nose, larynx, bronchi and bronchial tubes of the lungs and the trachea.

Fibrocartilage is strong and rigid and is located at the pubic symphysis (the site where the pubic bones meet) in the front of the pelvis.

Elastic cartilage helps to maintain the shapes of some organs such as the larynx, external ear and the Eustachian (auditory) tubes.

Bone is abundant in mineral salts, such as calcium phosphate and calcium carbonate, which are responsible for its hardness. Collagenous fibers make up about one-third of bone composition. Bones provide protection, leverage, mineral storage and the formation of blood cells.

Vascular tissue, blood, is part of the circulatory system. It is a transportation system of gases (oxygen and carbon dioxide), nutrients, waste products, hormones and enzymes. It controls pH (the acid-alkaline balance in the body), body temperature, water content of cells and helps fight disease.

connective tissue massage a hands-on system that works on the FASCIA, the membranous sheath surrounding muscles and organs. It is also called BINDEGEWEBSMASSAGE and was developed in Germany by Elisabeth Dicke in 1929.

The night before a scheduled amputation of her right leg, Dicke started massaging painful areas on her back. She found that by pulling a bent finger, with light pressure, across her lower back, the pain in her back subsided and eventually feeling returned to her leg. She recognized that by working on one area of the body, there could be far-reaching reactions. She created a system that treated many illnesses and organic imbalances through the use of her massage technique. This system recognized that particular surface areas of the body corresponded with specific organs.

Many clinical investigations on the same topic were going on about the time Dicke made her discovery. In 1898, English neurologist Dr. Henry Head described similar discoveries about the body's surface and its relation to specific viscera. In 1917, Dr. J. Mackenzie wrote of his observations that certain muscles shared the same nerve supply with ailing organs.

The layer of tissue between the body's most superficial layer, the skin, and the deepest layer, the muscles, is CONNECTIVE TISSUE proper. Tension within this tissue depends upon its vascularity and blood supply. Connective tissue massage takes place in this structure, yet it is not certain which elements are receiving the stimuli.[1]

Before treatment begins, an examination of the client is necessary to determine the affected connective tissue zones. They can be found by palpating suspected areas. Tension changes can be found between the skin and its underlying (subcutaneous) tissue and between the subcutaneous layer and fascia on the surface contour of the back.

The patient sits in a chair for the examination. Ideally, the client's back is straight and the pelvis is slightly tilted forward to shorten the muscles of the back and permit the skin to move. This is also the best position for overall treatment except for the legs. An adjustment must be made to accommodate the patient if the condition requires. The examination and treatment could then be provided with the patient lying on her side.

Visible examination reveals changes in the shape of the back. It also can indicate affected reflex zones in subcutaneous connective tissue. Changes in the connective tissue can be found in its corresponding body surface. On the right side are the liver, gall bladder, duodenum, ileum, appendix, ascending colon and hepatic flexure (bend) of the large intestines. The left side corresponds to the heart, stomach, pancreas, spleen, jejunum, transverse and descending colon and the rectum.

The bladder, uterus (or prostate) and head will show changes in the middle of the back, while any ailments associated with the lungs, bronchi, kidneys, adrenals and ovaries (or testicles) are found corresponding to where they are in the body. Nerve or blood vessel problems also manifest themselves on the back's surface at their location in the body.[2]

The practitioner looks for any number of changes in the skin of the back including drawn-in bands of tissue; drawn-in, flattened areas; elevated areas; muscle atrophy (shrinking); hypertrophy (excessive growth) of muscles; or bony deformities especially in the spine.[3]

A manual examination is also an important part of client assessment. This helps the practitioner ascertain the mobility of the different layers of the connective tissue as well as identify painful areas. Lifting the skin folds between thumb and fingers on both sides of the spine indicates skin mobility.

Another investigative technique tests localized areas. Slightly flexed fingers of both hands are placed and pressed on specific areas in a uniform pattern from the buttocks to the scapula. A third diagnostic technique is a stroking technique using a bent middle finger on either side of the spine. A fluid fold along the stroked area indicates mobile tissue. Tension in the underlying tissues will arrest the stroke. This provides valuable information about the circulatory response of the body.

Practitioners of connective tissue massage may interpret physiological responses to their investigative findings in several ways. Frequently, the patient comes for treatment with a definite diagnosed pathology and the physical changes of the examination correspond with the ailment. In this instance, as the treatment progresses, the symptoms and connective tissue improve simultaneously.

In other cases, even when the connective tissue relationship with the diagnosis is corroborative, the treatments might correct the ailment but the changes in the connective tissue do not improve to the same extent. Although the pathology has improved, it might be necessary to continue treatments until the tissue responds.

A final scenario suggests clients who not only exhibit corresponding zone involvement for a particular diagnosis, but additional ones as well. This could indicate the presence of earlier disturbances that currently show no corresponding disabilities, or manifest only under duress. Treatment will eliminate these underlying problems as well as the diagnosed ailment.

The technique for connective tissue massage is a **tensile strain.**[4] This means that tension, or pulling, provides the vascular response to effect change. It is performed mainly with the middle finger supported by the ring finger. Lubrication is never used because a certain finger adherence to the skin is required to produce a reaction. The client should not experience discomfort during the treatment, although the pressure is firm. The direction of the stroke is an important consideration. Along the spine, the stroke follows the direction of the **dermatomes,** segmentally spaced regions that correspond with the somatic component of the nerve supply to the skin. In the periphery, the direction follows the path of the muscle fibers or at right angles to fascial borders and the septum between muscles.

Connective tissue massage can be used to treat many ailments including osteo and rheumatoid arthritis, "pins and needles" from unknown causes (acroparesthesia), headaches, migraines, lower back pain, prolapsed intervertebral discs, sacroiliac strain, Raynaud's disease (coldness in the extremities), disorders of the connective tissue, peripheral vascular disease, venous circulation disturbances and some scar tissue.

Notes

[1] Ebner, Maria, *Connective Tissue Massage,* Robert E. Kreiger, Publishers, Huntington, N.Y., 1962, p. 4.

[2] Ibid., pp. 54–56.

[3] Ibid., p. 56.

[4] Ibid., p. 65.

Further Reading

Ebner, Maria, *Connective Tissue Massage—Theory and Therapeutic Application,* Robert E. Kreiger, Publishers, Huntington, N.Y., 1962. This clearly illustrated text provides the background of connective tissue massage and explains the techniques in depth. Detailed treatments are given for many illnesses and complaints. This book was the first, and finest, to describe connective tissue massage.

Constitutional Massage[SM] also called Holistic Massage[SM] both an assessment methodology and a framework for creating a massage plan tailored to the constitution of a client.

With Constitutional Assessment, the specific nature and qualities of the massage can be determined, a priori, for an individual, whether a sedentary worker, an obese person, a bodybuilder, a child or an elderly person. The massage plan chosen is created specifically for the client's condition at that moment in his life.

In the absence of Constitutional methods, the best scenario is the experienced therapist who knows which modalities and which strokes work for her client. With appropriate massage techniques, the client may be brought into better balance. However, without a methodology the therapist is left entirely to her perceptions and current experience level.

The more common scenario is a therapist who works in only one modality or who exercises the same patterns with everybody, regardless of their physical condition and needs.

For both the student of massage and the skilled professional, a methodology that includes assessment of energy status and the appropriate determination of modalities and/or strokes can significantly enhance results.

The method of assessment of Constitutional Massage adopts the **eight principles pattern** from CHINESE MEDICINE. The therapist evaluates four energy parameters along a continuum of polar opposites. These parameters are hot/cold, deficient/excess, internal/external and, ultimately, yin/yang. Prior to massage, these parameters can be easily identified by the therapist from an assessment sheet and follow-up questions. For example, it is easy to determine if the client tends toward cold limbs or is red-faced; whether he is tired or hyperactive and irritable; or whether his ailments are deep inside the body and chronic or mostly on the surface, as in musculoskeletal problems. Then the therapist can determine the predominance of yin or yang by the following description: yin is cold, deficient and internal, while yang is hot, excess and external.

Since each of these qualities is given a numerical value in Constitutional Massage, it is easy to determine how cold or hot, deficient or excess, internal or external and yin or yang a person is. On a scale of zero to ten, absolute yin is valued at zero, the middle range is five and absolute yang is ten.

Most people fall into the middle range, as in the standard bell curve, yet the massage treatment is vastly different for a person who measures mostly yin, than from one who is mostly yang.

With the Constitutional status determined, the therapist is ready to create her massage plan. The therapist will **tonify,** or build up, the client who tends to be more yin. She will **sedate** those who lean toward the yang disposition and will use **even methods** for the client who is right down the middle.

In applying Constitutional methods to circulatory massage (SWEDISH MASSAGE), the tonifying treatment would select among strokes such as FRICTION, PERCUSSION (TAPOTEMENT), VIBRATION, deep PETRISSAGE and appropriate ACUPRESSURE. For sedating effects, EFFLEURAGE, Swedish gymnastics, light touching, light friction and appropriate acupressure strokes could be employed.

The therapist will modify the strokes to bring out the tonifying or sedating qualities by varying the pressure, rhythm, duration, speed, sequencing and intent. Modifying factors may even be used to give a tonifying stroke predominantly sedating qualities, or vice versa.

The science of Constitutional Massage becomes the art of massage based on the skill of the therapist in the selection and refinement of strokes and modifying factors.

Since the client receives a massage based on his actual needs, the body is brought into improved balance. From there, regeneration is possible. Constitutional Massage can be readily adopted to conventional techniques and soon becomes an essential ingredient in high quality therapy.

Constitutional Massage may also be applied to other major fields of bodywork, just as it has been done in Swedish massage and some forms of Oriental bodywork.

This system was created by William Berry, R.M.T., L.Ac., in the late 1980s. Berry is the director of the Phoenix School of Holistic Health in Houston, Texas, and, along with the students, continues to develop Constitutional Massage. They have demonstrated remarkable success with over 3,000 client hours to date.

Constitutional Massage is a relatively new body therapy. To reach its fullest scope, especially in regard to systems other than Swedish massage therapy, it requires the creative input and healing currents of many talented therapists.

CORE Bodywork[SM] a multiphase myofascial[1] and structural somatic therapy that was organized by George P. Kousaleos, L.M.T., N.C.T.M.B., the founder and director of CORE Institute of Massage Therapy and Structural Bodywork. He has been an internationally renowned practitioner and teacher of STRUCTURAL INTEGRATION since 1989. This system is an integration of the most precise clinical techniques with an innovative approach to client-centered somatic education.

All four phases of CORE body therapy share a theory of structural alignment that recognizes an innate spiral in the entirety of the human body.

Working to achieve balance, flexibility and efficiency within the parameters of the spiral improves the function and the neurosomatic (body/mind) awareness of the client. The four phases are organized according to the level or layer of FASCIA, musculature and supporting soft tissues that are manipulated. They are: CORE Massage, CORE Extrinsic, CORE Intrinsic and CORE Integration.

CORE Massage is taught to licensed or nationally certified massage therapists as a basic form of structural therapy that focuses on the superficial levels of fascia and musculature. The client is introduced to full-body session, alignment awareness techniques and flexibility exercises.

CORE Extrinsic consists of the initial three sessions of specific MYOFASCIAL THERAPY that focus on the mechanisms of full breathing, balanced stance and highly improved range of motion.

CORE Intrinsic consists of four sessions that focus on the deepest level of intrinsic musculature and investing fascia. Inner structural balance of the client's legs, pelvis, back, neck and cranium is achieved.

CORE Integration is made up of three sessions that seek to integrate structure with function, body with mind and intellect with creativity. During these sessions, an ''inside/out'' approach to client-centered somatic education is pursued, along with myofascial techniques that support continuous improvement and efficiency of the human form.

CORE body therapy is taught by master faculty members George P. Kousaleos, William E. Bonney, Ph.D., L.M.T., and Gary N. Genna, B.A., L.M.T., N.C.T.M.B.

NOTE
[1] Fascia is a sheet or broad band of fibrous connective tissue beneath the skin, which envelopes the body, enclosing the muscles, muscle groups and organs. Myofascia is deep fascia, which separates the muscles into groups.

Core Energetics® a deep and powerful therapeutic process that integrates the mind, body, spirit and emotions. The release of emotional blocks, negative images and belief systems through work with the body restores energy and consciousness to the individual. When material suppressed in the body is brought to consciousness, a vast amount of energy is released, creating vitality and greater life fulfillment.

John Pierrakos, M.D., founder of Core Energetics, was a student of Wilhelm Reich. Pierrakos expanded on the energetic ideas of Reich in the development of BIOENERGETICS and then incorporated the spiritual principles of the Pathwork Guide lectures and founded Core Energetics.

Core Energetics is a deep process that addresses five levels of existence in the human entity. These are: the physical body, the feelings and emotions, the mind and thought, the will, and the spirit.

Core Energetics, through the dimensions of energy and consciousness, works to breakdown and transform the individual's defense system in order to reach the core, a level of consciousness that represents the higher qualities of life with love being the central expression. The core is the **''seat of love.''** This process enables the individual, by reaching the spiritual self, or core, to become creative, receptive and in touch with one's ''real self.'' Core Energetics is a powerful process that affects one's very ''being,'' first, through deep work with the body, and second, by expanding the consciousness so that the person can discover her main task in life.

The evolution of the personality depends on systematically working with, transforming and integrating the spiritual self with the five levels of existence. This cannot be accomplished by overlooking the different levels of the personality and dealing only with the level of the spirit, as in the case with many spiritual practices. Core Energetics does not separate and specialize in only one level, but instead, considers unifying the whole person.

The therapeutic work of this process is based on the following principles:

1. The person is a psychosomatic unity.
2. The source of healing and the capacity to love

is within the self and not in an outside agency, whether it be a physician prescribing drugs or one's idealization of the spiritual process.

3. All of existence forms a unity that moves toward a creative evolution, both of the whole and the countless components. In the human being, the evolution consists of deep transformation of the negative aspects of the personality into a creative whole.

The concept of the Core Energetic process developed through many stages, incorporating basic Reichian concepts, bioenergetics, insights from modern physics, an evolutionary path of many physical, mental and spiritual experiences, as well as the inspiring lectures delivered by Eva Pierrakos, which later expanded into the process of the Pathwork.

Core Energetics is experienced through varying levels of energy and consciousness. The energy is the living force that emanates from each level of consciousness. The main characteristics of life energy are: pulsation, motility, rhythm, abundance, flexibility and malleability. There is instantaneous knowledge of what the truth is in the now and without duality. Our consciousness becomes the sculptor of the plastic, abundant and benign human energies by sculpting the shape of the body and by determining the basic shape of human existence. The creative potential of our life energy is tremendous.

The HUMAN ENERGY BIO-FIELD manifests life's energy through the specific qualities of pulsation, frequency, rhythm and color. By observing the pulsation frequencies of color in human energy fields, it is possible to define the states of functioning relating to illness and health. Laboratory findings have given decisive evidence as to the existence of the life energy and its relationship to the states of functioning of the human entity. By working in the laboratory, as well as with the five different levels of existence, it is possible to reach a deeper understanding of the states of the dysfunction in the human body and

personality. In the long run, these create serious illnesses.

The work is directed toward transforming and dissolving obstacles, such as energetic blocks and their corresponding distorted feelings, that prevent the true function of the core. Character defenses, as manifested in fears and chronic negative attitudes, block inherent creativity on the physical as well as on the spiritual levels. The physical body is the laboratory of life and the vehicle through which emotions, thoughts and the spiritual self is expressed. Striking information is revealed by the physical structure. By working with the body to help confront the defensive reactions of emotions, core energy is released. Bodies are the most wonderful instruments for evolutionary progress. The focus is on releasing the life energy held within the body as a way to touch the essence of one's being, or core. The Core Energetic vision is to help individuals and groups transform the obstacles that block contact with the core, source of all healing, wisdom, joy and creativity, or in other words, to fulfill their destiny.

Further Reading

Pierrakos, John, Dr., *The Core Energetic Process,* Institute for the New Age, N.Y., 1977. This book describes in detail the Core Energetic process.

————, *The Core Energetic Process in Group Therapy,* Institute for the New Age, N.Y., 1975. In a group therapy session, the theories of the Core Energetic process are applied.

————, *The Energy Field in Man and Nature,* Institute for the New Age, N.Y, 1975. The author describes the function and meaning of the energy bio-field, which surrounds all living beings.

————, *Human Energy Systems Theory,* Institute for the New Age, N.Y, 1975. The relationship between health and the human energy bio-field is disclosed in this book.

————, *Life Functions of the Energy Centers of Man,* Institute for the New Age, N.Y, 1975. Each energy center is described with its physical and emotional components.

CranioSacral Therapy^{SM} a gentle manipulation, which locates and corrects imbalances in the craniosacral system. Sensory, motor or intellectual dysfunctions may result from these imbalances. The positive effects of this therapeutic system are realized, to a large extent, by the body's innate healing and self-correcting abilities.

The craniosacral system is made up of the brain, spinal cord, cerebrospinal fluid (which cushions and bathes the brain and spinal cord from skull to sacrum), dural membrane (which supports the brain), cranial bones and the sacrum. It is a closed hydraulic system that moves with a minimal but perceptible rhythmic fluctuation.

The craniosacral system exists in humans and all animals with a brain and spinal cord. It develops with the fetus and functions until death.

During the early part of this century, William G. Sutherland, an OSTEOPATHIC student, observed that the sutures of the cranium (skull) were not fixed, but were flexible and had movement. The changes in their positions and movements affected the brain and cerebrospinal fluid pressure, often causing serious, systemic physical problems. He noticed that the cranium moved in response to the production of the fluid within the brain ventricles and that the ventricles' pulsation altered the hydraulic pressure, causing the cranium to expand.

This fluid is filtered out of blood in a constantly driving feedback loop. Pressure builds as the fluid increases, forcing the fluid up and down the spinal cord. The skull and the membranes, which contain the fluid, also move, generally at a rate of 6 to 12 cycles per minute.[1]

Dr. Sutherland's system became known as cranial osteopathy. However, his unconventional treatment techniques lost favor with contemporary physicians and his findings were largely ignored.

In 1970, Dr. John E. Upledger, D.O., F.A.A.O., a major proponent of CranioSacral Therapy and director of the Upledger Institute, was witnessing neck surgery when he observed the rhythmic, pulsation of the membranes of the cerebrospinal fluid system. He recognized that a disturbance within this system could affect the brain, spinal cord and their associated organs. A

far-reaching physical effect might result from an imbalance.

At a seminar of cranial osteopathy in 1972, Dr. Upledger recognized that his findings were similar to those of Dr. Sutherland: a fluid system, encased within a membrane, that communicates with the skull and spinal cord. This became the basis for his CranioSacral Therapy.

Seeking to establish scientific data for this system, Upledger led an interdisciplinary team at the Department of Biomechanics at Michigan State University's College of Osteopathic Medicine in 1975. The results of the investigation validated Dr. Sutherland's thesis. Restrictions of the cerebrospinal rhythm caused migraines, depression, cerebral palsy and other ailments.

The evaluation of a patient is most efficacious in the cranium, sacrum and coccyx (tailbone) because of their membranous attachments, which contain the cerebrospinal fluid. A light touch of no more than 0.18 of an ounce (the weight of a nickel) can feel the rhythmic pulsations. Gentle manipulations at the sutures and subtle adjustments release tension from the membranes and the entire system, allowing the body to self-correct. Although the vertebrae, pelvis and jaw can also be used for the examination, it is more difficult to feel the fluid's pulsation since these bones are not directly involved with cerebrospinal flow.

A low amplitude of cerebrospinal rhythm indicates low vitality and low resistance to disease. A symmetry in the craniosacral rhythmical motion throughout the body is used to localize pathologies. Although this sign does not explain what the problem is or its cause, it will alert the practitioner where the problem lies.

CranioSacral Therapy is used to treat numerous ailments. Used alone or in conjunction with other bodywork therapies, it can treat TEMPOROMANDIBULAR joint disorders, headaches, eye and ear problems, stiff neck and spine, whiplash, fatigue, depression, pelvic disorders and gastrointestinal complaints. The pediatric application has been particularly successful in treating dyslexia and other learning disabilities, hyperactivity and cerebral palsy.

An easy **frontal lift** near the temples can relieve eye strain and sinus pressure. Hands of the practitioner placed inside the client's mouth help to balance the jaw and relieve the sinuses.

Another, more advanced, technique called **unwinding** helps free specific trauma by recreating the position of the body during the trauma and releasing the tension. The accompanying pain and organic dysfunction is usually eradicated. This work may evoke an emotional discharge as well, since a physical injury always has an emotional component.

CranioSacral Therapy is practiced by a small number of osteopaths. The Cranial Academy in Meridian, Idaho, had a membership of under 300 in 1989.[2] One reason the number is so small is that the palpatory skills of practitioners must be keenly developed. Another possible reason is that the treatment is time-consuming. Sessions generally last 45 minutes, enough time for a doctor to see two or three patients instead of one.

However, many licensed bodyworkers who spend an hour or more with their clients, such as massage therapists, chiropractors, physical therapists, doctors and acupuncturists, have started incorporating this system into their practice.

Notes

[1] Upledger, John E., D.O., F.A.A.O., D.Sc., "The Therapeutic Value of the CranioSacral System," Upledger Institute, Palm Beach Gardens, Fla., no date, p. 1.

[2] *Prevention Magazine,* "Hands on Healing," Rodale Press, Emmaus, Pa., 1989, p. 68. With 24,000 licensed osteopaths in 1989, fewer than 300 practice CranioSacral Therapy.

Further Reading

Manheim, Carol J., M.S., P.T., and Lavett, Diane K., Ph.D., *CranioSacral Therapy and Somato-Emotional Release,* Slack, Inc., Thorofare, N.J., 1989. This collaboration of physical therapy and psychotherapy explains chronic pain syndrome caused by posttraumatic stress disorder and presents philosophy and methods of treatment. Documented scientific explanations support the beneficial results of CranioSacral Therapy and Somato-Emotional Release.

Upledger, John E., D.O., F.A.A.O., D.Sc., with Vredevoogd, J.D., M.F.A., *CranioSacral Therapy,* Eastland Press, Seattle, 1983. This is the innovative text for the study of CranioSacral Therapy. Written by the director of the Upledger Institute, this book offers scientific evidence for the success of CranioSacral Therapy.

———, *CranioSacral Therapy II. Beyond the Dura,* Eastland Press, Seattle, 1987. Volume II of this text offers advanced treatments.

———, *Somato-Emotional Release and Beyond,* Upledger Institute Pub., Palm Beach Gardens, Fla., 1990. The theory and methods of Somato-Emotional Release are offered in this text, written by today's major proponent of the system.

———, *CranioSacral Therapy, Somato-Emotional Release: Your Inner Physician and You,* North Atlantic Books, Berkeley, Calif., 1991. This book describes how these systems can diagnose and provide treatment information about a large assortment of ailments and illnesses.

cross-fiber friction See CYRIAX MASSAGE.

cryotherapy See ICE THERAPY.

crystal healing also referred to as crystal or gem therapy, is the use of crystals or gemstones for healing purposes. Throughout history, gemstones were used to cure disease. They were placed on the body, usually corresponding with the CHAKRAS (vital force centers), to balance the flow of energy. Because crystals have electromagnetic properties with polarity and can emit vibrations, auras and frequencies, it is believed that they have a penetrating effect into the areas on which they are placed. Different crystals vibrate at different frequencies and even some from the same mineral composition have their own unique pattern.

Crystals may be worn as jewelry, carried as loose stones, placed on the body or left in the home. Crystal healing affects the mind, body and spirit by unblocking energy pathways and increasing the flow of energy. It is often used in conjunction with work on the human energy bio-field and the chakras.

In addition to healing purposes, crystals can be strategically placed in a room or the home to hold and clear the energy within. In treatment spaces, they are used to bring additional healing energy into the room, to collect dead orgone energy (DOR),[1] to protect the practitioner from absorbing negative energies and to stay grounded and to enhance the beauty of the space. In order to test the crystal to determine if it is in its optimum place, leave it for a few days in one spot. If it doesn't feel right in that area, move it around the room until it feels correctly placed.

Practitioners often use clear quartz crystals to improve their health, clear their minds, to increase their sensitivity to the energy bio-field and for protection before beginning to work. The crystal is held in both hands and a low vibratory energy is self-directed. The practitioner can also wear a quartz or amethyst pendant over the solar plexus to strengthen her energy bio-field. Rose quartz worn over the heart is protective of the heart.

The crystals that are worn should be selected carefully, making sure that they suit the wearer's body. A gem that has a vibration too strong for the user will eventually deplete his energy. Ideally, a stone that is only slightly stronger than the person will help enhance and fortify the energy field. If the stone is too weak and vibrates at a frequency that is too low, it can slow down the wearer's vibrations.

Old jewelry is usually imbued with the energy of the former owner and should be **cleared** for at least one week to purify it. The crystals at home or in the treatment room must also be cleared, or cleaned, because of accumulated vibrations and environmental effects such as sound, light, thoughts and emotions, which are also absorbed by the stone.

There are a number of ways to clean crystals. They can be kept outdoors in direct sunlight for a few days. If the owner lives near the beach, crystals may be buried in the sand under the water for a couple of hours. They can soak overnight in $\frac{1}{4}$ teaspoon of sea salt dissolved in one pint of spring water. They also may be passed through smoke or flames.

Crystals may be charged with healing energy and given to an individual who absorbs the energy from it. It is also possible for powerful practitioners to continue to charge the crystals from long distances, keeping the healing energy constant.

There are very few contraindications to crystal healing. Hypersensitive people who cannot tolerate the powers of crystals should stay away from them. In addition, people who undergo intense chakra balancing work should avoid using crystals, since their vibrations may disturb the previous work.

Crystals can attract or affect physiological and/or emotional changes because of their vibrations. Here is a partial list of crystals and their healing properties:

Agate—depth, courage, tone and strength

Amber—harmony and purification

Amethyst—spirituality, strength, the endocrine system and the immune system

Blue Sapphire—strength and hope

Citrine—prosperity, clarity, kidneys, colon, liver, gallbladder and heart

Clear Quartz—pineal, pituitary gland and brain stimulation

Fluorite—balance of the mind, body and spirit

Garnet—passion and general health

Golden Topaz—peace

Jade—long life

Lapis—courage, skeletal system, thyroid stimulation

Malachite—release of suppressed emotions, heart and circulatory system

Moonstone—stomach, spleen, pancreas and lymph

Onyx—centering and self-control, stress reduction and strengthens the bone marrow

Pearl—purity and integrity

Peridot—peace of mind

Pink Tourmaline—dynamic expression

Rose Quartz—self-love and healing, kidneys, fertility and circulatory system

Snowflake Obsidian—stress reduction, balances stomach and intestines

Tiger Eye—stability, grounding and centering, spleen, colon, pancreas

White Sapphire—justice and focus

Note

[1] Brennan, Barbara Ann, *Light Emerging*, Bantam Books, N.Y., 1993, p. 22. Dr. Wilhelm Reich coined this term to describe undercharged or low energy with the human energy field.

Further Reading

Bravo, Brett, *Crystal Healing,* Warner Books, N.Y., 1988. The author talks about the healing properties of many crystals and their application in treating illnesses.

Brennan, Barbara Ann, *Hands of Light,* Bantam Books, N.Y., 1987. This book, filled with clear illustrations, is a detailed text of the human energy field, chakras and auras. The author describes various ways to heal using high sense perception and crystal healing, clearing these layers of energy.

———— , *Light Emerging,* Bantam Books, N.Y., 1993. Many case histories involving healing the human energy field are cited in this text.

Chocron, Daya Sarai, *Healing with Crystals and Gemstones,* Weiser, York Beach, Me., 1986. This book explains the use of crystals in healing and the properties of each gemstone.

Kaplan, Miriam, *Crystal and Gemstone Windows,* Cassandra Press, San Rafael, Calif., 1987. The history of crystal healing is explained in this book along with healing methods using various gemstones.

Silby, Uma, *Complete Crystal Guidebook,* Bantam Books, N.Y., 1986. This extensive book details the healing properties of crystals and their application in treating many illnesses.

cupping an ancient technique that uses small jars, in which a vacuum has been created, to treat numerous diseases and soft tissue injuries that were caused due to the stagnation of CHI, blood and fluids.

Almost every culture has its own version of cupping. This healing technique was first described as the "horn method" in the *Zhou Hou Bei Ji Fana* (Prescriptions for Emergencies), written by Ko Hung during the first century A.D. The ancient name *jiaofa* was given to the cupping jars, which were initially made from animal horn. These cups can be made of glass, bamboo or ceramic and come in various sizes, depending on the surface area they will treat. Suction secures the jars.

Small jars are placed directly on the afflicted areas and a vacuum is created by heating the inside of the vessels with alcohol-treated cotton or paper. The cotton is either removed before placement or left in the jar to burn out. The skin

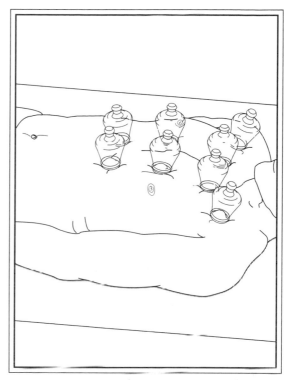

Cupping, the ancient healing technique of Chinese and Ayurvedic medicine, is used to lower blood pressure and reduce muscle spasms and pain. Glass jars are placed directly on the affected areas and a vacuum is created by heating the air inside.

and underlying tissues are pulled into the vacuum, which increases localized circulation, releasing the stagnation and thereby bringing blood and nutrients to the area.

The Chinese have several ways of heating the vessel and creating a vacuum. The combustion methods are: *tou hou fa,* which uses burning paper inside the cup as its heat source; *tie main fa* employs cotton wool moistened with alcohol; *shan huo fa* uses cotton wool moistened with alcohol. The inflamed cloth is moved around inside the cup with a pair of tweezers to create the vacuum, rather than left to burn out; and *jia huo fa,* another heat conduction method, which secures a piece of cloth in place by weighing it down with a coin. The burning cloth is then covered with the jar.

A noncombustion method uses boiling water to heat the cups for at least 10 minutes. Excess water is shaken off and the rim is tapped against a wet, cold cloth to avoid burning and placed on the skin.

Cups are kept in place for 3 to 10 minutes. The Chinese have different ways of using the cups. The first method is the **simple** method, placing the cups on the areas to be treated and left for several minutes. Another technique is the **migration** method were the suction cup is slowly moved around an area. Lubrication placed on its rim allows it to rotate and travel without breaking the seal. Cups may be **impregnated** with decoctions of herbs or filled with medication and placed over an afflicted area.

Cupping may also be done directly over an acupuncture needle to make the treatment even more powerful. **Scarification** is done to create bleeding. A triangular acupuncture needle is inserted into the area 10 to 40 times, depending upon cup size, until the blood flows. The heated cup is placed over the incisions and kept there as the blood collects. No more than .338 of a fluid ounce of blood should be lost in this process.

Further Reading

The Academy of Traditional Chinese Medicine, *An Outline of Chinese Acupuncture,* Foreign Language Press, Beijing, 1975. Included in this concise text of Chinese medicine is a detailed description of cupping methods and applications.

Auterole, B., et al., *Acupuncture and Moxibustion: A Guide to Clinical Practice,* Churchill Livingstone, Edinburgh, 1992.

An easy-to-understand, yet very thorough description of Chinese medicine, including a section on cupping and its applications.

Xinnong, Cheng, *Chinese Acupuncture and Moxibustion,* Foreign Language Press, Beijing, revised text, 1993. This detailed text describes the history and use of cupping in Chinese medicine.

Cyriax massage a deep, cross-fiber friction massage developed by English orthopedist Dr. James Cyriax for the treatment of injuries to the muscles, ligaments, tendons and joints of the body.

Deep friction works in many ways. It increases circulation, helps to diminish pain and promotes greater flexibility. The analgesic effects of the stroke result from deeper and more lasting hyperemia (localized blood flow).[1] The cross-fiber friction moves and separates fibers, allowing for increased mobility and a breakdown of adhesions (fibers sticking together) and scar tissue.

Deep friction may be applied with fingertips or thumbs, but the direction of the stroke is always across (transverse) the fibers.

Cyriax also promoted the use of deep EF-FLEURAGE to relieve edema (swelling) and congestion.

Note

[1] Tappan, Francis, *Healing Massage Techniques,* Reston Publishing Co., Inc., Reston, Va., 1980, p. 183. Localized, increased blood flow will supply oxygenated blood and hasten removal of waste products. The swelling, which often accompanies injury or trauma, is relieved, thereby reducing pain. Nerve endings are also calmed during deep massage.

D

dance injury massage a technique of very specific, deep, full bodywork based in MEDICAL MASSAGE. Its goal is to achieve full release for the athlete's or dancer's entire musculature from sprains, strains, inflammations, compensations due to injury, and the limits of constricting body armor on range of motion.

Medical massage is generally detailed work done only on the injured area for no more than 30 minutes. This time frame affords ample opportunity to address the chief complaint and its concomitant compensation. However, when the client is a highly trained athlete or artist who must continue to work in spite of injury, the whole body becomes involved. At this level of physical skill, daily exertions of the class and rehearsal schedule and the rigors of performance can actually define dance as a continued state of injury.

Dance injury massage was developed by massage therapist Thomas McCracken during the 1980s. He began working with members of the New York City Ballet and recognized that the demands placed on their bodies required a massage system that would offer them deep therapeutic work while they were still performing, since they could not take time off to rest their unremitting injuries. It was also important that the system be biomechanically efficient, allowing for several daily treatments without injury to the practitioner. The care of the therapist's hands, body, and spirit is carefully incorporated into a technique, which took McCracken 10 years to create.

All strokes begin with a floating center of gravity. Power, generated from the legs, is transmitted through the upper body (chest, shoulder and arms) and directed out the stabilized platform of the hands. The strokes are stylized from the Swedish massage technique. EFFLEURAGE type strokes include alternating hand, rolling knuckle, supported thumb and hooked finger.

KNEADING is patterned after the pressure/counterpressure sensation of a handshake. FRICTION, the most important stroke in dance injury massage, includes circular, cross-fiber and sliding strokes. Compressions, pulls, and stretches are utilized alone or in tandem with other strokes to produce distraction for the client. Since the mind usually focuses on one thing at a time, when two or three stimuli are used simultaneously, the client's focus cannot fixate on any one ache or pain. This allows the practitioner to work through problem areas quickly and thoroughly.

There are inherent physiological benefits from all massage strokes (see SWEDISH MASSAGE). In dance injury massage, the priority of each stroke is to help the practitioner locate a set of TRIGGER POINTS. These points are located using the hands as "homing devices," actually "listening" for their presence. As each point is located, it is systematically and repeatedly manipulated with friction, constituting a **"call and response"** sequence. It is as if each stroke asks a question and the response is heard through the hands as a quality of tissue resistance, the degree of alteration in breathing pattern, skin movement, or other discernible physiological signs. The therapist's talent, skill, focus, and innate understanding of the client determines how much information is available and if that information can be used effectively.

If the call and response dynamic creates a dialogue between the client and practitioner, the vocabulary for this conversation is pain. Pain acts like an airplane's altimeter since it establishes a relative reference point for the depth of pressure. Pain focuses the attention of both participants. It alerts the practitioner to areas of concern and reminds the client to open his mouth and breathe. This patterned breathing converts what appears to be passive acquiescence into active participation. Friction is applied at an accurate angle and with just enough natural force to allow palpation without the client pulling away. In other words, the work is performed just below the acceptable threshold of "comfortable pain." Working at this level of intimacy requires a client's trust. The technique cannot work effectively if a client does not possess the willingness to be vulnerable.

Dance injury massage encompasses the needs of the professional dancer or athlete who wishes to maximize his performance in spite of injury. Overall, the work is extremely useful for any client who desires articulate, deep work. It can further be utilized to disengage counterproductive body armor, which has become locked into posture. Regardless of the client's reasons for seeking the work, an inevitable result is that the client is more at home with pain.

McCracken has found that one of the great dangers in a long career in bodywork, or even just a long day, is repetition. With repetition of any activity comes the possibility of boredom. This begets slackened biomechanics, which may cause practitioner injury and/or client dissatisfaction. Dance injury massage builds an intuitive practice into "automatic pilot" where productive bodywork becomes a matter of course.

dance therapy the use of the creative art of dance as a movement therapy to help individuals experience their bodies, and consequently their feelings, more effectively and build self-esteem. It is often used in conjunction with other therapies, such as psychotherapy and PHYSICAL THERAPY.

Dance therapy can be used in the treatment of many conditions and employed in a variety of settings. In hospitals, nursing homes, clinics, and rehabilitation centers, this system is a pleasurable way to help those patients strengthen their motor skills, improve their range of motion, increase balance, and overcome physical disabilities. In day care centers, community mental health centers, and correctional facilities, social skills can be learned or relearned, behav-

ioral problems can be addressed, and substance abuse treated.

There are many different methods, which are currently used, but the most popular form of dance therapy is the circular form. The session usually begins with a simple warm-up set to music. Props, such as balls, scarves, fans, musical instruments, etc., may be used as participants move, jump, hop, run, walk and sway to the music. The participants' movements respond to the changing rhythm of the music.

The American Dance Therapy Association was formed in 1966 to establish professional standards and qualifications. A graduate degree is required to become a dance therapist.

deep massage a unique approach to bodywork distinct from DEEP TISSUE MASSAGE. With deep massage, the point is to greatly provide an opportunity for a powerful depth of response for the client. "Deep," therefore, refers to the depth of the client's positive experience, not just the amount of pressure.

The deep massage therapist utilizes over 50 advanced techniques to systematically free the upper and lower halves of the body as well as its **core.** These soft-tissue techniques involve the simultaneous touching of the client's structure and energy. The deep massage therapist also has an educated appreciation for the role of the nervous system in shaping bodies, intelligence and emotions. In the course of studying, the deep massage therapist learns more deeply about her own structure/energy, cultivating a high quality of contact, movement, care, empathy and wonder.

A typical session of deep massage involves the client and therapist meeting to elicit relevant history and to realize a working assumption regarding the appropriate theme or purpose for the work. The table work is then done with the client draped, usually focusing on one or two key regions of the body, and integrates each session with core work on the back, neck and shoulders. During the session, the therapist practices advanced observation skills to promote the structural/energetic connection for the client. Deep massage is effective for muscular and fascial strains and sprains, structural balance, realigning structure and energy, relieving emotional stress and evoking inner peace.

Deep massage was founded by David Lauterstein to overcome the dualistic approach of many bodywork forms, which aim exclusively at either the physical or the emotional sides of being. Developed out of 13 years teaching experience and 20 years of therapeutic study and practice, deep massage is an attempt to systematically answer one very important question: What are the elements that give rise to incredibly positive bodywork experiences? This has resulted in deep massage's emphasis on session design, the heightened presence of the therapist and the cultivation of advanced observation skills. Some of the major influences on this work are developments within modern philosophy and art, psychotherapy, structural bodywork, CRANIOSACRAL THERAPY and zero-balancing.

The certification process consists of four workshops: the Upper Pole, Lower Pole, the Core, the Advanced Seminar in Session Design as well as supportive practical and contemplative assignments.

deep tissue massage, also called deep muscle therapy or deep tissue therapy, is an umbrella term for bodywork systems that work deeply into the muscles and connective tissue to release chronic aches and pains.

The best known of the deep tissue massage is ROLFING, which focuses on bringing the body back into balance by working on the FASCIA. Rolfing has given rise to other deep tissue systems, such as HELLERWORK, which incorporates fascia work with movement exercises. Other systems include SPORTS MASSAGE, PFRIMMER METHOD OF DEEP MUSCLE THERAPY, and CONNECTIVE TISSUE MASSAGE, among many.

The work is generally localized and the client must be relaxed to permit the practitioner to work deeply. The pressure starts lightly, but progresses to the deepest level the client can tolerate. It is believed that physical correction takes place at the discomfort level.[1]

Deep tissue massage has been found effective in treating chronic pain, muscle adhesions (muscle fibers that stick together creating a knot or nodule), whiplash, lower back and neck pain, sciatica and circulatory problems. It can be either corrective or generally therapeutic.

Deep tissue massage is contraindicated on torn muscles, bruises, vascular weaknesses such as varicose veins, or if the client is pregnant, nursing or cannot tolerate the pain.

Note
[1] *Prevention Magazine,* "Hands-On Healing," Rodale Press, Emmaus, Pa., 1989, p. 77.

dō-in an ancient exercise and self-massage system designed to work the MERIDIANS, promote overall health and treat specific problems. Dō-in developed over the centuries within the Oriental religions of Shintoism, Hinduism, Taoism and Buddhism. Over 5,000 years ago, Taoist monks recognized the instinct to touch the site of pain or injury and called the system tao-yinn, or *tao,* meaning "the way," and *yinn,* meaning "gentle approach." It existed as a natural adaptation to the environment, and its ultimate goal is spiritual harmony with the universe.

Dō-in was introduced in the United States in 1968 by Michio Kushi, an authority on macrobiotics and president of the Kushi Foundation. These exercises, which often resemble YOGA asanas (postures), work all the meridians of the body and therefore affect the circulation of the vital QI (CHI) energy that flows through them. Because of the relationship of dō-in with the channels, proponents assert that this system can benefit most ailments.

One example of dō-in works the feet and toes, and another is for the eyes and all corresponding meridians. Lie on the back with knees bent, about two feet apart. Extend both legs and rub the foot top, sole and side with the first and second toes of the opposite foot at least 100 times, or until they are warm. Repeat on the other foot. This exercise stimulates the stomach, intestines, liver, spleen, bladder and kidney meridians (all the channels of the feet).

To treat eye strain, myopia, farsightedness, astigmatism, glaucoma and control circulation and heart rate, place both palms over the eyes (remove glasses). Breathe normally. After a few minutes, press into the top of the eye socket with the three middle fingers, three times. Close the eyes and carefully press into the top of the eyeball. Lightly vibrate. Repeat for the bottom of the eye. Press the closed eyes 10 times with the same three fingers. Grasp the upper lid and vibrate 50 to 100 times. Pinch the bridge of the nose between the thumb and index finger for two seconds. Release suddenly.

Supporters of dō-in hold that practicing these exercises and self-massage techniques will promote a healthier lifestyle on all levels.

Further Reading

Kuchi, Michio, *The Book of Dō-In: Exercises for Physical and Spiritual Development,* Japan Publications, Elmsford, N.Y., 1979. This book clearly illustrates the principles and exercises of dō-in. Treatments for specific ailments are offered.

drama therapy one of the creative arts used for therapeutic purposes. The world of the imagination, of make-believe, becomes a safe way to explore and disclose social, emotional and psychological problems.

Role-playing, which is also found in conventional psychotherapies such as GESTALT THERAPY and psychodrama, puts a greater emphasis on the theatricality of the drama. It uses props such as masks, puppets, scripted stories, etc., to help individuals express feelings.

Drama therapy, under the guidance of a professional drama therapist, has helped mentally disabled children improve their language and motor skills. In correctional facilities, role-playing and improvisation are used to prepare prison inmates for life on the outside.

This system is particularly helpful to emotionally and developmentally disturbed children and adults who can "play" certain behaviors and emotions in a nonthreatening environment. Taking on roles as other characters, frees many of these individuals to feel what they cannot in real life.

Storytelling, using a familiar tale or fable, affords people the opportunity to identify with certain characters or characteristics. How the individual enacts the part is very revealing and the drama therapist can interpret and discuss the significance of the performance with the individual.

In a geriatric setting, such as a nursing home, oral histories and storytelling provide the elderly with a sense of purpose and self-worth.

The National Association for Drama Therapy, incorporated in 1979, sets the standards for professionals and has developed national guidelines for master's and doctoral training.

E

ear therapy, or auriculotherapy, is a method of treating diseases by placing ACUPUNCTURE needles, thin sticks or finger pressure to certain areas of the ear. Two thousand years ago, the Chinese *Huangdi Nei Jing* (Canon of Medicine), c. 300–100 B.C., recognized the relationship between the ears and the MERIDIANS and internal organs. "The ear is the place where all the channels meet."[1]

The ear is representative of the fetus upside down in the womb, and the organs are mapped out following the physical pattern. The lobe, for example, represents the head. Pathological changes within the body manifest themselves with tenderness in the related ear points. These **auricular points,** or **reaction points,** are stimulation points for the therapy.

Oriental medicine, which considers the ear to be a major part of the body, believes that the bigger the ear, the longer the life and the greater the fortune. Representations of Buddha always characterize him with large ears and extremely long earlobes.

None of the 365 regular acupuncture points are actually on the ear itself, although some points are on the perimeter of the ear. The six YANG channels traverse or skirt the ear either directly or through branch channels (see ACUPUNCTURE). The six YIN channels also have no direct connections to the ear but are linked through the inner/outer relationship with the yang channels. "All the vessels congregate in the ear."[2]

Although there are traditional references to auricle manipulation,[3] the "map" of the ear is a recent development. In 1957, a French physician, Dr. Paul Nogier of Lyon, wrote about ear acupuncture in a German acupuncture periodical, which drew enormous attention to the relationship between points on the ear and various parts of the body. He detailed the points on the ear and his "map" is still used today. Chinese medical workers, after years of arduous study, had chartered 200 sites on the ear.

Ear points are named according to the associated anatomical relation, for example, kidney point. Locations on the ear only vary according to people's shapes and sizes.

There are a variety of ways for a therapist to choose the points for treatment. One way selects an ear point according to the associated anatomical region or organ. Another system might choose a point because of its physiological and/or pathologic association. For example, the point for the endocrine system might be stimulated to treat irregular menses. The CHINESE MEDICINE association of channel to organ could be another way to choose a point. Finally, points might be picked because of their clinical effectiveness.

Locating the points in the ear can be done in a variety of ways. Direct examination may reveal color or physical changes at an auricular point. Changes in shapes of the ear or the inability in wiping away ear accumulations may also indicate the site of the point.

Probing with a blunt-tipped probe pressed against the point may reveal a tenderness, which indicates the point to treat. Electrical resistance may also be used to find the exact points, which details skin's resistance to the impulses at various sites.

In addition to ear reflexology, which employs finger pressure on organ-related points, acupuncturists have numerous ways to treat the ear. Needling is the most common method of treatment. The area is located and cleaned with alcohol before the needle is inserted. Once it is in place, it may be turned to stimulate the QI energy, life's vital energy, and left for 30 to 60 minutes. In serious conditions, the needles can be left in place for up to two hours. Ten treatments are usually standard, although the client's condition will dictate whether more or fewer sessions are necessary. Three to five needles can be placed in the ear in one session. Usually, but not always, at least one point on

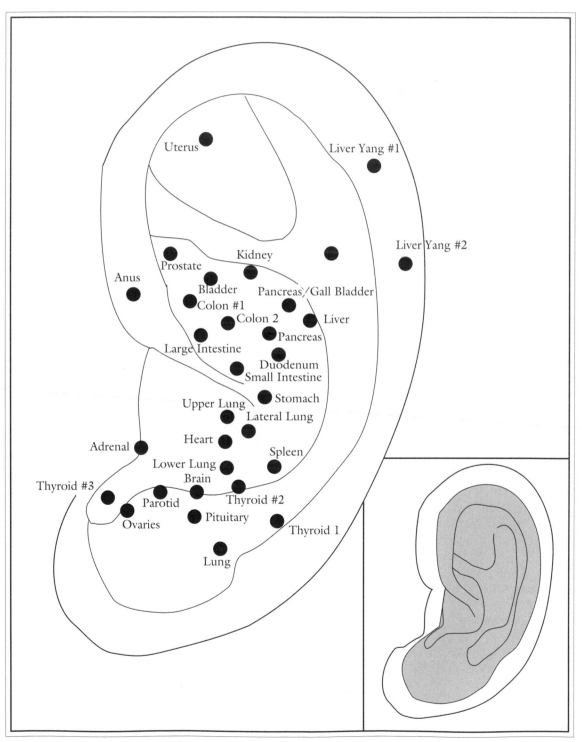

Patterned after the baby head-down in the womb, the acupuncture points found all over the ear relate to specific organs and glands throughout the body. Stimulation to an ear point affects its respective organ.

the ear that corresponds to an organ will be stimulated.

Another popular method is needle embedding, which secures special intradermal ear needles or tacks onto a specific point for long periods of time, usually one week or so. These needles should be pressed several times a day to stimulate *qi* and the underlying tissue. The needle sensation is important to maintain or the ear will adapt to the pressure. This treatment has become popular for people who are trying to give up smoking and other addictive behaviors.

MOXIBUSTION is used in ear therapy in cases of chronic rheumatism or cold diseases. The points are treated for three to five minutes.

Pricking auricular points with the tip of a needle to produce bleeding is used in acute inflammatory conditions. Three to five drops are usually produced a few times each day.

Electro-acupuncture using two needles with electrical stimulation is performed for 15 to 30 minutes. The amount of the stimulation is based on the client's tolerance and comfort.

Injection therapy injects remedies into the points and is used for pulmonary tuberculosis, bronchial asthma and as an anesthesia.

Notes

[1] Academy of Traditional Chinese Medicine, *Chinese Acupuncture and Moxibustion,* Foreign Language Press, Beijing, 1975, p. 269.

[2] Shanghai College of Traditional Medicine, *Acupuncture: A Comprehensive Text,* translated by John O'Connor and Dan Bensky, Eastland Press, Seattle, 1981, p. 472.

[3] Ibid., p. 472. During the Tang dynasty, the physician Sun Simo wrote in his *Thousand Prescriptions* about treating certain diseases with ear manipulation. *The Great Compendium of Acupuncture and Moxibustion,* a Ming dynasty classic, prescribed moxa on the ear.

Further Reading

Bourdiol, René J., Dr., *Elements of Auriculotherapy,* Maisonneuve, Moulins-les-Metz, France, 1980. This book presents a clinical approach to ear therapy. Many treatments are presented.

———, *Auriculo-Somatology,* Maisonneuve, Moulins-les-Metz, France, 1983. This book correlates auricular points with the treatment of many diseases.

Kropej, Helmut, M.D., *Fundamentals of Ear Acupuncture,* MedicinaBio., Portland, Oreg., 1991. This easy-to-follow book describes the history of ear therapy and many treatment points for common ailments.

Nogier, Paul, Dr., *From Auriculo Therapy to Auriculo Medicine,* Maisonneuve, Verdun, France, 1981. This book was written by the doctor who formalized the "map" of the ear, charting all the auricular points.

effleurage from the French meaning "flowerlike," is the introductory and final stroke in Swedish massage. It is the most common stroke used during general treatment. Effleurage is a long, gliding stroke, which is used to apply the lubrication, acquaint the client with the therapist's touch, is a valuable tool in evaluating the condition of the underlying tissue, prepares the body for deeper work and is the transitional stroke from one body part to another. Effleurage can be either a light touch or deep in pressure.

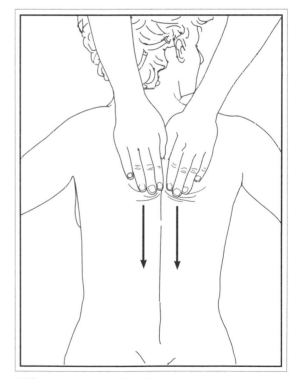

Effleurage is the Swedish massage stroke that begins each massage and massage sequence. It is used to spread the lubricant, evaluate the condition of the underlying tissues and enhance blood and lymph circulation.

The stroke can be performed using open palms, knuckles, forearms, elbows, fingertips or thumbs, depending upon the desired pressure and result. When effleurage is performed on the limbs, the pressure of the stroke is centripetal, or toward the heart, to assist venous blood and lymphatic circulation.

At the conclusion of the massage, or at the end of treatment to each body part, a very light fingertip, gliding stroke, called the **nerve stroke,** is often used. Since the pressure is extremely light, the direction of the stroke is incidental, but is often down toward the feet to "ground" the client and signal the end to the massage.

The physiological effects of effleurage are numerous, but the increased effect on the circulatory and lymphatic systems is its most important influence. Arterial blood, the rich, oxygenated blood, which flows to all tissues of the body, is circulated by the pumping action of the heart. Venous blood and lymphatic circulation, however, flow against gravity and are pushed back toward the heart through muscular contraction and mechanical stimulation. Effleurage is directly involved in promoting the return of venous and lymphatic circulation.

The action is actually a suction-pressure pump movement. As the veins are emptied by the pressure of the stroke, blood from peripheral veins is sucked into the emptied vessels with minimal force. The pressure does not affect the opposing arterial flow since arteries are deep within the body and their walls are more resistant.[1] Venous flow is enhanced due to the faster outflow of venous circulation and the reduction of venous pressure.

Lymph drainage is also stimulated through the use of the effleurage stroke. The lymph vessels are primarily noncontractile and rely upon outside forces to promote circulation. These influences include muscular contractions, pressure of the filtration of fluid from the capillaries and massage.[2] If the lymphatic system cannot drain excess fluid effectively, swelling of the extremities, or edema, often occurs. Mas-

sage, in particular effleurage, reduces the swelling and promotes increased reabsorption of lymph by shifting edematous fluid from the tissues to the blood, resulting in increased urinary volume and excretion of waste material.[3] Capillary pressure is also reduced from the action of effleurage.

As a direct result of increased circulation, metabolic waste product removal is promoted and oxygenated blood and nutrient delivery is enhanced. Localized circulation and temperature is increased, often creating a reaction called **hyperemia,** reddening of the skin from increased circulation.

Effleurage can counteract incipient inflammations by acting as an antiphlogistic (anti-inflammatory). Pain is thereby reduced from the release of the pressure of the inflammation.

In cases of delayed healing, poor circulation, traumatic injury or poor tissue nutrition, the application of effleurage is instrumental in preventing gangrene or mortification of a limb through its ability to increase circulation and lymph reabsorption.

Effleurage supplies a passive stretch to muscle tissues, reducing spasms and accompanying pain and can act as a restorative to tired muscles. Carbonic acid, lactic acid, phosphates, etc., are removed from the muscle tissues and are replaced by oxygen and nutrient-rich blood. Muscular strength and contractibility are increased from the application of effleurage.

Athletic performance and post-event recovery is improved with effleurage. Muscles massaged after fatigue sets in regain their strength faster and become stronger as a result of the treatment. Greater pliancy and flexibility are also reported to be a result of the massage.[4]

Light effleurage has a relaxing effect on the body, probably a result of its sedating effects on the sensory nerves of the skin.[5] It is also often used as the primary stroke in treating insomnia and general fatigue.

Effleurage on the visceral organs can stimulate activity. The contents of the stomach may empty faster and peristaltic (wavelike) movement of the large intestines may be stimulated. By massaging in a clockwise manner, following the direction of the large intestine, it is possible to assist the passage of fecal matter toward the descending colon. Intestinal gases may also be expelled with the application of effleurage to the large intestines.

Effleurage promotes relaxation which may result in the reduction of stress-related illnesses and improve a client's physical and emotional health.

Notes

[1] Yates, John, Ph.D., *A Physician's Guide to Therapeutic Massage: Its Physiological Effects and Their Application to Treatment,* Massage Therapy Association of British Columbia, Vancouver, Canada, 1990, p. 96.

[2] Jacobs, Miriam, M.S., "Massage for the Relief of Pain: Anatomical and Physiological Considerations," *The Physical Therapy Review,* Vol. 40, No. 2, 1960, p. 96.

[3] Yates, John, Ph.D., *A Physician's Guide to Therapeutic Massage: Its Physiological Effects and Their Application to Treatment,* Massage Therapy Association of British Columbia, Vancouver, Canada, 1990, p. 3.

[4] Ibid., p. 16.

[5] Scull, C. Wesler, Ph.D., "Massage—Physiologic Basis," *Archives Physical Medicine,* No. 26, March 1945, p. 163.

Egoscue Method® a diagnostic and therapeutic system that uses a specifically designed sequence of exercises to treat musculoskeletal pain and help athletes achieve top levels of performance.

Pete Egoscue, the developer of this system, believes that the body needs activity and motion in order to function efficiently. He purports that people in industrialized societies who lead predominantly sedentary lives, cannot achieve or maintain optimum health. Lack of movement and exercise causes deterioration.

Egoscue was a marine combat officer in Vietnam in the late 1960s when a bullet wound ended his tour of duty. While immobilized in the hospital, as part of his therapy, he realized that physical function was rapidly lost under such physical constraint. He believed that this lack of movement actually interfered with his healing abilities and contributed to dysfunction. This realization changed the direction of his life.

He trained as an anatomical functionalist with the belief that movement could restore function to the body. The Egoscue Method suggests a one-hour daily regimen of exercises in a special sequence. He also strongly maintains that the participant recognizes his own responsibility for his condition and his healing. Once responsibility is assumed, he believes that the Egoscue Method works every time.

This method is designed for people with musculoskeletal pain, injuries or those athletes who want to realize their maximum physical potentials and prevent future injury.

Egoscue defines fitness as "the positive control of one's environment on a daily basis without effort."[1] All the exercises ever done, vitamins consumed and dietary regimens followed amount to nothing if there is no control over the personal environment to fulfill one's physical and psychological needs.

Each session begins with an overview of anatomy and physiology so participants have a basic understanding of how the body works. Diagnosis, or self-diagnosis, follows as a description of four function/dysfunction categories. Egoscue believes that everyone falls into one of these categories.

Condition I assumes a body posture where the hips tilt forward, the feet evert (turn out) and the head is out of position (alignment). This posture is the source of much minor lower back pain.

Condition II reveals an upper torso rotation, which causes the shoulders and the hips to swing out of vertical and parallel alignment.

Condition III, the weakest body type, has the hips tilt under with the top of the pelvis tilting backward. This posture flattens out the natural S curve of the spine and can create many problems, aches and pains.

The fourth condition is not a dysfunction at all, but rather a state of perfect alignment and posture, which Egoscue calls **D-Lux.** The overall goal is to reach D Lux.

Once the categories have been diagnosed, the workout is performed daily to correct the dysfunction (or maintain health). Each category follows a specific sequence taken from 22 exercises.

Egoscue lists do's and don't's for performing the exercises:

1. Do remember proper alignment
2. Don't forget to breathe deeply
3. Do take off shoes
4. Don't forget to work both sides of the body equally
5. Do activate the muscles
6. Don't ignore pain
7. Do follow the sequence

On the subject of pain, Egoscue suggests that the symptoms must be addressed regardless of the diagnosed condition. Pain confirms that there is a problem. He recommends beginning the sequence with the **static back press** (laying on the floor with legs bent at 90° and supported from knees to ankles, flattening the spine), **supine groin stretch** (same position as static back press except one leg is placed at 90° while the other leg is extended straight on the floor with the foot propped on the outside to prevent outward eversion) and the **air bench** (back pressing against a wall with the knees bent at 90°, feet straight and shoulder distance apart) until the pain stops. Then begin the appropriate sequence.

The Egoscue Method has been used by many amateur and professional athletes, and it has helped people live healthier, pain-free lives and achieve complete fitness.

Note
[1]Egoscue, Pete, with Gittines, Roger, *The Egoscue Method of Health through Motion,* HarperCollins, N.Y., 1992, p. 45.

Further Reading
Egoscue, Pete, with Gittines, Roger, *The Egoscue Method of Health through Motion,* HarperCollins, N.Y., 1992. This book explains the Egoscue Method and how to self-diagnose your physical function/dysfunction. A series of clearly illustrated, carefully explained exercises demonstrate the method for regaining and maintaining physical fitness.

electrical current therapy   the use of one of three types of current for therapeutic purposes. The three types are galvanic, faradic and T.E.N.S.

Galvanic current is a steady, unidirectional current, which causes the muscle to contract even if the nerve supply to that muscle has been severed. It reduces pain because it increases blood flow and tissue metabolism. It also provides muscle stimulation when peripheral nerves have sustained injury, affording regeneration of the nerve.

Galvanic current produces a chemical reaction in the body. It breaks up molecules into their composite atoms and ions. At the point of entry, a positive charge collects and at the point of exit, a negative charge is collected. This polarity repels similar ions and attracts the opposite pole. The electrode pads, one positive, the other negative, must therefore be put in the correct place to ensure the appropriate result.

In order to determine the polarity, a litmus paper test can be used. Blue litmus paper will turn red in the presence of the positive pole. Red litmus paper will turn blue with the negative pole. Another test is the water test. With both poles placed under water, twice as many bubbles will collect at the negative pole than at the positive pole.

The applications of the current depend upon the desired results. The positive pole attracts oxygen, dehydrates, constricts blood vessels and causes ischemia (lack of blood), controls bleeding, is germicidal, sedates and relieves pain in instances of congestion. The negative pole attracts hydrogen, liquifies tissues, dilates blood vessels and causes hyperemia (presence of blood), promotes bleeding, stimulates and causes pain.

The electrodes should be very wet for use. Application and duration are determined by the practitioner based on the health of the client and the condition that is being treated. Generally, treatments should not exceed 30 minutes.

Faradic current is an alternating current most frequently used in physical therapy treatments. This current changes directions constantly and consists of two pulses, which follow each other in opposite directions. One pulse is a high intensity current of short duration and the second pulse is of longer duration and lower intensity. When a faradic impulse is placed on a motor point or anywhere along a nerve, a contraction results. Injured nerves or paralyzed muscles will not respond to a faradic current. It is primarily used to stimulate weak muscles with a normal nerve or to test for nerve degeneration.

T.E.N.S. (transcutaneous electrical nerve stimulation), is an electric current that is passed across the skin. T.E.N.S. apparatus is prescribed to control pain. It provides sensory, rather than motor, stimulation to reduce pain.

The electrodes are placed directly on the area of pain and if the pain radiates, an additional electrode may be placed along the nerve. Acupuncture points may also be stimulated within T.E.N.S.

T.E.N.S. is contraindicated with a demand-type pacemaker, directly on the heart in patients with arrhythmias (irregular heart beats) or myocardial disease, on open wounds and the pregnant uterus. It has proved to be a successful pain control system in cases of bursitis, cancer, multiple sclerosis, bowel stasis, labor, postoperative discomfort, migraine headaches, temporomandibular joint (TMJ) syndrome, whiplash, backaches, sciatica and frozen shoulders.

Further Reading

Gersh, Meryl, *Electrotherapy in Rehabilitation,* Davis Co., Philadelphia, Pa., 1992. This book is for physiotherapists who want to become more familiar with electrical current therapy.

Nelson, Roger M., *Clinical Electrotherapy,* Appleton & Lang, East Norwalk, Conn., 1991. This is a reference text for physical therapists. It is a technical book, which provides a comprehensive overview of the use of electrotherapeutic devices and procedures.

electromagnetics the use of the body's innate electromagnetics field and energetic bodywork systems or external fields for healing purposes. Electromagnetic healing methods vary greatly. They may include ACUPUNCTURE, HYPNOSIS, homeopathy, VISUALIZATION (guided imagery), PSYCHIC HEALING and ELECTROTHERAPY, to name a few systems that alter the body's energy bio-field.

Ancient healing systems acknowledged that life was endowed with a special energy, or life force, which was vital to existence. The Chinese called it *chi* or *qi,* the Japanese knew it as *ki* and the Sanskrit word for this essential force is *prana.* The dualistic forces of nature came from the connection of life energy to the natural forces of the environment. Health was attained when balances between the forces was achieved and disease, or death, resulting from an imbalance.

Modern technology is beginning to recognize the phenomenon and power of the electromagnetic field, which surrounds and penetrates the body, although they are just recognizing its application in healing.

The movement of electrons in an electrical current produces a similar field around the charge. If it is a DC current, the magnetic field is steady. The strength of the magnetic field depends upon the amount of current. Very large DC electromagnets can lift heavy objects. (The super trains currently being tested operate on this principle.)

Fluctuations in the electric current will produce the same effect on the magnetic current. The field is characterized in terms of frequency of fluctuation based on the term **hertz** (Hz), named after Heinrich Hertz who first studied this phenomena. Once per second translates to 1–Hz frequency, etc.

All electromagnetic fields are force fields, which carry energy, information and are capable of producing an action at a distance.[1]

Electromagnetic fields within the body control growth and healing, regulate the level of brain activity and produce vitally important biological cycles by receiving timing information from the earth's natural electromagnetic environment.[2]

Dr. Robert O. Becker, M.D., who has been studying the electromagnetic field for decades, explains the three types of energy medicine. In the first instance, there is no external energy administered to the body. These types of systems may include hypnosis, biofeedback or visualization. The treatment methods attempt only to activate preexisting energetic control systems. Becker calls these **minimal energy techniques.**

The second category includes those systems that administer external energy, but in amounts similar to those that the body itself uses in its energetic control systems. He refers to these as **energy-reinforcement techniques,** which might include acupuncture, homeopathy and some physical manipulation.

The third category, or the **high energy transfer techniques,** administers energy to the body in larger amounts than those that occur naturally. These are generally related to practices of technological medicine and may include electrotherapy, electrical current stimulation and high voltage therapy.[3]

Although these categories vary in the degree of energy they provide, the philosophy behind using them is the same: to provide enough energy to let the body heal itself.

Notes

[1] Becker, Rober O., M.D., *Cross Currents,* Jeremy P. Tarcher, Los Angeles, Calif., 1990, p. 69.

[2] Ibid., p. 86.

[3] Ibid., p. 93.

Further Reading

Becker, Robert O., M.D., and Selden, Gary, *The Body Electric, Electromagnetism and the Foundation of Life,* Quill, N.Y., 1985. This illustrated book presents the history that electromagnetic research advances may provide medicine with the ability to control and stimulate healing using the electromagnetic forces in the human body.

Becker, Robert O., M.D., *Cross Currents,* Jeremy P. Tarcher, Los Angeles, Calif., 1990. The emergence of electromagnetic medicine is discussed here. The author uses the model of the body electric to reveal the secrets of healing by popular alternative methods such as acupuncture, biofeedback, hypnosis and psychic healing.

Burr, Harold Saxton, *Blueprint for Immortality,* Beekman Publications, Woodstock, N.Y. Based on the theory that all organisms generate an electrodynamic field, this book explores its effect on individual cells of the biological system.

embodyment training a heart-centered and intuitive method of cocreative healing, which aims to integrate the body, emotions and soul. Bodies are shaped by experiences in life, which may include repressed memories and real or imagined traumas that are unconsciously held in the body. The embodyment process accesses the inner experience of sensations, images, feelings and energy as a way to work through old wounds and integrate new possibilities for ways of being.

These insights come directly from body-centered experiences. The embodyment process incorporates energy healing, dialoguing and movement techniques that, when used with developed sensitivity and listening of the facilitator, can lead to an individual's greater self-understanding. Freer movement, deeper breathing patterns and greater self-expression often result from this training method.

Embodyment training was founded by K. Douglas Brady (Balbdhadra), who received his M.Ed. in psychological counseling in 1978. He has studied many different bodywork systems, which reflects in his technique, such as MYOFASCIAL RELEASE, CRANIOSACRAL THERAPY, AURA and CHAKRA BALANCING, TRAGER, POLARITY THERAPY and KRIPALU YOGA.

Embodyment training consists of eight components. **Sacred touch** is a gentle, intuitive consciousness of touch that provides insight into acknowledging and accepting the internal experience. Sacred touch, combined with myofascial release, basic craniosacral balancing and tissue dialogue (palpation) comprise the embodyment hands-on approach.

Body journeying is a body-centered dialogue approach that uses physical sensations, gestures, sound, movement and touch to reach repressed memories and traumas and reconnect with the self.

Body reading is an in-depth system of observing the body's development and corresponding physical and emotional defense patterns. New options arise as an individual gains understanding of old habits and releases them.

Energy healing is a hands-on approach to clearing and energizing the auric field and major chakras. Through energy healing, individuals learn to access unordinary states of reality, work with their spirit guides and facilitate deep healing within the physical, emotional and spiritual body.

Intuitive development teaches individuals to validate and trust the images, feelings and guidance of the "inner voice." Intuition is the primary guide in embodyment sessions.

Movement and **sound** are a combination of kripalu yoga, dynamics partner yoga, dance, assisted myofascial stretching and primordial sounding to clear energy blocks and clear the chakras. It also awakens the capacity for joy and pleasure.

Cocreative rituals are open-ended experiences, which serve to reconnect the individuals with ancient energy sources, joy and creative expression and reestablish the connection to the earth's healing energies.

The **open forum** is offered in large and small discussion groups to explore issues that surface in therapeutic relationships, such as sexuality, intimacy, boundaries and ethical standards.

The embodyment community is dedicated to living life to the fullest in feeling, acceptance and expression.

emotional-kinesthetic psychotherapy an
integrative method that combines verbal dialogue, MEDITATION, touch with permission to facilitate the emotional process, working with silence and psychospiritual space, character analysis and actively building on the client-therapist relationship.

The work was developed by Linda Marks and builds on HAKOMI and psychosynthesis and incorporates elements that are parallel to FOCUSING. Central to emotional-kinesthetic psychotherapy is honoring the pace and nonverbal process of the client. The therapist **holds the space** through respectful and skillful application of technique to help the client increase emotional safety and find language from felt experience. Carefully and conscientiously exploring habitual ways of being, such as physical tensions, thought patterns, emotional habits or limitations, can unearth deeper parts of the self, which can then be met with appropriate responses.

Emotional-kinesthetic psychotherapy is heart-centered, using the heart both as an emotional anchor and a source of information about who we are and what we need. The therapist tracks the **emotional-kinesthetic charge,** which is an energetic signal, that changes as a person moves from one feeling state to another. Feelings have both physical and emotional components. For example, sadness may be experienced as a heavy heart, etc. By learning to find meaning from felt experience, a client can embody their power, find their voice, embrace their true nature and express it in relationships and work.

Emotional-kinesthetic psychotherapy is particularly powerful in healing trauma, abuse or neglect. It can also be used in a group therapy setting.

emotional release a form of bodywork that
addresses physical tensions that are basically emotional or psychological in origin. Dr. Wilhelm Reich (see REICHIAN GROWTH WORK) believed that the body's energy, which he called **orgone,** can become trapped in chronic muscle contractions, called **armor.** Within this armor, emotion as well as energy can be trapped. The purpose of emotional release work is to contact these blocked feelings and release them.

Emotional release work is often associated with BREATH THERAPY. Deep breathing exercises and hands-on work (this work can be any one of the numerous systems, such as SWEDISH MASSAGE or ROLFING, for example) on the rigid areas, individuals are encouraged to express suppressed feelings and free the body of constraints.

Fears, traumas, phobias and anxieties, which are locked in the body, may be relieved through emotional release, allowing the individual to let go of unwanted habits and unproductive behavior patterns.

energy bio-field work the balancing of the AURA, or human energy field, through various energy processes such as chelation, which is clearing the energy field by removing auric debris,[1] charging and clearing the aura, spinal cleaning, spiritual surgery, restructuring and vibrationally through COLOR THERAPY and SOUNDING.

Note
[1] Brennan, Barbara Ann, *Hands of Light,* Bantam Books, N.Y., 1988, p. 205.

Ericksonian hypnotherapy recognizes the hypnotic state as a natural human activity, which helps an individual reach his own storehouse of resources and possibilities within the unconscious mind. Dr. Milton H. Erickson believed that most of life is unconsciously determined and by reaching into that level of the mind through hypnotherapy, it would be possible to change unhealthy patterns and belief systems.

In Ericksonian hypnotherapy, the hypnotist functions as a compassionate guide, respecting each client and his unconscious mind. In the trance, the changes occur most effectively and on a permanent basis when the hypnotist concentrates on influencing the client's unconscious patterns, which often violate his values and basic emotional structure.

Erickson called the trance "a state in which learning and openness to change are most likely to occur."[1] He recognized that trances are natural phenomena, which happen to people on a regular basis in the form of daydreams, meditation, prayer and even during exercise. An indi-

vidual is not exactly in a somnolent state but rather can be deeply relaxed and may become aware of his mental and sensory experiences on a more acute level. During the trance state, clients often intuitively understand the meanings of their dreams, symbols and other forms of unconscious expression. With the understanding that people already possess a great deal of the information they will ever need, the trance state is simply a way to get to it.

Erickson's work has often been called magical. He used storytelling, while the client was in a trance, to provoke people to reach out in higher levels. These stories, which were sometimes majestic fairy tales, biblical references or stirring folk myths, or about Erickson himself or other real people, deeply affected his clients. They often identified with characters or situations in the stories and felt a sense of accomplishment and success as the stories came to satisfactory, victorious conclusions.

Erickson explained that the profound changes that happened to his clients occurred because of their trances. He believed that these teaching tales reinforced their strengths and evoked a powerful sense of accomplishment.

One of Erickson's theories was that **reparenting** took place within the context of the trance and the stories, which caused dramatic changes in his clients. Reparenting is a process that replaces previous parental prohibitions and injunctions with new ideas and experiences. Posthypnotic suggestions, where the client continues to respond positively to "hearing" the hypnotist's voice or suggestions, strengthens the client's desire to change.

Dr. Erickson died in March 1980. He was the founder of the American Society of Clinical Hypnosis, a life fellow of the American Psychiatric Association and a founding editor of the *American Journal of Clinical Hypnosis.*

Note
[1] Rosen, Sidney, ed., *My Voice Will Go with You: The Teaching Tales of Milton H. Erickson,* W.W. Norton & Co., N.Y., 1982, p. 27.

Further Reading

Erickson, Milton H., and Rossi, Ernest L., *Hypnotherapy: An Exploratory Casebook,* Irvington Publications, N.Y., 1979. Written the year before his death. Dr. Erickson explains his theories and cites many case histories of his hypnosis techniques.

Grindler, John, Delzier, Judith, and Bandler, Richard, *Patterns of the Hypnotic Techniques of M.H. Erickson, M.D.,* Vol. I, Meta Publishing, Cupertino, Calif., 1975, and Vol. II, 1977. These texts analyze the theories of Dr. Erickson and their applications in various therapeutic situations.

Haley, Jay, *Uncommon Therapy: The Psychiatric Technique of Milton H. Erickson, M.D.,* W.W. Norton, N.Y., 1973. Ground-breaking theories by Dr. Erickson are discussed in this book.

Havens, Ronald A., *The Wisdom of Milton H. Erickson, Vol. I: Hypnosis and Hypnotherapy,* Irvington Publications, N.Y., 1989. This book provides an insight into the history and philosophy of Ericksonian hypnosis.

Rosen, Sidney, ed., *My Voice Will Go with You: The Teaching Tales of Milton H. Erickson,* W.W. Norton, N.Y., 1982. This book represents many of Dr. Erickson's classes and group seminars and the stories he used for his hypnotherapy clients.

Esalen Massage a massage technique that is effective on three levels: slow, flowing strokes open a sense of ease in the recipient, specific muscle kneading releases tension; passive joint movement reaffirms the sensation of spaciousness; and a nurturing, supportive relation between client and practitioner encourages the recipient to consciously sense into himself, resulting in fuller breath and a deeply energized and relaxed state.

The approach is toward the whole person, seeking connections rather than disjointed parts. Flowing, light-oiled strokes are intrinsic; practitioners switch from employing hands to elbows or knees for deeper work and stretches. Light rocking or gentle holding concludes the personalized session, lasting approximately one hour and 15 minutes. The bodywork is widely effective whether the clients seek pain relief, sports massage, energy release or stress reduction.

At its home site, Esalen Institute, Big Sur, California, massages frequently take place in the open air, accompanied by the nearby ocean waves. Founded in 1963 by Michael Murphy and Richard Price to explore East-West thought, the institute's seminar program has promoted many innovative body/mind pioneers, such as Charlotte Selver (SENSORY AWARENESS), Ida Rolf (ROLFING), Moshe Feldenkrais (FELDENKRAIS METHOD), Fritz Perls (GESTALT THERAPY), Judith Aston (ASTON-PATTERNING) and Ilana Rubenfeld (RUBENFELD SYNERGY).

Esalen's Massage School offers professional level training and certification.

etheric release a bodywork system that recognizes that restricted emotional expression can create imbalances and malfunctions in the body. Forms of energy work, based on ALCHEMICAL SYNERGY are used to remove blockages and close the gaps in the energy flow channels.

The etheric layer of the human energy biofield is the physical plane and the first layer of seven. It corresponds with the first CHAKRA (root chakra) and comes from the word ether, signifying the state between energy and matter. It has the same structure as the physical body, including all anatomical parts and organs.

Eye-Robics® an eye exercise system that improves vision without the use of corrective lenses or surgery. Based on the Bates-Corbett method (see BATES METHOD OF VISION TRAINING), it was developed by Dr. Jerriann J. Taber, Ph.D., a former student and teacher of their method. In 1971, she founded the Vision Training Institute in El Cajon, California.

Dr. Bates, a noted New York ophthalmologist, recognized that vision was directly affected by tension. Relaxation is therefore a major component in correcting sight problems. Dr. Taber included self-growth techniques into her system, which acknowledge the physical, mental, emotional and spiritual wholeness of each individual.

The system works with the cause of the problem—tension, not the symptoms. Since it is an accepted belief that vision is not a fixed condition and can be remedied, the basis of the work concentrates on relaxing the muscles of the eye to reshape the lens.

Eye-Robics offers specific tools for relieving mental stress and muscular tension. It provides a comprehensive program of vision education including visualization techniques to stimulate the mind's eye, improved acuity, binocularity, centralization and peripheral awareness, convergence and accommodation.

Further Reading

Taber, Jerriann J., Ph.D., Eye-Robics: The Natural Alternative to Glasses, Contacts or Surgery, Eye-Care Publications Co., San Diego, Calif., 1986. The developer of the technique discusses ways to improve vision with eye exercises and relaxation techniques.

F

facial massage, or face-lift MASSAGE, is a natural approach to rejuvenating the skin and muscles of the face without plastic surgery. This system is a combination of facial exercises, self-massage, basic skin care, the use of sun-protective lotions and a healthy lifestyle.

The face can be damaged by overexposure to the sun,[1] smoking, excessive drug or alcohol use, poor dietary and nutritional habits, stress, temperature extremes, improper skin care, aging and gravity. Face-lift massage seeks to inhibit the influences that break down the integrity of the skin, soften and tighten it and tone the facial muscles.

Exercises should be performed for 15 minutes, three to four times per week. Belle Tuckerman, director of the Belavi Facelift Massage System, suggests beginning with an understanding of unconscious tension-holding patterns that wrinkle the skin and sag the muscles. She suggests placing a postage-stamp size piece of tape on brow lines, crow's feet by the eyes and the sides of the mouth. Sit quietly for a few minutes, keeping the face as calm as possible. When the areas tense, the presence of the tape will act as a reminder to relax. Gradually, those muscles will not react to tension as much because they can now consciously be released.

Her method commences by washing the face with a gentle, soap-free cleanser and applying a soothing, toning lotion over the throat and face, starting at the base of the neck. All the movements should be in an upward direction, counteracting gravity.

Massage each side of the neck with alternative hand strokes, lightly but rapidly to increase circulation.

The "full-face" stroke starts under the chin and continues over the jaw to the temples and up to the forehead. This fingertip stroke can be repeated up to 10 times.

Light circles around the eyes relax sensitive eye muscles. Press along the eyebrow ridge to relieve tension. The facial massage ends with a light fingertip tapping all over the face.

Acupuncturists have been performing "face-lifts" or rejuvenating treatments by inserting very small needles into the lines of the face (see ACUPUNCTURE). The increased blood flow tends to fill out the lines, making the face wrinkle free, relieves the skin of waste products and relaxes the underlying muscles. These treatments must be repeated often in order to produce effective an long-lasting effects.

ACUPRESSURE uses fingertip pressure at certain points, or **tsubos,** to relax and rejuvenate the face. Circulation is increased, bringing nutrients to the tissues and promoting waste removal.

Facial exercises are an important factor in toning facial muscles. Yawning and tensing and releasing throat muscles helps develop the front of the neck.

The lips may lose their wrinkles by opening the mouth and curling the lips inward, over the teeth, for five seconds and releasing. Raising and lowering the eyebrows tones the forehead.

Most professional massage therapists are trained in facial massage, which will bring increased circulation to facial tissues and relax tense muscles, providing a youthful appearance.

Note

[1] Tuckerman, Belle, "Saving Face: Facial Fitness," *Massage,* Issue 41, January/February 1993, p. 45. Researchers found that all damage to the skin by sun exposure is done by the time an individual is 18 years old. The damage doesn't show up until later in life, however.

Further Reading

Benz, Reinhold, *Facebuilding: The Daily 5-Minute Program for a Beautiful, Wrinkle-Free Face,* Sterling Publications, Co., N.Y., 1991. Clear, color photographs of facial exercises are matched with illustrations of facial muscles to demonstrate how to perform the exercises and exactly which muscles are being affected.

Clark, Linda, *New Faces,* Keats Publications, Inc., New Canaan, Conn., 1973. This book explains facial skin care including dietary considerations, illustrated wrinkle prevention exercises for the face and neck and facial massage treatments.

fascia the tough, loose (areolar) CONNECTIVE TISSUE that binds muscle fibers together, links muscles and bones (tendons) and covers the organs, nerves and blood vessels. It shapes, supports the body and holds the bones in place. Fascia spreads throughout the body in a three-dimensional network from head to toe without interruption.

Healthy fascia is loose and moist. When the body is healthy, fascia facilitates movement between different body parts. Under stress, trauma or disuse, fascia loses its flexibility and becomes rigid. The layers of fascia sometimes adhere (stick) together, forming palpable "knots."

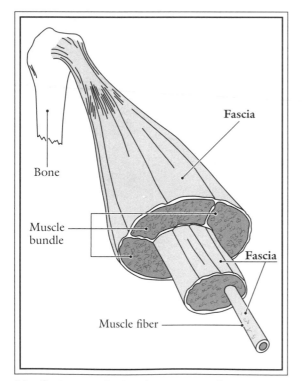

Myofascia, or fascia that covers the muscles, shapes, supports and separates the muscles. Fascia is the connective tissue found throughout the body. It covers all of the muscles, organs, nerves, blood vessels and cells of the body.

There are three types of fascia: superficial, deep and subserosa. The superficial, or subcutaneous, layer is directly under the skin. It covers the whole interior body and is made of an adipose layer and a loose connective tissue layer. In between is a network of arteries, veins, lymphatics, nerves, the mammary glands of the breasts and fascial muscles. It functions as a storehouse of fat and water, insulation for the body from heat loss, protector of the body from injuries and provides pathways for nerves and blood vessels.

The deep fascia is the most extensive fascia of the body. It is composed of dense connective tissue and lines the body wall and extremities and holds the muscles together in functioning groups. It permits the free movement of muscles, carries nerves and blood vessels, inhabits the spaces between the muscles and is sometimes the origin or insertion for muscles (points of attachment).

The subserosa fascia is found between the deep fascia and a serous membrane. Serous membranes line the cavities of the body that do not open to the exterior and they cover the organs within those spaces. The subserosa fascia protects the external surfaces of the viscera in the thoracic and abdominal cavities.

fascial kinetics, formerly called the Bowen Technique, is a series of gentle, cross-fiber massages used to manipulate the CONNECTIVE TISSUE and realign the body to promote balanced energy flow.

The term was coined by Russell Sturgess and based on the work of Australian practitioner, Tom Bowen. Bowen, a self-taught practitioner, never felt qualified to teach fascial kinetics, yet he was able to treat as many as 13,000 clients a year toward the end of his long career. It wasn't until after his death in the mid-1980s that a coworker inaugurated a program based on his work.

The system incorporates subtle movements, joint tapping in the extremities and some hydrotherapy as it is used in physical therapy. It is extremely gentle to receive and easy on the practitioner's body to perform. Superficial FASCIA[1] and connective tissue are the structures addressed in fascial kinetics.

A series of light, transverse manipulations applied to the superficial fascia results in the same significant changes deep and painful stroking provides. The treatment is generally followed by a two- to five-minute rest, providing adequate time for neuromuscular reeducation. Once the fascia releases, there is an increase in circulation and lymphatic drainage. Usually a tingling sensation or heat follows the treatment.

Sturgess purports that the attitude the practitioner brings to the therapy is as important as the technique. He suggests a **love-centered connectedness** between client and practitioner, which he believes is healing to both.

Fascial kinetics can be used whenever fascia is contracted, especially in cases of chronic pain, neck and lower back tightness, carpal tunnel syndrome and TMJ (temporomandibular joint) dysfunction. It is also effective in cases of specific injuries or illnesses.

Note
[1] Fascia is a sheet or flat band of loose connective tissue beneath the skin, around the muscles and organs.

fascial mobilization a hands-on system that releases restrictions in all layers of the FASCIAL system including the superficial layer, deep layer and core layer.

The fascia is a continuous, membranous sheath of CONNECTIVE TISSUE that spreads all over the body and plays an intricate role in the function of the body. It wraps around organs, blood vessels, bones and the nerves.

Restrictions in the fascia may cause pain, discomfort and limited movement. The techniques of fascial mobilization seek to balance, mobilize and provide symmetry to the body within the skeletal, soft tissue and craniosacral systems.

Each of the three layers of fascia is individually addressed. The superficial layer mobilizes soft tissue, releasing muscle contractions and spasms. The deep technique stretches and releases the fascia, and the core technique incorporates craniosacral therapy with extradural techniques of the superficial and deep layers.

Feldenkrais Method® an educational system, which uses movement to bring about more effective ways to function. It is an application of principles and exercises that help the body program the brain to benefit the entire body-mind system. First a student[1] is taught to become aware of his existing patterns of action and then the student is guided in the discovery of additional possibilities for action.

The Feldenkrais Method* has a broad range of applications. It can be used to reveal and change habitual behaviors that are responsible for chronic tension and pain. Recovery of movement from injury or trauma is also a result of this system. Athletes, dancers, musicians, etc., may improve their skills by using the principles of this method. It is designed to help students live fuller and more effectively by expanding their movements and actions.

The Feldenkrais Method is offered in two forms: through group lessons called **Awareness Through Movement®** and the one-to-one lesson called **Functional Integration®**. Each session lasts 45 to 60 minutes.

Awareness Through Movement is the verbally directed form of the Feldenkrais Method, which consists of the gentle exploration of highly sophisticated movement sequences organized around specific activities, such as reaching, sitting, walking, etc. The lessons evolve from basic movements to complex skills. The goal is to increase a student's awareness of multiple possibilities of action and achieve greater coordination.

These lessons, which are usually taught in a group setting, direct the class's attention to a

*FELDENKRAIS®, FELDENKRAIS METHOD®, AWARENESS THROUGH MOVEMENT®, FUNCTIONAL INTEGRATION® and the FELDENKRAIS GUILD® ARE REGISTERED SERVICE MARKS OF THE FELDENKRAIS GUILD.

slow, delicate exploration of an action. The students can be in a variety of positions: standing, sitting or lying on the floor.

For example, when lying on the floor, the students are asked to notice how their bodies touch the floor, which areas are tight or tense and the differences between each side of the body. The exercises, synchronized with breathing, start out as very small, easy movements.

Thinking, sensory perception and (guided) imagery are also involved in examining each movement. The complexity of the lessons depends upon the movement abilities of the students. The process is gradual and supportive to encourage successful learning. The lessons can eventually be done independently.

Functional Integration consists of a practitioner using verbal commands and noninvasive touch to guide individual students to an awareness of existing and alternative movement patterns.

The student may lay on a Feldenkrais table with the practitioner guiding his body through a variety of movements. The touch of Functional Integration is intended to communicate, not to correct or be curative. It evolves out of the immediate need to relay information to the student and is designed to enhance personal awareness and provide alternative movement choices. New sensory experiences and motor organization patterns are developed, which the student learns to recreate on his own.

The student is clothed and can be lying, sitting, standing, kneeling or in motion during the Functional Integration session. The instruction may be organized around a specific activity, as in Awareness Through Movement.

Practitioners of the Feldenkrais Method must spend four years (800 hours) studying a repertoire of movements and learn to be acutely aware of the finest details. They are also taught to recognize complex psychological, biological and neurological components of the learning process and have highly trained, sensitive hands.

Moshe Feldenkrais (1904–1984), a Russian-born Israeli, was a physicist, mechanical and electrical engineer before developing his movement theories. He received his science doctorate at the Sorbonne in Paris, studied with Frederic Joliot-Curie and worked on the French atomic research program and the British antisubmarine program. He was also a judo master and soccer player.

During the 1940s, a painful, recurring soccer knee injury propelled him to apply his scientific mind to the mechanics of the body and the brain.

The motor cortex has numerous connections and neurons (nerve cells) that correspond to specific muscles. If the same muscle patterns are constantly being repeated, then those areas of the brain also stay in fixed patterns. Feldenkrais believed that the more thoroughly an individual stimulates the entire muscular apparatus, the more the brain will be activated and the newly vitalized areas will stimulate adjacent regions. Potentially, the whole brain will function if more regions are used.

He created a system with thousands of exercises to bring about muscular and brain stimulation. Feldenkrais believed that people are aware of the front and upper parts of their bodies, but disconnected to the back and lower limbs. He strived for total body awareness, including the joints, skeletal structure and the influences of gravity.

This system has helped accident victims, people with polio, cerebral palsy, multiple sclerosis, as well as athletes and musicians who benefit from a greater range of movement. In addition to the physiological changes, improvements are made in digestion, sleep, alertness, flexibility, reduced stress and relieved hypertension. With this heightened awareness, bodies can move with lightness and freedom and function at a level much closer to true potential.

Note
[1] Rosenfeld, Albert, "Teaching the Body How to Program the Brain Is Moshe's Miracle," *Smithsonian Magazine*, January 1981. Moshe Feldenkrais claimed that he was a teacher; he had students, never patients, and did not provide treatments, but lessons.

Further Reading

Feldenkrais, Moshe, *Body and Mature Behavior,* Harper & Row, N.Y., 1972. The first book of Feldenkrais's was first published in 1949. It is a classic text describing, in neuropsychological terms, how patterns of movement and posture are acquired and then relate to sexual and social life. He says that improvements will come with a greater kinesthetic sense.

———, *Awareness through Movement,* Harper & Row, N.Y., 1972. This self-help guide explains how to improve posture, flexibility, breathing, health and functioning through 12 Awareness Through Movement lessons.

———, *The Case of Nora,* Harper & Row, N.Y., 1977. A case study of Functional Integration. Nora is taught to see, read, walk and function again after a severe stroke.

———, *The Elusive Obvious,* Meta Publications, N.Y., 1981. This book sums up 40 years of theory and practice of Functional Integration and Awareness Through Movement.

———, *The Master Moves,* Meta Publications, N.Y., 1984. This is a transcript of his five-day public workshop at Mann Ranch, in California in 1979.

———, *The Potent Self,* Harper & Row, N.Y., 1985. Written for the general public, this book explains the theory behind the Feldenkrais Method and offers lessons to achieve potency, self-awareness and spontaneity.

five element shiatsu an American adaptation of Oriental bodywork. The system emphasizes assessment and treatment strategy over specific techniques. Practitioners of five element shiatsu may have studied a variety of SHIATSU forms. However, the common core of this approach is that the FIVE ELEMENT THEORY paradigm is used in determining the primary pattern of disharmony within the MERIDIAN system (energy pathways, which run throughout the body).

The five elements of CHINESE MEDICINE are wood, earth, fire, water and metal. Each element relates to a specific organ, emotion, color, etc.

The use of the Chinese medicine's four examinations is employed for evaluation purposes. They are touching, listening, asking questions and observation. Reading the radial PULSES usually provides the most critical and detailed information about a client's condition. Confirmation of the assessment comes from palpation of the back and/or abdomen (see HARA). Abdominal assessment may include a variety of systems, including

mu (or *ma*) points (one point per meridian found on the abdomen and used for assessment and treatment), a five element pattern or *hara* evaluation. Visual observation of the face, ears and hands are considered along with diet and lifestyle.

Practitioners usually include the eight principle patterns in their examination, which categorizes physical disharmony in terms of internal/external, hot/cold, yin/yang and excess/deficiency.

The detailed analysis of each client's condition reveals a complete pattern of disharmony and illuminates a number of areas that might be pivotal in restoring energetic balance.

Any excesses of an external pathogen (heat or cold, damp, wind) are dealt with first or in lieu of a shiatsu session. Following that, the treatment would begin by tonifying the meridian of greatest deficiency. Techniques such as using light and rapid pressure with thumbs and hands are used to tonify. Elbows, knees or feet would be most appropriate for sedating or dispersing.

The ability to use specific points for tonification and sedation is very important. This usually includes use of the five elemental points on each meridian (along every meridian are points that directly correspond with the five elements). These are used to harmonize the quality of a particular element.

Treatments generally end with the meridian(s) having the greatest excess using sedating techniques, such as slow, deep pressure with the knees, elbows or feet. Points that sedate or disperse QI and elemental sedation points are important for this purpose.

Pressure varies according to the practitioner and adjunctive therapies, such as MOXIBUSTION, CUPPING, dietary guidance of home remedies or MAGNET THERAPY are often incorporated into five element shiatsu.

Five element shiatsu was defined as a specific category of Oriental bodywork by Cindy Banker, B.A., M.A., in the mid-1980s for the American Shiatsu Association. This original description was published in the A.S.A. pamphlet and

Massage Magazine. As the A.S.A. continued to network with other teachers, it became clear that other shiatsu teachers had come to similar theoretical conclusions. The most notable of these is Robbee Fian, L.Ac., Ms. Fian developed a form of five element shiatsu in the late 1970s and began teaching it in the early 1980s. Eventually, Fian and a number of her students joined the A.S.A. Both she and Banker continued to refine the definition of this system into the current form used by the American Oriental Bodywork Therapy Association.

Five Element Theory an ancient CHINESE MEDICINE theory that recognizes the relationship of the human being with nature. As in nature, people live according to the laws of the universe and flow with the changes that occur. The Five Element Theory maintains that people go through inner seasonal cycles and the elements are recreated within us.

The Chinese medical system is comprised of examination, diagnosis and treatment based on natural rhythms and processes. Life energy, or CHI, is vital to the concept of health. The five elements are descriptions, along with the concepts of YIN and YANG, of cyclical transformations. The ancients used these principles to diagnose illness. Health is considered to be the harmonious interaction of the elements.

The five elements are wood, fire, earth, metal and water. Each element is related to an anatomical organ as well as color, sound, smell, emotion, time of day, season, number, flavor, planet, moon phase, climate, food and MERIDIAN.

Wood creates fire (wood is the fuel for fire); fire creates earth (the ashes decompose to produce earth); earth creates metal (from compression in the center of the earth); metal creates water (the minerals of the metals compose water); water creates wood (irrigation creates trees); and the cycle continues ad infinitum.

All of the elements exist because of each other. This is also true of the related physiological functions within the body.

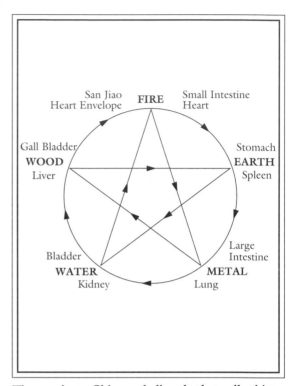

The ancient Chinese believed that all things in nature are composed of five elements: wood, fire, earth, metal, water. Each element interacts with the others to form a cycle of creation or destruction. The outer circle indicates the creative cycle, while the inner lines show the destructive cycle.

The wood element is closely associated with the idea of a tree. In health, a person's energy is strong and rooted. When this element is out of balance, the result is a person who exhibits symptoms of gnarled limbs (arthritis), nightmares, weakened limbs and spinal problems.

Chinese medicine uses examination as an important aspect of a person's evaluation. A subtle hue, or color, may appear on a person's face that will indicate which element, and therefore which organs, etc., are out of balance. The color of wood is green, especially in the spring, which is this element's season. The liver and gall bladder are the organs of wood.

	Wood	*Fire*	*Earth*	*Metal*	*Water*
Yin:	Liver	Heart	Spleen	Lung	Kidney
Time:	1–3 A.M.	11–1 P.M.	9–11 A.M.	3–5 A.M.	5–7 P.M.
	Heart C. (7–9 P.M.)				
Yang:	Gall bladder	Small Intestine	Stomach	Large Intestine	Bladder
Time:	11–1 A.M.	1–3 P.M.	7–9 A.M.	5–7 A.M.	3–5 P.M.
	T. Heater (9–11 P.M.)				
Organ:	Eyes	Tongue	Mouth	Nose	Ears
Color:	Green	Red	Yellow	White	Black
Taste:	Sour	Bitter	Sweet	Spicy	Salty
Climate:	Wind	Heat	Humidity	Dryness	Cold
Season:	Spring	Summer	Mid-Summer	Autumn	Winter
Emotion:	Anger	Joy	Worry	Grief	Fear
Expression:	Shout	Laugh	Sing	Weep	Groan

Fire has power, heat and light. In a balanced state, a person will exhibit warmth, which they can share with others. Those people lacking fire will be cold physically and emotionally. They may experience poor circulation, tend toward developing varicose veins, hot flushes, heartburn and digestive problems. The color of fire is red, and the organs are the heart and the small intestines.

Earth is special among the elements because it is their source.[1] Fertility and fullness are associated with this element. An imbalance will manifest itself in the cycles of life, losing their rhythm, such as menstruation, sleeping, breathing, coordination, body harmony, etc. Eating disorders such as anorexia, obesity, vomiting, hyperacidity are all related to the imbalance of this element. Sterility, or the inability to plant one's seed, is associated with the earth. The color that will manifest is yellow, and the organs are the stomach and spleen.

Metal is the most difficult element to experience in nature. It produces minerals and gems and provides substance, strength and structure in one's life. The life-sustaining aspects of this element are the networks that enable us to absorb food and air, to assimilate what we need, make use of the fuel and eliminate what is unnecessary. People with imbalances may experience rheumatic pains, a stiff back, lack of emotional strength, trembling and throat spasms. The color of this element is white, and its related organs are the lungs and large intestine.

The human body is composed of more than 70 percent water, so all the fluid systems of the body (the blood and lymph circulation, endocrine fluidity, saliva, urine, tears, sexual secretions and lactation) are all influenced by this element. An imbalance would result in those conditions that manifest in dryness, such as joint brittleness, thirst, excess or deficient perspiration, feelings of fear and inundation and being overwhelmed by life. Its color is blue, and the organs associated with the element of water are the kidneys and bladder.

Notes
[1] Connelly, Dianne M., Ph.D., M.Ac., *Traditional Acupuncture: The Law of the Five Elements,* The Center for Traditional Acupuncture, Inc., Columbia, Md., 1979, p. 51.
[2] Ibid., p. 63 (chart).

Further Reading
Connelly, Dianne, Ph.D., M.Ac., *Traditional Acupuncture: The Law of the Five Elements,* The Centre for Traditional Acupuncture, Inc., Columbia, Md., 1979. The five elements are clearly explained in this easy-to-read text. Examination and treatment procedures, along with case histories, are included.
Matsumoto, Kiiko, and Birch, Stephen, *Five Elements and Ten Stems,* Paradigm Books, Brookline, Mass., 1983. This book provides an in-depth study of the Five Element Theory and acupuncture.

Worsely, J.R., *Law of Five Elements Chart*. This laminated chart, 20 by 30 inches, clearly illustrates the relationship between each element and its organ function and Chinese pulses.

flotation, also referred to as sensory deprivation, is a concept that has gone through a complete metamorphosis. What was once regarded as a brain-washing technique[1] has grown in popularity and favor as an effortless way to experience profound relaxation.

Flotation (wet) tanks and isolation (dry) chambers are now used for therapeutic purposes as well as recreation. The therapeutic and preferred term for sensory deprivation is called REST, **Restricted Environmental Stimulation Therapy.** Flotation provides a safe environment for physical and emotional release.

The origins of the tank can be traced to Dr. John C. Lilly who believed, contrary to earlier theories, that by eliminating external stimulation, the human brain would create its own. He tested his principle by immersing himself in a dark, soundproof water tank and described his experience as profoundly relaxing and an "elaborate inner experience."[2]

After showering, the floater enters a sound and lightproof flotation tank filled with 10 inches of epsom salt-saturated water (1,000 lbs.). The water temperature remains a constant 94°F, which is the same as skin temperature. Free from the pull of gravity or any external stimuli, the participant floats effortlessly on the surface of the water. Breathing becomes deeper and areas of physical, emotional and mental tensions release.

The tanks may vary in size and design but are generally 5 to 7 feet high and 4 feet wide. Many tanks are equipped with underwater stereosystems, which can play music or educational tapes. In this extremely relaxed, highly receptive state, learning is much easier.[3] Controls for sound and light are handled by the participant within the tank. Very often, gentle music will be piped into the tank to signal the end of the session.

Since most sensory stimulation is removed, flotation often produces a meditative state, which relieves mental stress. Studies have shown that theta brain waves, those responsible for deep relaxation, are increased during a one-hour float session. Blood pressure is lowered, cellular waste removal is increased, stress is reduced and healing is accelerated.[4]

Flotation tanks are free from pathogenic organisms. The salt maintains a bacteria-free environment, and the tank water is often filtered and injected with ozone, an effective water purifier, between uses.

Dry tanks provide a similar feeling with the water. A participant lies on a body-conforming mattress, like a water bed, in an enclosed chamber. These rooms can sometimes be rather large, providing enough room to move around. They are often preferred to flotation tanks for treatment in changing unhealthy behavioral habits, such as addictions, because the participant can stay for longer periods of time, as long as 24 to 48 hours.

Notes
[1] Reader's Digest, *Guide to Natural Medicine: How to Stay Healthy the Natural Way,* Reader's Digest Association, Inc., Pleasantville, N.Y., 1993, p. 110. During the Korean conflict, American prisoners of war were placed in isolation tanks as a form of torture. It was believed that human consciousness could not function without external stimuli.
[2] Ibid., p. 110.
[3] Blue Light Flotation pamphlet, N.Y., no date, p. 2.
[4] Budzynski, Thomas, "Brain Lateralization and Rescripting," *Somatics,* Spring/Summer, 1981, p. 4. This study indicated that most of the "absorption of information" occurred within the initial stages of sleep characterized by a brain wave pattern of theta waves (4–7 Hz) with occasional bursts of alpha waves (8–12 Hz).

focusing a quiet, meditative, six-step process that uses bodily **felt sense** to let personal life issues surface and become clearer and amenable to change. Developed by Eugene Gendlin, focusing teaches a radical shift in attitude from talking at oneself to listening attentively to oneself.

Focusing allows an individual to go beyond

self-controlling habits and access deeper wisdom found in the body. The focusing process of finding exact words or images that fit emerging feelings and sensations can lead to important insights and significant stress reduction.

Focusing can be used whenever an individual is seeking healing, understanding or the wisdom of the body. It can be used in conjunction with counseling and psychotherapy, working with illnesses, in problem solving and spiritual awareness. Focusing is also useful for increasing creativity.

Further Reading
Gendlin, Eugene, *Focusing,* Bantam Books, N.Y., 1982. The developer of the technique explains the theory of focusing.

friction   one of the five standard SWEDISH MASSAGE strokes, among EFFLEURAGE, PETRISSAGE, TAPOTEMENT, and VIBRATION. It is the most penetrating of all the strokes and is used often in MEDICAL MASSAGE situations.

Friction can be performed with the thumbs or fingertips in two ways: transversely across the muscle fibers and CONNECTIVE TISSUE, or circularly into joints or around bony prominences. An open hand can also be used for broader surfaces, such as across the back. Friction is a deep stroke, which is followed by effleurage to promote reabsorption of waste products released by the application of friction.

Friction increases the glandular activity of the skin and speeds up lymph and blood flow to the area under treatment. Local temperature increases, which promotes fluid absorption.

Dry skin becomes moist and oily because perspiration and sebaceous (oil) secretion is increased. The skin's temperature is raised by increased heat production.

Friction is a valuable stroke for breaking up inflammatory products, so it is often used in the latter treatment of joint injuries, chronic rheumatism and fibrositis (inflammation of white connective tissue anywhere in the body).

Following the course of the large intestine, friction strengthens its walls and promotes peristalsis, which helps relieve constipation.

Friction around articulations provides greater flexibility and elasticity to the joints. It facilitates the breakdown of adhesions (fibers which stick together creating nodules) and granulation rendering the muscle tissues and joints more supple.

Like effleurage, friction has an effect on circulation. It promotes absorption of inflammatory products by spreading them over a wide area and increasing drainage into the lymph vessels. Light friction over a deep organ diminishes its blood supply by increasing the activity of the overlying vessels. This causes blood to go around rather than through the organ. Light friction will act on superficial veins by accelerating the flow of blood and lymph to the parts being treated and the subcutaneous capillaries.

Neurologically, friction can excite languid nerves or reduce swelling after nerve inflammation. This is particularly important when treating sciatica or any nerve irritation. The reflex action upon the vasomotor centers causes small vessels of the skin to dilate and increase the activity of the peripheral circulation.

Scar tissue can be loosened with friction.[1] Friction can also prevent fibrosis and edema (swelling) following an injury.

Note
[1] Massage over a keloid scar, those thick, ropy, raised scars, is contraindicated. Connective tissue scarring is not relieved with massage.

G

g-jo acupressure a simplified form of ACU-PRESSURE, which translates to "first aid" in its native Chinese. It was first used in the battle-fields of ancient China to treat the wounded soldiers. There are 116 small *g-jo* acupressure points that bring immediate relief from many common ailments. These points, which may also be needled in ACUPUNCTURE treatments, corre-spond to particular bodily areas or functions.

When pain arises, the appropriate point is located then massaged for a short period of time. The massage is a deep, goading stimulation lasting for 10 to 15 seconds. The point should be tender but the discomfort level should be toler-able. It is important to work bilaterally, on both sides of the body, with the same points for maximum results. One side may be more sensi-tive than the other, indicating the side to focus on. The points should be massaged as soon as the symptoms manifest themselves, thus stimu-lating the body's own healing powers.

There are some contraindications to the use of *g-jo* points: People taking daily medication for serious ailments, such as diabetes; pregnant women; and those individuals wearing pace-makers or any artificial energy-regulating devices should avoid *g-jo* acupressure.

Further Reading
Blate, Michael, *Natural Healer's Acupressure Handbook: Basic G-Jo, Vol. 1,* Owl Books, Henry Holt and Co., N.Y., 1976. This book provides readers with first-aid fingertip techniques and provides self-help points for treating common ailments.
———, *The Natural Healer's Acupressure Handbook: Vol. II, Advanced G-Jo,* Falkynor Books, Davie, Fla., 1978. Ad-vanced **g-jo** techniques for finding and healing internal organs with acupressure.

gall bladder meridian a **yang** meridian, which runs bilaterally from the outside corners of the eyes down the sides of the body to the fourth toes. It distributes nutrients throughout the body and balances the internal energy with the aid of hormones and internal secretions such as bile, saliva, gastric acid, insulin and intestinal hormones. There are 44 ACUPUNCTURE points along the gall bladder meridian. According to the FIVE ELEMENT THEORY, wood is the element of this channel.

Geriatric Massage a massage system that em-phasizes treating specific physiological and psy-chological conditions associated with the aging process with the expectation of improving the condition. Geriatrics is a medical term that refers to the health disabilities and impairments of old age.

This system recognizes, however, that the standard age of 65, which is considered to be the entry point into old age, is very much an arbitrary designation. There are no prototypes of old age and there is a large variable in the conditions of the elderly. Aging is an individual process, which can see robust octogenarians as well as frail, bedridden sexagenarians.

The 1993 United States census reports that the elderly make up 16 percent of the popula-tion, which translates to 32 million people who are 65 years and older. Out of this group, only 5 percent, or 1.6 million, live in nursing homes.[1] The frailest portion of this population is gener-ally over 85 years old, and there is a shortage of doctors trained to meet their special needs.[2]

Geriatric Massage is a new specialty pioneered by Dietrich W. Miesler, M.A., at the Day-Break Geriatric Massage Project in Guerneville, Califor-nia. Practitioners learn to recognize the changes that occur as a natural part of the aging process and those that result from injuries and illnesses. The massage is performed with each individual's condition in mind to promote improved health.

It is advisable for the practitioner to consult the client's physician so that the doctor may be informed of the work, which will affect his patient's health and may interfere with the effectiveness of medication. It affords an opportunity for both health care providers to share information about the client's condition.

As a normal part of the aging process, the metabolism slows down; constipation may result; there are psychological, muscular and connective tissue problems, which may be caused by stress, injury, wear and tear or poor nutrition; there is a loss in muscle tone;[3] illnesses associated with longer life, such as cancer, are more prevalent; and emotional traumas from personal losses may have a devastating effect upon a person's physical and emotional outlook.

The skin loses its moisture and becomes dry. Bedridden clients may develop bedsores or pressure sores, which must be carefully and lightly moisturized; joints may become stiff, arthritic and painful; bone mass is reduced, often leading to osteoporosis and brittle bones; high blood pressure, heart disease, arteriosclerosis (hardening of the arteries) and atherosclerosis (narrowing of the arteries) are some of the possible circulatory complications and respiratory diseases, such as smoking-related problems, asthma or bronchitis, are more severe in older people.

Geriatric Massage can effectively treat many of these frailties associated with aging. The system employs a variety of massage techniques, particularly SWEDISH MASSAGE and TRAGER. The massage can be active or passive in nature, depending on the needs and physical condition of the geriatric client.

The active techniques use the five strokes of Swedish massage[4] and combinations of them called **hybrid strokes** to stimulate circulation, flex joints and reduce pain. The passive techniques are especially useful for bedridden or frail clients. They include the gentle rocking motion of Trager massage to loosen fasciae (network of connective tissue that encloses muscles, muscle groups and internal organs) and relax muscles.

Geriatric Massage differs from regular massage because modifications must be made to suit the needs of the older population. It is not unlike SPORTS MASSAGE, however, where a physical assessment of the client is imperative to the ensuing care and where improvement of the condition is sought. Yet the beneficial effects of massage are equally applicable to Geriatric Massage, even when special considerations are required.

Circulation is improved, blood pressure is lowered, cells are detoxified more efficiently, edema (swelling) of the extremities is reduced as lymphatic drainage is promoted, pain decreases, muscles gain strength, joints become more flexible, depressions are lifted and clients regain a sense of well-being. Sedentary or bedridden clients respond to a light touch, which treats the physical symptoms as well as depression.

Very often, improvisation is required of the practitioner. The working environment may not always be the norm, such as working in a hospital or nursing facility, and clients may need assistance getting undressed, getting on and off the table and putting their clothes back on. Often, clients have to be treated while in bed, wheelchair or geri chair. This is all part of the individual attention paid to Geriatric Massage.

It is important to recognize that incorrect work can be harmful and sometimes deleterious, so a qualified assessment must be made before the work commences. Clients are rated as to their overall condition: robust, age appropriate or frail. A detailed medical history is taken and the attending physician(s) may be contacted.

The overall goals of the client and the treatment are discussed to ensure that reasonable expectations are sought. A robust client usually can tolerate a normal massage. The age appropriate candidate should be treated for no longer than 30 minutes, and the frail client should receive up to 15 minutes for the first treatment. Reactions to the massage are carefully monitored so adjustments to the treatments, or longer treatments can be made.

Many conditions respond well to Geriatric Massage: arthritis,[5] rheumatism, joint problems including hip replacements, poor circulation, spinal anomalies such as kyphosis (Marie Strumpel's disease) or scoliosis[6] and senility and Alzheimer's disease.

There are certain contraindications of massage that require either total avoidance of treatment or a physician's clearance: severe heart and respiratory conditions, acute phlebitis (inflammation of a vein) or thrombophlebitis (phlebitis caused by a blood clot), severe pain, acute arthritis, extreme swelling and edema, bone disease, cirrhosis of the liver, uncontrolled diabetes, contagious skin diseases, aortal aneurysms (dilation due to pressure of the blood on weakened tissues forming a sac of clotted blood), lumps, cysts, fevers, directly on hernias, low platelet counts and under heavy medication. However, contraindications are more directed at specific techniques than at hands-on work in general.

A study conducted by the Touch Research Institute found that elderly volunteers who massage needy babies, those suffering from prematurity, drug exposure or abuse, received as much benefit from the massage as the babies. The babies slept better, had calmer dispositions and lower stress levels. The volunteers expressed reduced anxiety levels, increased self-esteem, greater social contacts and visited their doctors less frequently.[7] Receiving as well as giving has its rewards.

Notes

1 Miesler, Dietrich, M.A., C.M.T., "Geriatric Massage—the Day-Break Way," *Massage and Bodywork Quarterly,* Evergreen, Colo., Fall 1993, p. 63.
2 Fein, Esther B., "Gaps in Geriatric Medicine Alarm Health Professionals," *New York Times,* May 16, 1994.
3 "To Find a Way to Age in Health," *Insight,* April 10, 1989, pp. 12–13. Starting an exercise program even in advanced years will increase muscle mass and strength. "Study Shows That Weight Training Can Benefit Very Old," *New York Times,* June 23, 1994, p. 16. Frail people in their 80s and 90s have actually thrown away their walkers after a few weeks of leg strengthening weight exercises.
4 The five strokes of Swedish massage are effleurage, petrissage, friction, vibration and tapotement.
5 Miesler, Dietrich, W. M.A., "Geriatric Massage: The Problem with Contraindications?" *Day-Break Yearbook,* Guerneville, Calif., 1994, p. 21, cited from *The Merck*

Manual of Geriatrics, Merck & Co., Inc., Rahway, N.J., 1990, pp. 1123–1124. Osteoarthritis is the degeneration of the joint cartilage. In advance cases, painful bone spurs develop in the joints. Women develop this condition more than men. Osteoarthritis afflicts 4 percent of people under 59 and up to 40 percent of people over 60. One million people over 55 are totally incapacitated by this disease.
6 Kyphosis is an excessive curve of the thoracic vertebrae, which produces a hunchback posture. Scoliosis is an abnormal lateral curve of the spine.
7 O'Sullivan, William, "The Gift of Touch," *Common Boundary,* May/June 1994, p. 12. The Touch Research Institute is located at the University of Miami, School of Medicine, Department of Pediatrics (D–820), P.O. Box 016820, Miami, Fla. 33101.

Further Reading

Day-Break Yearbook, 1994, Day-Break Productions, Guerneville, Calif., 1994. This book is compiled by the pioneers of Geriatric Massage, the Day-Break Geriatric Project, from numerous articles and studies about the care of the elderly. It includes guides to treatments, contraindications of massage, case histories and their instruction schedule.
The Merck Handbook of Geriatrics, Merck & Co., Inc., Rahway, N.J., 1990. This text details illnesses and treatments for geriatric patients.

Gestalt therapy a form of psychotherapy that promotes healing the neurotic split of mind and body and restores wholeness. It is existential in philosophy (emphasizing our ability to take responsibility and make choices) and experiential in both focus and method. By attending to process, rather than analyzing content, this work supports the growth of the self.

Gestalt, a German word, which loosely translates to mean "pattern," was developed by Dr. Frederick (Fritz) S. Perls, M.D., Ph.D. (1894–1970) and his wife Laura Perls, during the 1950s. The Perlses founded the New York Institute for Gestalt Therapy in New York in 1952. Fritz Perls also taught at the Esalen Institute in Big Sur, California, a holistic center, which continues to attract some of the most avant garde and innovative thinkers of the day.

This work was influenced by Gestalt psychology, Zen meditation practices, and the many body-oriented therapies that were being developed during the 1950s and 1960s, including

SENSORY AWARENESS work, psychodrama, etc. It is a departure from Reichian work in that bodily defenses and **armor** are not seen as resistances to be broken through, but as disowned energies of the client that need to be integrated.

Perls adapted the Eastern concept of "the here and now" to Western psychotherapy. He learned from Gestalt psychology that people need to go back to what they leave unfinished, and he maintained that people carry their pasts with them as **unfinished business,** or incomplete gestalten. Addressing what is unfinished allows us to truly live in the present. From an existential point of view, the present is all that exists—the past and future being a thought or fantasy that we are having now.

Gestalt is about "now and how." Being fully present with the experience of the moment allows us to create a more satisfying experience. Gestalt therapy theory addresses the "how," providing a model of contact and its interruptions. In a Gestalt therapy session, a client is directed to be aware of his emotions, sensations and quality of experiencing, with the therapy itself looked at as an experimental situation. Participants are not considered patients but individuals actively consenting to work and play in awareness. By paying attention to "how" a client sits, speaks, presents himself, etc., and not "what" he is talking about, Gestalt work remains nonjudgmental and also empowering.

A fundamental aspect of Gestalt therapy is body-oriented work. Gestalt therapy addresses the entire organism, and not just some of its parts (another meaning of the word Gestalt), and seeks to restore wholeness and heal splits. The split of mind and body is characteristic of our cultural neurosis. Working with breathing is one important approach. Breathing is fundamental to life and respiration patterns reflect habits of relating to the world. Awareness of breath supports excitement, instead of anxiety, and brings the participant into the present—the now—and creates the potential for change.

One of the areas in which Gestalt work has

developed since the 1950s is in its use of techniques from different somatic modalities. It is possible now to find Gestalt therapists who are also trained in bodywork modalities and who apply them with awareness and with attention paid to contact. The Gestalt Institute of Cleveland offers a body process concentration in its training program, and the Center for Gestalt Somatics™ in New York City provides training for bodyworkers in Gestalt theory and for psychotherapists in Gestalt somatic work.

Gestalt therapy has influenced many modern body/mind modalities such as HAKOMI, RUBENFELD SYNERGY and others.

Further Reading
Kepner, James, *Body Process: A Gestalt Approach to Working with the Body in Psychotherapy,* Gestalt Institute of Cleveland Press, Gardner Press, N.Y., 1987. A description of the body-based application of Gestalt therapy by the head of the body process concentration of the Gestalt Institute of Cleveland's Training Program.
Perls, Frederick, M.D., Ph.D., *The Gestalt Approach,* Science & Behavior, Palo Alto, Calif., 1973. This book explains the theory and application of Perls's psychological system.
———, *Eyewitness to Therapy,* Science & Behavior, Palo Alto, Calif., 1973. This book describes case histories using the Gestalt therapy approach to integrating the person.
———, *Gestalt Therapy Verbatim,* Bantam Books, N.Y., 1969. Most of the material in this book was edited from audio tapes recorded at dreamwork seminars by Dr. Perls at Esalen Institute, Big Sur, California, from 1966 to 1968.
Smith, Edward W.L., *The Body in Psychotherapy,* McFarland & Co., Inc., Jefferson, N.C., 1985. A survey of some major schools of body-based therapies from the perspective of a Gestalt therapist.

governing vessel meridian a **yang** meridian whose function is to regulate all the yang meridians and yang energy. It is called the "sea of yang." The governing vessel meridian is a unilateral meridian that begins between the anus and coccyx, goes up the spine, over the head and ends inside the mouth, under the upper lip.

There are 28 ACUPUNCTURE points in this meridian. Those points on the back are located between the vertebrae.

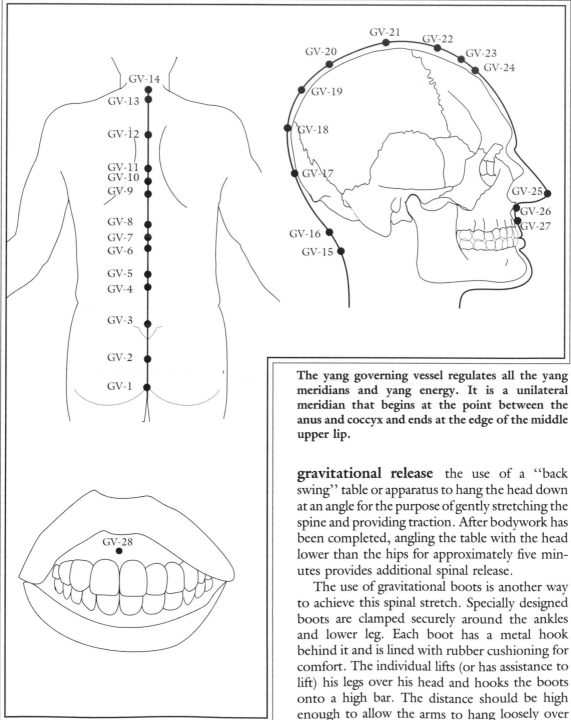

The yang governing vessel regulates all the yang meridians and yang energy. It is a unilateral meridian that begins at the point between the anus and coccyx and ends at the edge of the middle upper lip.

gravitational release the use of a "back swing" table or apparatus to hang the head down at an angle for the purpose of gently stretching the spine and providing traction. After bodywork has been completed, angling the table with the head lower than the hips for approximately five minutes provides additional spinal release.

The use of gravitational boots is another way to achieve this spinal stretch. Specially designed boots are clamped securely around the ankles and lower leg. Each boot has a metal hook behind it and is lined with rubber cushioning for comfort. The individual lifts (or has assistance to lift) his legs over his head and hooks the boots onto a high bar. The distance should be high enough to allow the arms to hang loosely over his head without the fingers touching the floor.

Another type of apparatus is a short bench that positions the individual's thighs between padded rollers and a moveable cushion. This cushion, placed at his hips, inverts, turning him over, hips in the air, while the rollers secure his position.

Gravitational release stretches the spine, releases pressure between the intervertebral discs, lifts internal organs against gravity's pull, increases blood flow to the head and face, which can help purify facial skin and is relaxing.

Some people experience lightheadedness the first few attempts at gravitational release but quickly become inured to the sensation. For safety, it is advisable to perform these maneuvers in the presence of another person.

guided imagery a relaxation system that uses imagination, thoughts, visualizations and other techniques to promote physical, mental and emotional health. It is also called visualization (interactive), creative or mental imagery.

Positive thoughts can have positive effects on a person's life, health and relationships, while negative thoughts can have equally powerful but adverse effects. The theory behind guided imagery is that whatever is imagined in the mind's eye has physiological consequences, which impacts on a person's health.

Guided imagery has been used as a therapeutic tool to help people fight diseases, addiction and to stimulate innate healing capabilities. It may provide conscious control over the physical system. Many seriously ill patients have used visualizations to imagine the destruction of their diseases.

In addition to imagining the annihilation of the disease, many patients are encouraged to draw the disease and their feelings about it. As the visualizations get stronger and the patients get better, or more in touch with their feelings, the change is exhibited in their pictures.

Athletes have also used imagery in competition by visualizing their goal and imagining themselves performing them perfectly. Olympic Gold Medalist diver Greg Louganis and Silver Medalist skater Elizabeth Manley have reported using this system to perfect their skills.

The imagery, which can be performed in the privacy of one's home with a leader or in a group setting, begins with relaxation, which is followed by creating a mental picture. In one technique, known as **palming,** the eyes are closed and covered with the palms. The individual concentrates on the color black and tries to expand it outward, eliminating any interference. In one case, to reduce stress, the color often associated with stress is conjured up and then replaced by a color associated with relaxation.

Guided imagery can also be an interactive process, which may be used in conjunction with briefer, solution-focused therapy. This process may include the use of **ideal modeling imagery, dialoguing, evocative imagery, inner advisor** or **regression.** By introducing these powerful inner resources, the imagery guide can empower the client at an early stage of the therapeutic relationship, promoting greater self-reliance by the client. The inner advisor technique also helps to minimize and/or clarify transference issues early and sets the stage for completion of therapy as clients learn to depend more upon their own inner guidance.

Interactive Guided Imagery℠ was developed by the Academy For Guided Imagery, Mill Valley, California. Founded in 1989, this organization has taught nearly 500 health professionals to incorporate Interactive Guided Imagery with other forms of therapies. This system allows therapy to proceed very quickly without having to sacrifice the emotional depth that is so necessary to resolution and healing. It helps clients to quickly identify, strengthen and utilize their own inherent healing resources, encouraging self-management and autonomy.

Through guided imagery, deep internal resources can be motivated to provide the insight allowing change.

Further Reading
Bresler, David, Ph.D., *Free Yourself from Pain,* Simon & Schuster, N.Y., 1979. This book describes how pain can

be overcome. Methods explore why we hurt, what the pain means and what can be done to alleviate it.

Rossman, Martin L., M.D., *Healing Yourself: A Step by Step Program for Better Health through Imagery,* Pocket Books, N.Y., 1987. Dr. Rossman, a director of the Academy for Guided Imagery, along with Dr. David Bresler, shows how to invoke the body's capacity to resist and fight disease through the use of imagery.

Wells, Valerie, *The Joy of Visualization,* Chronicle Books, San Francisco, Calif., 1990. This easy-to-follow book offers various visualization exercises for desired results.

H

Haelan Work™ which stems from the Old English *haelan,* meaning "to be or to become whole," is a combination of THERAPEUTIC TOUCH, psychotherapy and counseling, which facilitates the healing process of the whole person, including those nearing death. This system was developed by Janet F. Quinn, Ph.D., R.N., who is an associate professor of nursing at the University of Colorado. She is a practitioner, researcher and teacher of therapeutic touch and is certified in Stanislav Grof's HOLOTROPIC BREATHWORK. She created Haelan Work as a result of working with people with cancer, AIDS and other physical and/or psychosomatic illnesses.

Quinn believes that the integration of body/mind/spirit may be difficult for some people to achieve if they are primarily focused on a physical illness or emotional/psychological issues. Often, the physical pain and discomfort may be so great, that, although patients may want to explore emotional and spiritual matters, they are prevented from doing so.

Haelan Work evolved out of more than 20 years of clinical and theoretical work and is based on three fundamental assumptions: That we are not responsible for our illnesses, but we are called to be responsive to them; that all curing and healing emerges from within our own unique body/mind/spirit, at times assisted by medicines, surgery and/or other therapies; and the acknowledgment that the integrity of body/mind/spirit is always about mystery unfolding, that the healing is fundamentally mysterious, beyond our control yet open to our conscious participation and intention.

Therapeutic touch, which is the hands-on process of Haelan Work, is derived from the ancient practice of LAYING ON HANDS but is devoid of any religious connotation. Since therapeutic touch works with the HUMAN ENERGY BIO-FIELD, it may be practiced with or without physical contact. This makes it particularly helpful in working with patients for whom physical touch may not be appropriate or helpful.

Therapeutic touch has been shown to reduce pain, induce deep relaxation and accelerate wound healing. In addition, there are powerful psychological, emotional and spiritual benefits derived from this work.

Holotropic Breathwork, developed by Stanislav and Christina Grof after 30 years of research, is a powerful experiential process that can mobilize the spontaneous healing potential of the human psyche using accelerated breathing, evocative music and carefully applied bodywork.

Centering prayers/meditations are methods that support the whole person through the psychospiritual dimension. This may also be used as a daily self-care practice.

Haelan Work can assist people with physical illness to participate in their healing from a holistic and integrated perspective. In addition, those people interested in growth-oriented psychotherapy or who are working with other therapists find this work extremely useful.

Dr. Janet F. Quinn earned a Ph.D. in nursing at New York University, New York City. She is an associate professor and senior scholar/clinician at the Center for Human Caring, a Fellow of the American Academy of Nursing, and a member of the teaching staffs at Esalen and Omega Institutes. She is trained in HAKOMI body-centered psychotherapy, therapeutic touch and Holotropic Breathwork.

Hakomi Integrative Somatics® a personal growth and transformation system, which revises ideas that an individual has about himself and his world through a variety of processes. It is a synthesis of Western psychotherapy and bodywork methods. Eastern philosophies and contemporary science, which studies body/mind patterns of **core beliefs.** Core beliefs are self-limiting notions, which were formed early in life and stored in the subconscious. Hakomi purports that an individual had certain feelings, thoughts and sensations as a child, which were powerful enough to create a set of ideas about himself. The work traces these core beliefs back to childhood events where the responses were first created.

Hakomi therapy was developed during the late 1970s by Ron Kurtz. He was greatly influenced by the innovative body/mind integrative works of FELDENKRAIS, GESTALT, BIOENERGETICS, ROLFING, REICH, ERICKSONIAN HYPNOSIS, NEUROLINGUISTIC PROGRAMMING and the traditional Eastern philosophies of Buddhism and Taoism. The Hakomi Institute was founded in 1980.

Hakomi is an ancient Hopi (Native American) word, which literally translates to "how do you stand in relation to these many realms?" In common vernacular, it means "who are you?"

Hakomi Integrative Somatics, a branch of the Hakomi Institute, created by Pat Ogden, is made up of bodywork and therapy that recognizes the holism of body/mind/spirit. The body is considered to be a source of enormous information, which can be used to create change. The bodywork incorporates MASSAGE, DEEP TISSUE work, structural work, movement and body awareness. Through this hands-on system, awareness of sensation—physical and emotional—is heightened, and it is possible that deeply hidden memories and beliefs may emerge. The Hakomi Integrative Somatics therapist is conscious to work through the body as a resource of personal information and not on it, to create change.

Hakomi therapy is done during an altered state of consciousness called **mindfulness.** This is a place of deep knowing and acute awareness. Mindfulness encourages open communication between the conscious and unconscious minds. It is possible for an individual to observe his experiences without interference or judgment. The therapy is an exploration of the limiting choices a person has made and provides him with the ability to make new, self-affirming ones.

There are five principles in the Hakomi method: mindfulness, unity, nonviolence, organicity and mind/body holism. The therapist seeks to build a relationship that maximizes safety and the cooperation of the unconscious. Then the client is assisted in focusing on and studying how he organizes his core experiences. Since most behavior is habit and automatically organized by this core material, the client is guided to come into contact with those reactions.

At the heart of the method is the deliberate study of the organization of the experience in the moment. In Hakomi Integrative Somatics, the therapist evokes experiences, through the bodywork and psychotherapeutic procedures, that lead to the core material and then assists in processing the experience, all while the client is in a state of mindfulness. The client might be asked to recapture an experience and feel it in his body. He may discover certain physical patterns and find meaning in that physical response.

Advice and problem solving are not offered by the therapist. Instead, the therapist "befriends" the unconscious and creates an environment where the unfolding can take place. There is also little value in having the client talk about the past, since the emphasis is in the moment.

Hakomi Integrative Somatics does not only seek to rediscover negative experiences. It is equally important for an individual to reestablish contact with his strengths, talents and resources.

Whether this system is on an individual basis or group workshop, clients experience greater self-awareness, self-acceptance, personal freedom, empathy and compassion for others.

Further Reading

Johanson, Greg and Kurtz, Ron, *Grace Unfolding,* Crown Publishing Group, N.Y., 1994. This book applied the spirit and principles of Lao Tsu's *I Ching* to the practice of contemporary psychotherapy. It is a book that explains the roles people play in the therapeutic process. It discusses the relationship between the therapist and the client, the use of the body in therapy and the meaning of nonviolence and nondoing.

Kurtz, Ron, *Body-Centered Psychotherapy: The Hakomi Method,* Life Rhythm, Mendocino, Calif., 1990. The history and theories of Hakomi are explained in this book.

Kurtz, Ron, and Prestera, Hector, *The Body Reveals,* Harper & Row, N.Y., 1976. This illustrated book describes physical holding patterns and explains their emotional significance.

hama massage or hamma, a Japanese massage technique, based on SHIATSU, that is designed specifically for the visually impaired and blind. In Japan, the blind put their highly developed sense of touch to good use and become massage practitioners. Hama massage was created to take advantage of their acute tactile perceptions and palpation skills.

hand reflexology the treatment of the reflex points on the hands to effect changes in their corresponding body parts. The hands contain the same reflexes as the feet but their locations are different. (See [FOOT] REFLEXOLOGY.) The manipulation of these reflex points may bring relief from a vast array of symptoms, increase vitality and promote general well-being.

Dr. William Fitzgerald is credited with rediscovering the ancient healing technique of reflexology. In 1913, he wrote, "Zone Therapy (as it was called) has been practiced and taught by some of the most noted doctors in America."[1] ZONE THERAPY practitioners believe that body parts can be affected by pressure anywhere along the related zone.

Hand reflexology can be self-administered at any time. Both the hands and feet contain reflex points that are associated with organs and glands. When the reflexes are massaged, a stimulating message is carried to that body region,

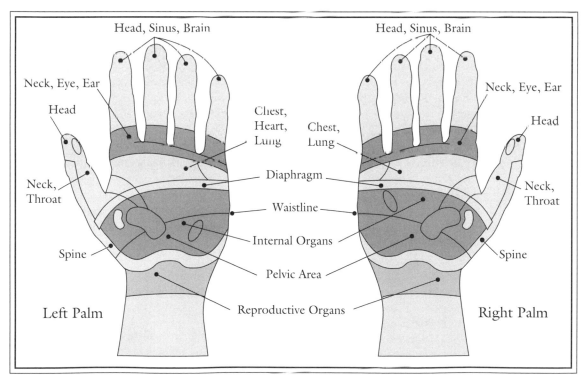

Organs of the body are reflected on specific points and areas of the hands, just as they are on the feet. Reflexologists agree that pressure to a particular point will affect its corresponding organ.

often correcting imbalances and/or maintaining optimum health. Reflexology, both hands and feet, breaks down energy blockages and restores its free flow throughout the body.

The body is divided into 10 zones, or 10 vertical lines, 5 on each side of the body, starting from the fingertips and ending at the toes. All reflex points found along a particular line in the hands correspond with organs or glands found within the same line. For example, the head corresponds to the thumb and all the glands in the head, such as pituitary, can be stimulated by massaging the reflex in the thumb.

The hands can be further divided in half, which would conform with the upper and lower halves of the body and the organs within those regions. Unlike ACUPUNCTURE's regular MERIDI-ANS, which are predominately bilateral (found on both sides of the body), hand and foot reflexes are found only on the extremity that relates to where an organ is located. For example, the liver, found on the right side of the body, is only found in the right hand and foot.

Pressing and massaging can be performed anywhere, at any time. There are no special tools required through reflex clamps, combs or hand massagers can be used for long-term pressure on a particular region.

The massage technique of hand reflexology uses the thumb or the fingers to press into the hand over a particular point. The hand is pressed deeply enough so the underlying bone or muscles can be felt. A "walking" movement of the thumb (pressing and rolling combines with pressing and pulling) seeks out sore areas. Each reflex is pressed for a few minutes.

Another technique uses the thumb on the palm of the hand and the fingers pressing into the reflexes on the back of the hand. This method stimulates a reverse electrical (energy) flow throughout the body. Massage should also be done on sore spots found on the back of the hand. Except for reflexes to the vital organs in the center of the hands, any sore spots can be returned to as often as necessary.

A general hand reflexology treatment begins with a massage of the thumb region, front and back, starting at the tip and working down the finger. Press with the index finger and thumb of the opposite hand. Reflexes along this finger stimulate the head, pituitary and pineal glands, throat, neck and sinuses. The same procedure continues with the rest of the fingers. The reflexes in the second finger stimulate the sinuses at the tip and the eyes at the base. The middle finger reflexes treat colds, nervous conditions and the eyes, at the finger's base. The fourth finger treats ear problems and nervous conditions, while the little finger also treats ear problems.

Once the fingers have been massaged on each side, the massage proceeds to the hand. The treatment continues with stimulation to the "ball" of the hand, or the joints where the fingers attach to the hand. Any sore spot on a reflex indicates a malfunctioning in the body regardless of its distance from the hand. Hand reflexology indicates that if a reflex hurts, "rub it out."[2]

Specific reflexes are now treated in the hand, starting with the lungs, stomach, solar plexus, thyroid, adrenals and kidneys, liver, heart, spleen, gallbladder, appendix, pancreas, lower back and lymph glands. A chart would be most helpful in locating the exact sites of these reflexes.

The webbing between the fingers also contains important reflexes, such as the throat, neck, spine, stomach, thyroid and internal organs, and should be included in the overall treatment.

Notes

[1] Carter, Mildred, *Hand Reflexology: Key to Perfect Health,* Parker Publishing Co., West Nyack, N.Y., 1975, p. 9.

[2] Ibid., p. 58.

Further Reading

Carter, Mildred, *Hand Reflexology: Key to Perfect Health,* Parker Publishing Co., West Nyack, N.Y., 1975. This innovative book is filled with illustrations, reflex charts and photographs depicting the proper technique of hand reflexology. Several chapters detail specific treatment techniques for dozens of ailments.

Kunz, Kevin and Barbara, *Hand and Foot Reflexology*, Reflexology Research Project, Albuquerque, N.Mex. A guide for working on hands and feet with a directory for treating specific symptoms.

Hanna Somatic Education™

an education system that teaches voluntary, conscious control of the neuromuscular system to individuals who suffer from muscular disorders of an involuntary nature. It provides hands-on somatic work (recognition of the integration of body and mind) and a series of somatic exercises, which increases a client's flexibility and range of motion, relaxes chronically contracted muscles, eases pain and restores control over voluntary neuromuscular junctions. "Soma" infers an awareness of internal feelings and movements as a sentient being. The bodywork and exercises supply new sensory information into the sensory-motor feedback loop, which became a closed loop due to constant stress and traumatic injury.

Thomas Hanna called this **sensory-motor-amnesia**. Prolonged injury causes loss of muscle control and we forget how to relax them. This new information, provided by sensory stimulation, "tells" the muscles to relax. Hanna believed that sensory-motor-amnesia is a pathology that is neither medical nor surgical. This is why it can't be diagnosed or treated within conventional medical practices. Sensory-motor-amnesia is a practice of learning and education, not one of treatment. Exercises are repeated at home to reinforce the conditioning.

Thomas Hanna (1929–1990) was born in Waco, Texas, and graduated in 1949 from Texas Christian University with degrees in music and philosophy. He received a master's degree in divinity and a Ph.D. in philosophy from the University of Chicago. While working at the University of Florida Medical School as a philosophy professor, he took some classes in neurophysiology, which laid the groundwork for his somatics theories.

He moved to San Francisco in 1973 and became a faculty member and then the director of the Humanistic Psychology Institute. There he arranged Moshe FELDENKRAIS's first training programs in the United States. As a result of this meeting, Hanna became interested and influenced by Feldenkrais's work. Hanna was also influenced by Hans Seyle, an endocrinologist and medical researcher who recognized that diseases could be caused by stress. The bodywork and exercises of somatic education are derived from Seyle's and Feldenkrais's theories and principles of BIOFEEDBACK. In 1975, Hanna organized the Novato Institute for Somatic Research.

He believed that the body's deterioration as we age is not inevitable. He said that decreased activity causes muscle atrophy (shrinkage) and weakening, causing sensory amnesia. He firmly believed that it could be reversed.

Hanna felt that as many as 75 percent of adult Americans suffer from sensory-motor-amnesia due to the relentless onslaught of traumas and stresses in our modern society. These traumas trigger any of the three specific reflexes that lead to habitual muscle contraction and weakness.

The **red light** reflex is the response of fear. This withdrawal manifests itself by tightening the jaw, face, abdomen and lifting the shoulders. The **green light** reflex is the assertive response to stress, which causes people to stick out their chests, pull back the shoulders and develop a sway back. The **trauma reflex** is usually found around an area of injury or surgery. In this reaction, there is a spastic contraction at that point.

These responses become so imbedded in our bodies and central nervous system, that people lose the ability to relax. It becomes compounded over time resulting in general stiffness, soreness, limited range of motion and premature aging.

Hanna's point of view was that, as sentient beings, we can be aware of our movements and intentions. This is why he didn't manipulate people, rather he educated them to move freely again.

An individual lies down, fully clothed, on a low, padded table. Information is offered to the client in two ways: pushing and pulling parts of the body to suggest how to move beyond present limitations and directing the client to actively extend and flex certain muscle groups and slowly release the contractions. Follow-up exercises are performed at home to habituate the muscles to a new pattern of movement. Hanna believed that these exercises offer faster results than the hands-on work.

Hanna rejected the idea held by Reich and many other bodyworkers that memories are stored in the body. If the body relaxes, the memories flood to the surface where an emotional, psychological expression of that release takes place. Rather than accepting the theory of energy release, Hanna based his ideas on the sensory-motor ability to control the body.[1]

Hanna Somatic Education should be a lifetime commitment in order to stay flexible and contain muscle atrophy.

Note
[1] Knaster, Mirka, "Thomas Hanna: Mind over Movement," *East-West Journal of Natural Health and Living,* February 1989, pp. 63–64. Of all the many different bodywork systems Hanna studied, he said that he only found three that were innovative and solid: biofeedback, Feldenkrais and acupuncture.

Further Reading
Hanna, Thomas, *Bodies in Revolt: A Primer in Somatic Thinking,* Free Person Press, Novato, Calif., 1970. Hanna's first book discusses his theories about somatics, voluntary control and the aging process.
_____ , *Somatics: Reawakening the Mind's Control of Movement, Flexibility and Health,* Addison-Wesley Publishing Co., Inc., N.Y., 1988. This book, written two years before his death, provides a detailed description of the somatic exercise program.

hara, according to Oriental healing systems, is the energy center of the body. The body's strength and energy stems from this abdominal region. The actual ACUPUNCTURE point is found on the CONCEPTION VESSEL, a unilateral YIN MERIDIAN, which runs up the midline of the front of the body, $1\frac{1}{2}$ inches below the navel. The point is CV 6, also called *tan den*. It is believed that the life force (QI) originates from this point. In Japanese, it is called *kikai* and in Chinese, *qihai,* or "ocean of ki energy."

In Japan, the hara has a sacredness that is echoed in its language and culture. Japanese massage, SHIATSU, includes a specialized massage system, called AMPAKU, which is used to diagnose and treat the *hara.* Diagnostically, the *hara* is considered to be the measuring tool by which the health of the client is assessed. The condition of the meridians, or energy pathways, can be determined and corrected in the *hara.*

The organs of the body are represented on specific areas of the *hara,* not unlike the way organs are mapped out on the feet in reflexology. Clients lie supine on a padded mat with their knees bent. This helps to relax the abdominal muscles and allows for deeper work.[1]

The practitioner places her hands on the *hara* and gently palpates the area. A *hara* is considered healthy if the area below the navel is muscular and protrudes slightly more than the upper hara.[2] The practitioner feels for tightening, intestinal gas, and/or temperature changes, which may indicate health problems. Since each meridian is also represented in the *hara,* the health of these energy pathways can also be determined. A deeper examination of the *hara* assesses the condition of the internal organs.

Ampaku pulse diagnosis can also be made from feeling the aorta, which leads from the heart into the abdomen. The pulse should be strong but not so resonant that it can be felt up the practitioner's arm. A weak pulse also indicates illness. Care must be taken not to press too deeply directly on the aorta, since vessel walls may be weak.

The meridian/organ relationship starts under the ribs. Directly in the middle, under the xiphoid process of the sternum, is the heart meridian. In descending order on the right is the gall bladder, liver and lung. In descending order on the left is the stomach, triple heater and lung. Directly under the heart is the heart constrictor, followed by the spleen, the kidney, which semicircles upward, the bladder below. The small intestine crosses diagonally toward the hipbones on both sides from the edge of the spleen, through the kidney, bladder, and large intestine. The large intestine stretches on both sides above the hipbones, from the iliac crest to the pubic bones.

Hara massage is always done with both hands. One hand, the **mother,** is in contact with the abdomen at all times. The other hand, the **son** or **wanderer,** moves around the *hara*. The massage may be performed with open palms for light pressure, sides of the hands, four, three, two, or one finger for deeper work. Thumbs provide the deepest amount of pressure.

The practitioner starts with a gentle rocking to relax the *hara* and prepare it for deeper work. The *hara* may then be squeezed, using the sides of the hands, following the rhythm of the breath and a clockwise direction. There is a release on inhalation and pressure during the exhalation.

Deeper work follows as the mother hand is stationary on the *hara* and the son presses into the meridians/organs of the abdomen using any combinations of fingers or thumb.

Practitioners often divide the *hara* into upper and lower halves and massage one portion at a time. Or the practitioner might follow a circular pattern, tracing the outside meridians/organs and spiraling in toward the center.

The end of the treatment is signaled by another gentle rocking or by placing open hands on the abdomen. *Hara* massage can be very relaxing, sometimes trancelike, and provides stimulation and energy to the visceral organs and major meridians.

Notes
[1] If the female client has an intrauterine device or is pregnant, deep ampaku massage is contraindicated.
[2] Traditional statues of Buddha always display a large belly indicating a healthy, robust *hara*.

Further Reading
Durckheim, Karl Fried, *Hara: The Vital Centre of Man,* Samuel Weiser, Inc., N.Y., 1962. This book provides an historical analysis of the *hara* in many cultures.
Masunaga, Shizuto, *Zen Shiatsu,* Japan Press, N.Y., 1990. Considered by many to be an expert in his field, this book describes the principles of Zen shiatsu and includes a detailed analysis of *hara* diagnosis.
Matsumoto, Kiiko, and Birch, Stephen, *Hara Diagnosis,* Paradigm Books, Brookline, Mass., 1988. A concise book describing the significance of the *hara* in diagnosing illnesses.
Ohashi, Waturu, *Do-It-Yourself Shiatsu,* E.P. Dutton, N.Y., 1976. This photographed and illustrated book explains self-massage procedures and has a chapter for *hara* massage and diagnosis.

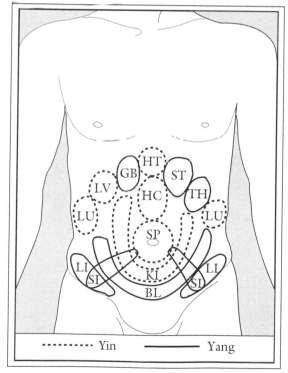

------- Yin   ——— Yang

Considered to be the center of vital energy, or *qi*, in Chinese medicine, the *hara* is located in the abdominal area. It is used as an evaluation and diagnostic region of the body.

Hawaiian bodywork (see LOMILOMI) also called Hawaiian temple bodywork or Kahuna bodywork.

heart constrictor meridian   also called pericardium, is a YIN meridian whose element is fire. The organ relation of this meridian is the parietal pericardium, or the pericardial sac, which envelopes the heart. It supplements the function of the HEART meridian as it relates to circulation. It governs the heart organ, including the cardiac artery and the system of veins and arteries. The heart constrictor also participates in nutrition.

It flows bilaterally up the middle of the inside of the arms from the side of the nipples to the radial side of the third fingers. There are nine ACUPUNCTURE points found along this meridian.

heart meridian a YIN meridian whose element is fire. It governs emotions and spirits as well as blood and circulation, and houses the mind. It also functions as a mechanism that adapts external stimuli to the body's internal environment.

The heart meridian reflects in the face and is involved in mental activities such as thought, memory or sleep. It flows bilaterally up the inside of the arms, on the ulnar surface, from the center of the axillae to the inner tips of the little fingers. There are nine ACUPUNCTURE points found along the heart meridian.

heliotherapy from helio meaning "sun," is another name for the use of ULTRAVIOLET and INFRARED light.

Hellerworkᔆᴹ a series of 11 90-minute sessions of deep tissue bodywork, movement education and dialogue designed to realign the body and release chronic tension and stress. It is an integrated system, which seeks to align the entire body. It is not a remedy for illness, rather it is a process in which people experience relief from chronic stress and tension as well as more ease and flexibility in movement.

The hands-on bodywork, which is rooted in the ROLFING TECHNIQUE, is a deep tissue muscle therapy that manipulates the CONNECTIVE TISSUE, focusing on the FASCIA (connective tissue that wraps around the muscles) to reduce tension and realign the body. The realignment takes place on

two levels: with gravity, involving earth's gravitational field and being (kinesthetically), aware of the body's position.

Movement education is based on ASTON-PATTERNING and the purpose of the dialogue between client and practitioner is to get people to realize the connection between their lives and its effects on their bodies.

Hellerwork was created in 1978. Joseph Heller (not the *Catch 22* author) was born in Poland in 1940. He emigrated with his family to Los Angeles, California in 1957. He received a degree in mathematics from the California Institute of Technology in 1962 and spent 10 years as an aerospace engineer at the Jet Propulsion Lab in Pasadena, California.

Heller started going to encounter groups and weekend workshops as his involvement with humanistic psychology intensified. He studied Rolfing with Ida Rolf and became a certified Rolfer in 1972. In 1976, Heller was elected the first president of the Rolf Institute.

He met Judith Aston during his tenure at the institute and became a structural patterner, based on her teachings, in 1973. It was from these two influential women that he extracted the bodywork and movement education he incorporated into Hellerwork.

Heller recognized that bodies store emotions and attitudes and when certain body parts are touched, people talk about specific subjects. The dialogue is used to assist the client in becoming aware of emotional stress that may be related to a particular physical tension. It explores how the body affects the mind, and vice versa.

The deep connective tissue bodywork is designed to release tension within the connective tissue network and return the body systematically to an aligned position. The fascia is stretched back to its normal position. The hands-on aspect of Hellerwork accounts for about one hour of the 90-minute session.

The Hellerwork movement education program makes the client profoundly aware of his body and movement patterns. Simple suggestions and visualizations are used to rebalance movements for optimum alignment and fluidity.

The focus of the movement education is the use of the body during daily activities. The work is done while the client is sitting, standing, walking and moving in normal patterns as well as in those movements of particular sports and activities he engages in. Video feedback is often used as an educational tool.

The verbal dialogue component of Hellerwork allows the client to become aware of the connection between emotion and its effects on the body. The focus of the dialogue begins with, but is not limited to, the theme of each section. Becoming aware of these emotional forces begins the process of change.

Hellerwork recognizes three causes of accumulated tension: physical, emotional and misuse. The goal of the work is to become free of set patterns, mentally and physically, and to promote the ability to adapt to life's changes in new, easier ways.

Each practitioner has their client fill out a questionnaire on the initial visit, which rates, on a scale of zero to ten, certain aspects of health and life. The practitioner focuses on those areas that have the lowest score. Photographs are taken with the client against a grid and a plumb line down the front of the body to demonstrate the changes that occur throughout the 11 sessions.

Each of these 11 sessions focuses on a different part of the body in a prearranged sequence. The preferred treatment schedule is once a week but clients can adjust that timetable according to their needs. The number of sessions can vary from person to person. Each of the 11 sessions can take more than one treatment to accomplish the desired result.

The first three sections of Hellerwork, **Inspiration, Standing On Your Own Two Feet** and **Reaching Out,** focus on the surface or superficial layers of the body's connective tissue and those muscles that are near the surface of the body, called the **sleeve muscles.** Developmen-

tally, the superficial sections deal with issues of infancy and childhood such as breathing, standing up and reaching out.

Sections four through seven are called the **core sections: Control and Surrender, The Guts, Holding Back** and **Losing Your Head.** These refer to the deeper musculature (intrinsic muscles) and connective tissue. These muscles help us perform fine motor skills. The core sections focus on developmental issues of adolescence, as listed above.

The final sections, numbers 8 through 11, are organized to integrate the core and the sleeve muscles. The practitioner balances and aligns the unique patterns of each client's body. The final section does not necessarily include bodywork, it integrates the Hellerwork series with the client's life. Developmentally, this section focuses on issues of maturity: **Masculine** and **Feminine** styles, **Integration** and **Coming Out** into the world.

Each session (section) is comprised of five components: the purpose, theme (attitudes and emotions), involved anatomy and structure, movement goals and between session activities and experiences.

Section one is Inspiration. The purpose is to open up the breathing and align the rib cage over the pelvis. Its theme is inspiration or "drawing in the spirit." Anatomically, all the body parts involved with deep breathing are addressed. The movements also involve uninhibited free breathing and clients are taught proper sitting and standing techniques. Between sessions, clients are asked to notice those things that are inspirational and depressing and observe if breathing patterns change.

Section two, Standing On Your Own Two Feet, aligns the legs, horizontalizes the knee and ankle joints and distributes body weight over the arches of the feet. The theme examines issues of security, self-support and sufficiency. The superficial musculature and the connective tissue of the legs and feet are the focus of the bodywork, and the related movement is walking in a balanced manner. Between sessions, clients are asked to consider their stability in the world, financially, emotionally and interpersonally.

Section three, Reaching Out, focuses on releasing tension in the shoulders, arms and sides and to bring vertical alignment to the sides of the torso. The context of reaching out means giving and receiving as well as aggression and expressions of anger. The bodywork concentrates on the anatomy of the arms and sides. The movement calls for more freedom in lateral, sideways breathing. Between sessions, clients are asked to notice what happens when they don't reach for what they want.

Section four, Control and Surrender, releases the bottom of the core and brings alignment to the midline of the inner leg. Control issues include "keeping things together" and surrender signifies the healthy balance between control and giving up. Anatomically, the focus is on the insides of the legs and the muscles of the pelvic floor (the control of toilet training). The movement requires relaxation of the pelvic floor and a lengthened core. Between sessions, clients are asked to consider things they feel must dominate in contrast to those things that they have surrendered. Concentration is on how these emotional issues are reflected in the muscles of the inner legs and pelvic floor.

Section five, The Guts, lengthens the front of the core and releases the deep pelvic muscles. The emotional issues are those of courage and strength and the process of energy. The muscles that are worked on are the abdominals, psoas and iliacus, deep in the pelvis. The movement goal is to be more relaxed in the core. Between sessions, clients are asked to pay attention to feelings in their guts.

Section six, Holding Back, lengthens the back of the core. Tension in the back is the theme and holding back emotionally is the emotional component. The muscles of the back are worked on and a fluid and flexible spine is the movement goal. Clients are asked to see what happens when they are withholding.

Section seven, Losing Your Head, releases the top of the core. The theme concentrates on excessive attention to the analytic, mental and inner processes of the mind. The head, neck and face are the focus of the bodywork. Movement goals of lengthening the top of the core and relaxation are desired. Clients are asked to notice what happens to them when things "go into their heads."

Section eight, the Feminine, is for men and women. This section releases rotations in the lower half of the body. The feminine way manifests itself in the power of attraction, beauty and well-being. The anatomical focus is on the legs, feet and pelvis. Balance of core and sleeve movement is sought as well as the application of learned activities to more complex tasks. Between sessions, clients are asked to consider the role of the feminine principle in their lives.

Section nine, the Masculine, releases rotations in the upper half of the body. The masculine principle of doing and achieving is this section's theme. The bodywork focus is on the arms, shoulders, rib cage and neck and the movement education involves integrating more complex movements in the upper half of the body. Between sessions, clients are asked to notice and perform areas of penetrating action, with ease, in the upper torso.

Section ten, Integration, establishes the overall integrity of the body by working with the joints. The theme reveals present integrity and uncovering balance in the body. The joints, which reflex maturity, are the concentrated areas of treatment. Movement exercises include moving as a whole, with fluidity, in all activities. Clients are asked to notice integrity and separation in their lives and how it feels.

The final, eleventh, section, Coming Out, is concerned with completion, self-expression and empowerment. Bodywork is not necessarily a part of this section. The theme infers taking what the client has learned out into the world and allowing full self-expression to radiate throughout the body. This is the time to tie up loose ends and express the feelings about Hellerwork.

After the work is completed, the body is more aligned and balanced, and is freer in movement. Changes may still occur as long as one year after the work.

Further Reading
Heller, Joseph and Henkin, William A., *Bodywise,* Winbow Press, Oakland, Calif., 1986. This book details the Hellerwork approach, including an analysis of each section.

HEMME APPROACH™ a problem-solving approach of soft tissue (muscles, fascia, tendons and ligaments) therapy. The letters in the acronym stand for: H—History; E—Evaluation; M—Modalities; M—Manipulation and E—Exercise.

History and evaluation define the problem, which is treated by the use of modalities, manipulation and exercise.

Dave Leflet, M.S., L.M.T., developed this system in 1986. It is derived from aspects of osteopathy, physical medicine, chiropractic and physical therapy. HEMME seeks to relieve pain, restore alignment and improve myofascial dysfunction by working on spasms and contractures (permanent contractions caused by spasms or paralysis), TRIGGER POINTS and muscle weaknesses.

The initial step in the HEMME APPROACH is taking the client's medical history. This *history* provides the practitioner with the information needed to identify contraindications and to develop a treatment plan.

The physical *evaluation* is also instrumental in assessing the client's health. HEMME uses four types of evaluation: palpation, observation, auscultation (listening) and percussion. Palpation is most useful in ascertaining the condition of the underlying soft tissue. Information about tissue temperature, moisture and resistance to pressure is gathered through this sensitive touch.

Observation of the client during rest, active movement and passive movement is helpful in determining areas of pain and dysfunction. Auscultation, or listening for abnormal sounds, will aid the practitioner in locating areas of tension. In this system, percussion is a light but sharp tapping used to determine the condition of the tissues.

The *modalities* of the HEMME APPROACH prepare the body for the ensuing manipulation. They reduce pain, facilitate reabsorption of the excess lymphatic fluid, which causes edema, relieve muscle spasm, decrease tissue viscosity and can either stimulate or sedate the metabolism. The modalities used in the HEMME APPROACH are **thermotherapy** and **cryotherapy** (heat and cold) and mechanical vibrators.

Thermotherapy usually involves the application of moist heat directly over the area of tension. However, there are other heat-producing agents that are equally effective: gel packs, whirlpools, paraffin baths and infrared lamps. Contraindications for thermotherapy include bleeding, inflammation, cancerous tumors, edema, burns, fevers, debilitating heart disease and general weakness.

Cryotherapy, or ICE THERAPY, can treat spasms and activated trigger points. Smooth-edged ice cubes are placed locally on pain areas until burning or numbness occurs. A local, analgesic effect is provided by the ice. Cold is vasoconstricting and is beneficial to decrease bleeding, inflammation, control edema and increase muscle tone. Ice is contraindicated in people with sensitivity to cold, heart disease, Raynaud's disease (abnormal vasoconstriction of the extremities when exposed to cold temperatures) and client tolerance.

Mechanical vibrators relax muscle spasms, relieve pain, increase circulation and provide an effective substitute for those clients who cannot tolerate compression or stretching.

The *manipulations* of this system are gentle push-pull movements, which work to reposition the soft tissues. Practitioners use the minimum amount of force needed to achieve this goal and to avoid pain or harm to the client. The manipulations most often used are trigger point therapy to contain pain, neuromuscular therapy to minimize muscle spasms and strengthen muscles, connective tissue therapy to break down adhesions and range of motion stretching to restore muscle tone and elasticity of joints.

Exercises are necessary to relieve pain, restore spinal alignment and strengthen the musculature. The level and duration of the exercises should be based on the client's ability and physical condition.

The HEMME APPROACH has had much success in treating chronic low back pain and soft tissue injury.

Further Reading
Home study manuals are available directly from HEMME APPROACH. Each book clearly defines the technique and its applications. All courses are offered for continuing education credits.
Leflet, David H., *HEMME APPROACH to Managing Low Back Pain,* HEMME APPROACH Publications, Bonifay, Fla., 1994.
_____ , *HEMME APPROACH to Soft Tissue Therapy,* HEMME APPROACH Publications, Bonifay, Fla., 1992.
_____ , *The AIDS Virus,* HEMME APPROACH Publications, Bonifay, Fla., 1994.

herbal body wraps   See BODY WRAPS.

Hoffa massage technique uses the five SWEDISH MASSAGE strokes that were adapted by Albert J. Hoffa to his particular style. Like traditional Swedish massage, the pressure followed venous blood flow, toward the heart except on the back. However, unlike this classic system, Hoffa's strokes were always gentle and light, and he minimized his sessions to under one half hour.

Hoffa advocated an anatomical approach to the work, following larger blood vessels and massaging muscle groups in a specific order, from distal (the farthest) to proximal (closest to the torso). He believed that the client's joints should be half-flexed, providing optimum relaxation during the treatment. Healthy tissue should be massaged first, followed by work on injured areas. He also believed that the body part being massaged should be free of hair.

Hoffa's EFFLEURAGE stroke begins and ends each treatment and is made up of several variations: light and deep stroking, knuckling, circular, thumb, alternate hand stroking and simultaneous stroking. The pressure always follows venous and lymph flow. The light and deep effleurages differ only in the amount of pressure being used.

Knuckling has often been associated with Hoffa's style. This variation penetrates deeper than basic effleurage and is used in treating thick fascia (connective tissue sheath, which envelopes organs, muscles and muscles groups). The first interphalangeal joints are used and the pressure of the stroke alternates from light to deep, back to light again. Circular effleurage provides alternative fingertip circles, while the thumbs are primarily used on the foot.

His PETRISSAGE technique is made up of a one-handed stroke on small limbs to lift and squeeze the muscle between fingers and thumbs. The two-handed petrissage is an alternating, back and forth, pickup of the muscle. His two-finger stroke is a pick up of muscle between thumbs and forefingers.

Hoffa used thumbs, index fingers or both for FRICTION and suggested that the skin should be moved under the finger. Hacking, or the TAPOTEMENT stroke, using the ulnar surface of the opened hand, was used lightly on the back. VIBRATION was performed with fingertips or flat, open palms.

Further Reading
Tappan, Francis M., *Healing Massage Techniques,* Reston Publishing Co., Inc., N.Y., 1980. This illustrated book clearly describes and compares many of the more popular massage techniques.

Hoffman Quadrinity Process® a program committed to healing the wounds of childhood, which reflect in negative adult behaviors and attitudes and replacing them with self-acceptance, self-esteem and unconditional love.

This system was developed in 1967 by Bob Hoffman, a former Oakland businessman who gave psychic readings as a hobby. He conceived the Quadrinity Process after a profound meditation.

This seven-day residential intensive integrates the participant on four levels—the Quadrinity: emotionally, spiritually, intellectually and physically. Practitioners are called teachers and participants are called students. The teacher-student ratio is one to eight, limited to a maximum of 22 students.

The process is a structured combination of journal keeping, GUIDED IMAGERY, mind revelations and cathartic work similar to aspects of GESTALT psychology, transactional analysis and spiritual work.

Hoffman maintains that all adult actions are deeply rooted in childhood because of the **negative love syndrome.** In an attempt to receive unconditional love and approval from parents, children unconsciously adopt parental behaviors, attitudes and moods, both good and bad. As adults, however, the negative aspects of this conditioning (or programming), creates conflict and tensions in our lives. Additionally, the individual, in order to assert himself, rebels against some of the adoptive, programmed behavior, creating different but equally ineffective traits.

The inner, emotional child does not experience unconditional parental love, and the adult is struggling to protect those painful, learned feelings of unloveableness and inadequacy. The physical body becomes the battleground for this conflict, eventually breaking down and getting sick. All this negativity is an expression of the disintegration and lack of harmony between the four aspects of self: emotion, intellect, spirit and body.

The process begins with a **preprocess assignment,** where the student learns to connect current adult problems with past negative programming. During the week, a supportive environment continues with a deeper examination of the negative programming in a series of nine carefully delineated steps.

The **prosecution of mother and father** is an examination of the negative aspects of each parent or parental figure. Guided imagery focuses on repressed childhood emotions, such as anger, shame, fear and the behavior that was adopted and the consequent problems exhibited in adulthood. Physical and emotional release allows the student to express and disconnect from these painful feelings.

The **defense of mother and father** permits the student to fully understand the early experiences of his own parents in order to see that unconditional love was also unavailable to them. They too were victims of the negative love syndrome from their parents. Deep **compassion** and **forgiveness** for one's parents and oneself follows.

A remarkable **truce** between the student's intellect and emotions then becomes possible. Deeper forms of unconditional love are experienced as the student learns to release vindictiveness and other resentments, which have been accumulating during his life.

This is followed by **recycling,** which teaches the student to access his inherent spiritual wisdom to change negative patterned behavior into positive expressive ones. **Play day** allows the student to reclaim, more fully, the natural spontaneity, innocence and joy that has been dormant for so long.

Toward the end of the week, the positive side of the intellect is **empowered** over the negative side during a profound cathartic experience. **Closure** allows the inner child to grow to adulthood, bringing with it the childlike joys of youth and leaving behind the childish, negative patterning.

The new emotional self couples with the adult intellect into a partnership of equals. The spiritual self can now fully be recognized, and it joins with the intellect, emotions and physical body to become one accepting, loving, holistic self: an integrated Quadrinity.

Further Reading
Hoffman, Bob, *No One Is to Blame: Freedom from Compulsive Self-Defeating Behavior,* Hoffman Institute, San Anselmo, Calif., 1981. This book outlines the Hoffman Quadrinity

Process and offers individuals a unique way to free themselves from unhealthy behavior patterns and lead a more joyous life.

holistic (wholistic) refers to the inseparability of body/mind/spirit to create the whole person. This term also refers to healing practices that treat the whole person rather than just the injured part or symptom and provides the means for the body to heal itself. The word comes from the Greek *holos* meaning "complete" or "total."

Holotropic Breathwork® a powerful and comprehensive approach to self-exploration and healing, which includes physical, psychological and spiritual dimensions. It is based on mobilizing the spontaneous healing potential of the psyche and the body that becomes available in unordinary states of consciousness. These states are brought on by breathing, stimulating music and energy-release bodywork.

Holotropic Breathwork was developed in 1976 by Stanislav and Christina Grof, leaders on TRANSPERSONAL PSYCHOLOGY. The term comes from the Greek *holos,* meaning "whole" or "complete" and *trepein* meaning "to move in the direction of." The translation is therefore "moving toward wholeness."

Stanislav Grof, M.D., is a psychiatrist who has been researching psychotherapy and unordinary states of consciousness for 30 years. He is one of the founders and chief theoreticians of transpersonal psychology. Christina Grof is a cocreator of Holotropic Breathwork and the founder of the Spiritual Emergence Network.

Holotropic Breathwork is offered in different formats. It can be practiced individually, in therapeutic groups, and as one day, weekend or five-day workshops. It is compatible with traditional therapeutic approaches and spiritual practices.

Participants lie on the floor while certified facilitators guide breathing techniques as evocative music or rhythmic drumming is played. In addition to the breathing, focused bodywork and mandala drawing, symbolic designs of Buddhist rituals, are integral parts of the process.

During the sessions, the participants alternate between experiencing and "sitting" (a supporting and assisting function).

Holotropic Breathwork sessions are two to four hours long. The system mediates to access all levels of human experience, including unfinished issues from postnatal biography, sequences of psychological death and rebirth and the entire spectrum of transpersonal phenomena. Blocked memories are recalled and relived, freeing the individual from unhealthy behavior patterns and negative emotions.

This work is highly experiential, emotionally demanding and physically strenuous. As a result, Holotropic Breathwork is contraindicated in cases of severe mental illness, pregnancy, cardiovascular ailments, glaucoma, epilepsy or recent surgeries.

Further Reading

Grof, Christina, *Thirst for Wholeness: Addiction, Attachments and the Spiritual Path,* HarperCollins, N.Y., 1993. The cofounder of Holotropic Breathwork discusses breaking unhealthy behaviors and addictions through spirituality.

Grof, Stanislav, M.D., and Grof, Christina, *The Stormy Search for Self,* J.P. Tarcher, Los Angeles, Calif., 1990. Self-exploration and self-healing are discussed in this book.

Grof, Stanislav, M.D., *Beyond the Brain: Birth, Death and Transcendence in Psychotherapy,* SUNY Press, Albany, N.Y., 1985. The author discusses the search for self.

———, *The Adventure of Self-Discovery,* SUNY Press, Albany, N.Y., 1987. The path of self-enlightenment is the subject of this text.

———, *The Holotropic Mind,* HarperCollins, N.Y., 1992. The philosophy and theory of Holotropic Breathwork is discussed in this book by the creator of the system.

homeostasis comes from the Greek *homeo,* meaning "same" and *stasis,* meaning "standing." It was coined by the American physiologist Walter B. Cannon (1871–1945).[1] It is the condition of the body where the internal environment remains relatively balanced. The body has unique regulating devices to protect itself against stress factors.

External temperature changes never affect the internal body temperature because one can produce perspiration in heat to keep cool and contract the skin (goose bumps) in the cold to stay warm. Heart activity increases to satisfy the need for fresh blood and nutrients during strenuous activity, and the respiration rate changes to accommodate physical demands.

Homeostasis is controlled by the nervous and endocrine systems. The nervous system detects physical changes and quickly sends messages to the appropriate organs to oppose the stress. The endocrine system, made up of glands that secrete hormones into the blood, slowly issues chemical regulators to provide homeostatic balance.

Note
[1] Tortora, Gerald J., and Anagnostakos, Nicholas P., *Principles of Anatomy and Physiology,* Harper & Row, N.Y., 3d ed., 1981, p. 25.

Hoshino Therapy® the art and science of hand therapy developed by Professor Tomezo Hoshino, born in Japan in 1910. As a doctor of ACUPUNCTURE, he found that in cases of **arthrosis,** acupuncture offered only temporary relief. He originated a unique therapy that integrates the principles of acupuncture with the art of hand therapy.

Arthrosis is a painful and disabling condition of soft tissue, which affects the moving parts of the body. These problems, which arise with advancing age, are also influenced by a sedentary lifestyle and habits of poor posture and inadequate exercise. People may develop uncoordinated movement patterns that cause muscles, tendons and ligaments to contract and harden.

Arthrosis is the condition that underlies soft tissue disorders such as bursitis, tendinitis, back pain and muscular tension. When left uncorrected for many years, such conditions may eventually lead to degenerative joint diseases such as osteoarthritis and spinal disk disorders.

Individuals of almost any age group whose movement is restricted, impaired or misused may find relief with Hoshino Therapy.

Hoshino Therapy, recognizing that arthrosis is the cause of soft tissue disorders, works to correct the underlying cause of the pain and disability. As movement patterns begin to return, the conditions that create irritation and stress are relieved

and the symptoms naturally disappear. The revitalizing of soft tissue, the foundation of this system, is accomplished exclusively through the hands. There is an evaluation of 250 "vital" points, using digital (thumb) pressure, to enable the therapist to detect hardened tendons and ligaments and the early stages of calcification long before they show up on X rays. This evaluation also reveals other abnormalities of the tissue such as muscle atrophy (shrinking and weakening), as well as deformed or immobile joints. In this way, the therapist discovers the true location of the body disequilibrium that has brought on the pain or disability.

When Mr. Hoshino was 16 years old, he lost his sight in a motorcycle accident. As a result of this incident, he studied HAMA MASSAGE, a Japanese massage system designed for the blind, as his livelihood. A year and a half after his accident, a blow to the head knocked him out. When he regained consciousness, his vision returned. He continued his studies by learning acupuncture from 1935 to 1939. His travels took him to Argentina where acupuncture was not a recognized therapy. So he began working with his hands once again, putting together a massage technique that combined his knowledge of the Oriental healing arts.

The practitioner's palpation skills are very keen, intrinsic to this technique and a result of Hoshino's initial blindness.

The dosage is the art of applying deep, yet agreeable pressure to revitalize soft tissues without causing discomfort to the client. This is especially important when treating painful areas. The skillful and sensitive hands of the therapist stimulate selected points to create a deep, soothing heat and increased blood flow that counteracts the cold rigidity of the affected parts. As tissue activity improves and stress on tissues is relieved, pain tends to disappear.

Coordination is restored in the final phase of the therapy. As movement patterns return to normal, stress on tissues and joints is minimized. Muscles regain their elasticity, tendons and ligaments are drawn into their normal positioning and a normal range of movement is restored to the joints.

On the initial visit, clients receive a complete evaluation, and the therapist will advise if he can successfully treat the problem and the approximate number of treatments required. Treatments last 30 to 40 minutes and relief from the original symptoms, along with improved flexibility, is usually experienced within the first three or four sessions.

Hoshino Therapy may be indicated for disorders such as osteoarthritis, bursitis, tendinitis, nontraumatic disk disorders and sciatica, as well as for nonspecific complaints such as headache, muscular pain and tension, fatigue, nausea, numbness, dizziness and back pain.

human energy bio-field (see AURA) the energy field, or emanations, which surround and penetrate the physical body.

hydrotherapy the use of water in any of its three forms, solid, liquid or vapor, internally or externally, to treat disease, injury or trauma. In hydrotherapy, the environment of the body is changed by using water at varying temperatures and applied in any number of mechanical means. Physiological changes and responses are in direct proportion to the extent of the environmental changes. Water, which is a versatile therapeutic agent, can alter physiological responses by changing its temperature.

Hydrotherapy is one of the oldest types of healing practices. It comes from the Greek word *hudor,* "water" and *therapeutikos,* "to heal" and has a distinguished and ancient history. Hippocrates, considered to be the father of modern medicine, made use of salubrious waters in the fifth century B.C. Sanskrit texts dating to C. 4000 B.C., mention the use of baths and remedies. Babylonians, Cretans, Egyptians and Persians used water and baths very frequently. Ancient Romans built luxurious baths, some of which still stand in Europe and Africa. Emperor Augustus of Rome is reported to have been one of the most famous patients who recovered from illness through a water cure when other known forms of medicine failed.

Native Americans used vapors in the form of sweat lodges, followed by a cold plunge, to treat disease and for purification. During the 15th century, Turks in Constantinople, now Istanbul, popularized a hot air bath called the Turkish bath. In 1776, John Wesley, the evangelist and founder of the Methodist Church, published *Primitive Physick: Easy and Natural Method of Curing Most Diseases,* which practiced cold water bathing to treat a myriad of ailments.

Father Sebstian Kneipp, who was regarded as the renowned water doctor, developed hot and cold contrast baths and cold water washes followed by warm BODY WRAPS. His book, *My Water Cure,* published in 1890, popularized his theories, which made their way to sanitariums and treatment facilities in the United States.

In the United States, Drs. Simon Baruch, who published *The Principles and Practice of Hydrotherapy* in 1899 and John H. Kellogg, who wrote *Rational Hydrotherapy* in 1900 and developed the heated cabinet, were major champions of the use of hydrotherapy.

Throughout history and all over the world, people have sought the healing properties of natural springs. Warm baths, to which aromatic oils may be added (see AROMATHERAPY), can relax and sedate, increase circulation and relax muscle spasms. Hot baths can treat arthritis, rheumatism, neuritis and gout. Short, cold baths can ward off fatigue, reduce swelling and pain. Sitz baths are used for localized healing.

Minerals added to the baths, such as sulfur, pine, Epsom salts and other mineral salts, increase the effects of the hydrotherapy as these minerals are absorbed into the system through the skin or mucous membranes.

Internally, water cleanses the body through drinking, colonics, enemas or douches.

Vapor and steam baths stimulate cleansing and promote elimination through the skin, lungs and kidneys.

In its solid form, ice packs are used topically to reduce swelling, anesthetize an area, reduce inflammation and control pain.

There are many variations of hydrotherapy, some of which are now installed in the home. General applications of hydrotherapy include whirlpools (Jacuzzis), hot tubs, steam cabinets, THALASSOTHERAPY (a massage while submerged in water), contrast bathing, Turkish baths (hot, dry air) and Russian steam baths (a steam room or cabinet with a hole for the head to stick out, heated up to 130°F). These forms of hydrotherapy may be used for either general or therapeutic purposes.

Localized use is more commonly associated with therapy and may include fomentations (hot, wet packs specifically placed), sitz baths (a tub of hip-level water heated to 105° to 115°F or cold at 55° to 75°F), hydrocollator (preheated chemical pack of silica gel) and hot footbaths (heated to 100° to 115°F).

Hydrotherapy can treat muscle soreness, athletic injuries (ice pack within the first 24 to 48 hours for twenty-minute intervals every few hours), arthritis, and be sedating and/or invigorating.

Contraindications to the extreme temperatures of hydrotherapy include high blood pressure, recent surgeries, pregnancy and cardiac problems.

Further Reading

Thrash, Agatha, M.D., and Thrash, Calvin, M.D., *Home Remedies,* New Life Style Books, Seale, Ala., 1981. This book includes many types of home remedies, including hydrotherapy, to treat many common ailments.

hypnotherapy the use of hypnosis for therapeutic purposes, is a highly relaxed, altered state of awareness or consciousness where the mind is focused and receptive to suggestions. When it is used for specific physical or psychological purposes, it is called **clinical hypnosis.** Hypnotherapy is a safe procedure, which leaves the client feeling refreshed and alert.

Hypnosis has been used since ancient time. Egyptian priests used incense with incantations to induce healing, hypnotic states. In tribal societies, shamans, medicine men and witch doctors created hypnotic trances for rituals and healing.

The oldest therapeutic form of hypnotherapy is called **suggestive therapy.** Modern clinical hypnosis dates from the time of Franz Anton Mesmer (1734–1815). He called his system "animal magnetism" and believed that the human body had a magnetic polarity that was surrounded by a force field.

The word hypnosis was coined by a Scottish doctor, James Braid, M.D., in 1841. It continued to gain popularity in Europe. In Vienna, Drs. Sigmund Freud (1856–1939) and Joseph Bauer (1842–1925) used hypnosis with their patients in their psychotherapy sessions. Later, however, Freud abandoned hypnotherapy in favor of free association and other psychological methods.

Hypnotherapy is now recognized as a valuable medical system by the American Medical Association and the British Medical Association. Practitioners must be doctors or qualified hypnosis professionals in order to practice.

A session generally begins with a complete medical history to determine if the procedure is contraindicated (i.e., serious heart conditions) or if other forms of therapy would be more appropriate. The length of a treatment series varies according to the severity of the problem and the client's cooperation. Treatment can last anywhere from one session to several. It is often used in conjunction with other forms of psychotherapy or bodywork.

Contrary to popular misconceptions, the trancelike state is not a loss of consciousness, will or control. The session can be terminated at any point by the client by simply opening the eyes.

It generally takes about 15 minutes to achieve maximum relaxation, although practice will shorten that time. The client is seated comfortably in a dimly lit room. The hypnotherapist asks the client to concentrate on an object or the sound of his voice, all the while making suggestions, not commands, about the eyelids feeling heavy, etc. The client is gently guided into a state of relaxation. Another way of quieting the mind is by counting backward. In hypnosis, the sense of time is distorted and a great deal seems to happen in a short amount of time.

It is not difficult for most people to achieve the **light stage** of hypnosis. In this state, limbs may feel heavy and be difficult to lift. On a **deeper level,** total anesthesia may be possible[1] or the ability to control involuntary body functions.

A study by Frumkin, Ripley and Cox in 1978, indicated that under hypnosis, the usual left-brain domain for verbal material was reduced. They concluded that the right cerebral hemisphere's participation was greater during altered states of consciousness. When this transition occurs, the right brain "hears" messages, which can transform the body.[2]

Self-hypnosis is a natural phenomena, which often occurs naturally throughout the day. Daydreaming, for example, is a hypnotic state. It helps overcome stress, control pain, break habits and alleviate other problems. Self-hypnosis has also been used in labor to relax the mother, reduce pain, eliminate or reduce medicated births and keep the mother and baby alert. Self-hypnosis, however, is best taught under the initial supervision of a professional.

While sitting in a comfortable position, focus your eyes on an object, point on the wall or a lit candle. Make auto-suggestions to relax. Breathe deeply and sigh on the exhalations. As your eyes start to close, tell yourself to relax. It will take a lot of practice to induce hypnosis. A pleasant image or color will enhance the process.

Once your eyes are closed, concentrate on relaxing the body, one muscle group at a time, by contracting and releasing each group. Mental exercises, such as counting backward or imagining yourself descending stairs, deepens the hypnotic state. To confirm that you are "under," pinch yourself. There should be a sensation of pressure, but no pain.

To reverse the state, count forward from one to five, gradually getting more alert and refreshed. When you reach five, you will be completely awake.

Hypnosis has helped people overcome many physical and psychological problems. It has successfully been used to treat addictions of smoking and drinking, weight control, phobias, speech disorders such as stuttering, posttraumatic stress disorder and pain, and to reveal deeply suppressed experiences. Hypnosis has also been used in forensic work with witnesses. Posthypnotic suggestions, which usually diminish within a few days, are useful in relieving postoperative pain and cancer pain.

Notes
[1] Reader's Digest, *Family Guide To Natural Medicine,* Reader's Digest Association, Inc., Pleasantville, N.Y., 1993, p. 124. Dental surgeon Dr. Victor Rausch successfully used self-hypnotherapy instead of anesthesia during surgery to remove his gallbladder. He received no premedication and walked back to his room after the final sutures were in place.
[2] Budzynski, Thomas, "Brain Lateralization and Rescripting," *Somatics,* Spring/Summer, 1981, pp. 6–7.

Further Reading
Alman, Brian, Ph.D., and Lambrou, Peter, M.D., *Self-Hypnosis: The Complete Manual for Health and Self-Change,* Brunner/Mazel, Inc., N.Y., 1992. This text teaches self-hypnosis and discusses expectations and definitions of hypnosis. It moves from relaxation and guided imagery to posthypnotic suggestions.
Bowers, Kenneth S., Ph.D., *Hypnosis for the Seriously Curious,* W.W. Norton & Co., Inc., N.Y., 1976. This introduction to hypnosis reviews the basic concepts and provides some hypnotic treatments.
Hammond, Corydon D., Ph.D., *Manual for Self Hypnosis,* A.S.C.H., Des Plaines, Ill., 1987. This book was written for individuals who will be learning self-hypnosis from a trained professional. It discusses hypnosis, the most effective use of language and the construction of hypnotic suggestions.
Hunter, Marlene E., M.D., *Psych Yourself in Hypnosis and Health,* SeaWalk Press, Ltd., West Vancouver, B.C., 1987. The use of hypnosis in the medical field is discussed. The author talks about methods of helping patients feel more in control and responsible for their health.
Spiegel, Herbert, M.D., and Spiegel, David, M.D., *Trance and Treatment,* American Psychiatric Press, Inc., Washington, D.C., 1987. Part I of the advanced text discusses the

definitions of hypnosis and the Hypnotic Induction Profile (HIP). Part II reviews HIP research and Part III presents clinical applications.

Wester, William C., II, Ed.D., *Clinical Hypnosis: A Case Management Approach,* Behavioral Science Center, Dallas, 1987. This basic/intermediate text provides information on the history of hypnosis, induction techniques and advanced clinical applications.

I

ice therapy or cryotherapy, is the application of cold HYDROTHERAPY on localized areas of the body for therapeutic purposes. Cold causes blood vessels to contract thereby reducing blood flow, swelling and inflammation. It can also reduce fever and control pain.

Ice packs are generally the first aid remedy to musculoskeletal injuries when applied within the first 24 to 48 hours after the trauma for approximately 20-minute intervals every couple of hours. Packs are also effective remedies for headaches, nosebleeds, muscle spasms, sprains, acute bursitis, acute joint inflammation, rheumatoid arthritis and as an immediate treatment for burns.

Cold water immersions are used for larger surfaces, such as limbs, and for the relief of fatigue, fevers and heat exhaustion.

Used alternatively with heat, cold can increase localized circulation, which supplies oxygenated blood and removes waste products from an injured area.

Further Reading
Packman, Harold, *Ice Therapy—Understanding Its Application,* Harold Packman, Whitestone, N.Y., 1977. This book gives the history of hydrotherapy and the application of ice therapy as a painless, drugless therapy.

infant massage a modified SWEDISH MASSAGE program specifically designed for babies from the age of one month until they become toddlers.

Unlike other mammals who lick and clean their newborns immediately after birth to stimulate respiration, human infants receive that same stimulation on their voyage through the birth canal. The infant's first massage actually begins in utero, with the contractions of labor. These contractions stimulate the baby's skin—like the licking of the animals—which activates the autonomic nervous system, signaling the beginning of respiration.[1] Babies delivered by Caesarean section do not get this cutaneous (skin) stimulation and can benefit tremendously from massage.

Babies need to be touched in order to survive and develop into loving adults. There are many benefits of infant massage, to the baby as well as the new parents or nonrelative provider.[2]

Daily massage can relax new parents and baby. For those parents who work, massage offers concentrated time to be with the baby. Bonding becomes stronger as love is communicated through touch and parental attachment strengthens. Massage contains all the essential elements of bonding: eye-to-eye contact, skin-to-skin contact, smiles, laughter, soothing sounds, cuddling, smell, responsiveness and communication.

Daily massage for the newborn can ease the trauma of birth. The baby's soft bones are compressed as she passes through the birth canal and its muscles are strained. According to Bonnie Prudden, the developer of TRIGGER POINT THERAPY, trigger points, or hypersensitive "knots" found within the muscles, may have originated from being squeezed through the birth canal. If they are not treated and released early in life, they can continue to cause pain and discomfort throughout adulthood.

Sleep is promoted because the baby is more relaxed. The baby's immune system is strengthened and the increase in endorphin output, compounds which promote a sense of well-being, reduces pain and tension. Premature babies and those who were exposed to drugs and/or abuse, show lower stress levels and sleep better with daily massage.[3]

Massage stimulates a child's circulation and internal organs. Colic and intestinal gas can be comfortably relieved through a light abdominal massage.

A study at the Rainbow Babies' and Children's Hospital in Cleveland, Ohio, showed that early touch enhanced children's intellectual de-

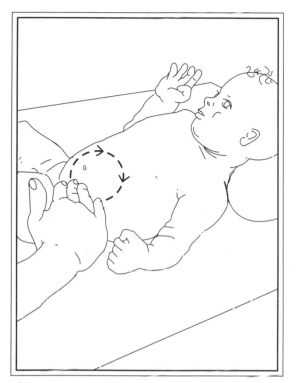

This nurturing massage is an ideal and relaxing way for parents to bond with their child. It provides many psychological benefits to the newborn, such as stress reduction and improved sleep, as well as to the provider. A light abdominal massage in a clockwise direction can relieve gas and treat colic.

velopment, raised language skills, reading scores and IQs.[4]

Parents also receive benefits from massaging their infants. Their parenting skills and nurturing abilities are increased. Fathers enjoy the opportunity to be caregivers and nurturers. Nursing mothers are more successful in breast-feeding, since the response to massaging her child actually increases the secretion of prolactin, the hormone necessary for milk production.

Infant massage is not a new phenomena. Many tribal societies practiced infant massage to promote the child's ability to survive against some of nature's harshest living conditions. It also ensured closeness within the tribe, which was often vital for survival.

Daily infant massage should begin when a newborn is one month old and should last up to 30 minutes. When the baby starts to crawl, massages may become less frequent, perhaps two to three times a week.

There are a few contraindications to infant massage. Immediately after a feeding is an inappropriate time to massage, since it could upset the baby's digestion. Wait at least one hour before massaging. If the baby is extremely fussy or crying hard, perhaps another form of succor would be more effective.

It is contraindicated to massage anyone when a fever is present. This rule applies to the infant as well. The legs or arms should be avoided after a vaccination shot.

Infant massage can be taught to new parents by certified or licensed massage therapists.

Notes

[1] Stillerman, Elaine, L.M.T., *MotherMassage: A Handbook for Relieving the Discomforts of Pregnancy,* Dell Publications, N.Y., 1992, pp. 111–112.

[2] O'Sullivan, William, "The Gift of Touch," *Common Boundary,* May/June 1994, p. 12. A study conducted by the Touch Research Institute at the University of Miami School of Medicine showed that elderly people may actually benefit more from administering infant massage than from receiving their own daily treatments. The self-report questionnaires indicated that anxiety and depression declined, they saw their doctors less frequently, their social contacts increased and their self-esteem increased.

[3] Ibid., p. 12.

[4] Stillerman, Elaine, L.M.T., *MotherMassage: A Handbook for Relieving the Discomforts of Pregnancy,* Dell Publications, Inc., N.Y., 1992, p. 112.

Further Reading

LeBoyer, Frederick, *Loving Hands: The Traditional Indian Art of Baby Massage,* Alfred A. Knopf, Inc., N.Y., 1976. A beautifully photographed account of Indian infant massage.

Schneider-McClure, Vimala, *Infant Massage: A Handbook for Loving Parents,* Bantam Books, N.Y., 1982. An easy-to-follow photographed book on the art of infant massage. The benefits to child and parent are explained.

Stillerman, Elaine, L.M.T., *MotherMassage: A Handbook for Relieving the Discomforts of Pregnancy,* Dell Publications, N.Y., 1992. This book clearly explains the benefits of prenatal and postpartum massage and has a beautifully illustrated chapter on infant massage.

infrared radiation therapy uses energy in the form of waves or rays. Rays travel through the air, or ether, until they come upon a source that can absorb them. Upon absorption, these rays are converted into different energy sources and create certain reactions. Infrared rays produce heat when the body absorbs them.

Many heat sources emit infrared rays, including the sun, hot water, pipes, gas, coal, etc. When used for therapeutic purposes, these rays are divided into two groups; **nonluminous** or **long rays,** and **luminous** or **short** infrared rays.

Nonluminous rays do not exhibit bright light or glare, and they require a short period of time to heat up before maximum intensity is reached. They are beneficial for use on peripheral blood vessels, nerve receptors, lymphatics and other subcutaneous structures.

Luminous rays are produced by incandescent lamps with a red (glass) filter added to absorb the visible and ultraviolet rays. They penetrate to deeper muscle layers than the nonluminous kinds.

Infrared radiation is an effective treatment in conjunction with other therapies. It is often used in cases of nonacute arthritis, muscle spasms, sprains and strains after the initial 36- to 72-hour period, stiff joints, restricted range of motion and peripheral neuropathy.

Infrared rays increase metabolism, dilate blood vessels, reduce blood pressure, relieve pain, relax muscle spasms, increase the activity of sweat glands and produce a localized rise in temperature.

Each session generally lasts 20 to 30 minutes, although shortened treatments can be done several times a day. The recipient is lying down comfortably with the area of treatment exposed. The rays of the lamp should be aimed at a right angle to the skin for maximum absorption and at a distance of 18 to 24 inches away from the skin's surface. The recipient's eyes should be averted from the rays or shielded with a covering.

The use of infrared rays is contraindicated in cases of malignancies, high fevers, hemorrhages, defective arterial blood supply and for individuals who cannot communicate due to age or physical disability.

Integrative Acupressure™ a comprehensive, highly effective system for health work, which combines an in-depth energetic approach based on the Oriental medical model with unique structurally based techniques. The integration of these two approaches serves to increase the effectiveness of either approach by itself.

The energetic aspect of the Integrative Acupressure system is based on the Oriental approach to health. However, this system is optimized for finger pressure and manipulation instead of needling, as in ACUPUNCTURE or MOXIBUSTION, the use of heated herbs on acupuncture points.

The system combines this energetic method with a sophisticated method of nonforceful structural release and balancing. This system incorporates neurological repatterning techniques to prevent recurrent loss of alignment.

Also unique to this system is acupressure lymphatic drainage, which serves to augment the functioning of the lymphatic system thereby supporting the immune, reparative and eliminative functions on a cellular level.

Additionally, the Integrative Acupressure system is designed to be modular. Other techniques and modalities can be integrated using the overview and understanding afforded by the Integrative Acupressure system. Several Western alternative techniques are included and practitioners are encouraged to develop their own techniques by using the systems with which they are familiar.

Integrative Acupressure was developed by Samuel McClellan, Director of the New England Institute for Integrative Acupressure in Haydenville, Massachusetts.

integrative eclectic shiatsu a variation of the SHIATSU Japanese massage system, which combines CHINESE MEDICINE methods and Japanese *komo anma* techniques[1] with Eastern and Western SPORTS MASSAGE procedures.

Integrative eclectic shiatsu was developed by Toshiko Phipps who studied and practiced sports massage and Oriental healing methods in her native Japan. In 1936, she worked at the Japanese Winter Olympics Ski Training Center. She came to the United States in 1950 to continue her studies. She opened her own school, the Nippon Shiatsu Daigaku, in Putney, Vermont, and was a founding member of the American Oriental Bodywork Therapy Association (A.O.B.T.A.) in 1990.

Integrative eclectic shiatsu is a healing and preventive art, which integrates and promotes healthy functioning of the body/mind/spirit. It is a synthesis of Japanese shiatsu, which uses the MERIDIAN system and ACUPUNCTURE points, and Western and Eastern manipulations.

The effects of this system often restores the normal flow of energy within the meridians, blood and lymph vessels. Shiatsu pressure along the spine relieves entrapped nerves and, consequently, strengthens the corresponding organs. It is most beneficial in treating problems that are functional, such as lethargy, poor circulation, numbness, neuralgia, back pain, insomnia, digestive and elimination discomforts, PMS and menstrual cramps and breathing difficulties.

There are over 3,000 hand techniques in *koho anma*. These are some of the most frequently used movements in integrative eclectic shiatsu: *hirate-no-te,* a gentle touch used to evaluate and treat. It is performed with either one or both hands. **Rubbing** is gentle pressure in a circular motion. **Kneading,** just like kneading bread dough, is performed by grasping the muscle with firm pressure. **Tapotement** is a percussive stroke performed with a variety of finger or hand positions. **Pressing** provides finger or hand pressure directly into the center of the body or toward the meridian flow. **Stretching** puts pressure following the meridian lines to work for energy, or from the origin to insertion (the attachment points) of a muscle to work on them

by elongating the underlying tissue. **Vibration** can be done with the hand, fingers or thumbs. *K'yokude* is a form of tapotement where the striking surfaces are the joints of the hands. **Mobilization** is a form of joint range of motion, which can include stretching, pushing, pulling or shaking.

Five forms of pressure are incorporated into the strokes of integrative eclectic shiatsu. *Shiatsu* is gentle touch used primarily to evaluate and heal. The pressure of **shiatsu**, three pounds in the head and neck region and 17 to 20 pounds for the rest of the body, can be done with fingers, hands or thumbs and held at a comfortable level for three to five seconds. Shiatsu pressure moves the KI energy and provides deep relaxation. *Hakuatsu* is forceful pressure done with fingers, thumbs, hands, knuckles, elbows, knees, feet or magnet tools. The stroke is performed in short, quick motions that are held for 5 to 10 seconds. Longer pressure, from 30 to 60 seconds, may be used until the release of energy is felt. *Kiatsu* directs *ki* energy into the body and may be done with fingers, thumbs or palms, using an extremely gentle touch. The acupuncture point is held until the energy block is released. *Yokuatsu* is used exclusively around the navel to regulate high and low blood pressure and reduce fever. It moderates the aortic pulse, which stabilizes the heartbeat. The pads of three fingers are gently pressed into the aortic pulse and held for one minute. The five-pound pressure is released for two seconds and then repeated. This process, called *sairin yokuatsu,* may continue for 10 to 20 minutes, or as long as one hour, until balance is restored.

The sequence of a full-body treatment begins with the head and follows the YANG meridians down the back of the body to the feet. With the client in a supine position, the practitioner begins on the feet and proceeds upward with the YIN energy to the head.

Note
[1]Phipps, Toshiko, *American Oriental Bodywork Therapy Association Education Program: Integrative Eclectic Shiatsu,* Putney, Vt., no date, p. 1. *Koho anma* is one of the traditional

ancient Chinese massage methods. *An* means pressure, which represents sedation, while *ma* implies rubbing and represents tonification. This system is used to regulate the condition of the *ki* (*qi*) energy and blood.

integrative psychotherapy a psychotherapeutic process, which incorporates several different approaches to psychotherapy and body therapy, developed by psychologist Joel Ziff after 15 years of study and personal growth work. His training included doctoral work in developmental psychology, RUBENFELD SYNERGY family systems, GESTALT, transactional analysis, classical HYPNOSIS and ERICKSONIAN HYPNOSIS.

The focus of integrative psychotherapy is the concept of **habituation.** Ziff believes that people develop habitual ways of responding, which becomes unconscious. They may become habits of posture and movement, spirit, beliefs and ways of relating to ourselves and others.

The therapeutic process begins by creating a safe environment in order to heighten the awareness of these habits, build on strengths and expand an individual's range of choices. Focus can be shifted according to what is most efficient and effective through the course of the work. Decision making is based on dialogue and mutuality between the client and the therapist.

internal organ massage See CHI NEI TSANG.

iridology, or eye diagnosis, is the study of the markings of the iris to diagnose specific illnesses. It correlates areas of the iris (the colored, contractile membrane of the eye around the pupil) with specific body parts. Iridology can also be used to determine the presence of toxins, drugs or dietary deficiencies.

Iridology is based on a system devised by Hungarian physician Ignatz von Peczely during the 19th century and adapted by American chiropractor Dr. Bernard Jensen in the 1950s. As a young man, Peczely was playing with an owl when he inadvertently broke its leg. He happened to look into the bird's eye and saw a black line developing in the lower region of its iris. He cured the bird (which incidentally stayed

with him) and, over the years, the streak faded to a white line.

As a physician, Peczely used the opportunity to notate the eye markings of his patients in regards to their relationship with the physical problem. In 1881, he published his findings, complete with charts, which correlated body parts to specific regions of the iris. A Swedish homeopath, Nils Liljequist, improved many of the diagnostic techniques.

Dr. Jensen's theory divides the iris into six regions, or zones, and relates them to body systems and organs. The innermost zone, the one surrounding the pupil, relates to the stomach. Proceeding outward, the second zone relates to the intestines, the third to the blood and lymph systems, the fourth to organs and glands, the fifth to the muscular and skeletal systems and the sixth to the skin and organs of elimination.

The iris is further divided into upper and lower halves. The upper half corresponds with the top of the body including the brain, face, neck, lungs and throat. The lower half of the eye relates to the lower half of the body. The right eye represents the right side of the body and the left eye, the left side. Jensen assigned every organ a particular location on one or both irises.

Iridologists also make distinctions in the lightness or darkness of the iris, which indicates the level of drug toxicity, and any unusual markings that may appear in any region. A dark rim around the iris may signify sluggish elimination of waste products, which might affect the skin. White marks may indicate stress or inflammation on the respective organ, while dark marks may explain sluggishness and poor nutrition.

The fibers within the iris are also examined for their texture. A strong constitution is represented by a fine-grained pattern, while loosely woven fibers may signify general weakness.

Iridologists theorize that the hundred thousand nerve endings in the iris connect to organs and nerve systems through the optic nerve and spinal cord. Dr. Jensen recognizes that iridology is not all-inclusive, but that as a diagnostic tool,

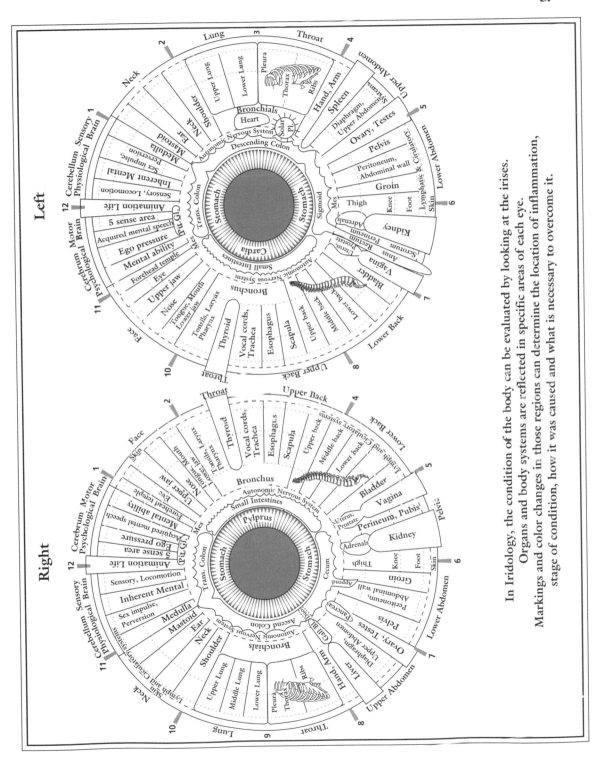

In Iridology, the condition of the body can be evaluated by looking at the irises. Organs and body systems are reflected in specific areas of each eye. Markings and color changes in those regions can determine the location of inflammation, stage of condition, how it was caused and what is necessary to overcome it.

it has a definite place in preventive health care.[1] He maintains that its advantages over conventional forms of diagnosis are numerous. The inherent structure and working capacity of an organ can be determined through iris diagnosis, environmental strain can be recognized, blood circulation and nerve force can be ascertained and pressure systems, such as prolapsus, can be detected early.

The iris of the eye can reveal acute, subacute, chronic and destructive phases in the body[2] as well as functional weaknesses. It reveals the suppression of diseases, possibly from incorrect medication, and indicates when tissues are or are not healing. Iridologists use this diagnostic skill to forewarn their clients of impending disease, in time, perhaps, to prevent their occurrence.

Iris analysis is performed by photographing the eyes with a specialized camera. These pictures are enlarged and examined by the iridologist.

The National Iridology Research Association was created in 1982 to promote the knowledge of iridology and provide a source of information and research.

Notes

[1] Jensen, Bernard, D.C., N.D., *The Science and Practice of Iridology,* BiWorld Publications, Inc., Provo, Utah, 1952, p. ii.

[2] The iris is constructed in four layers. According to iridology, each layer represents a particular stage of a disease, from the superficial acute stage, to the deepest, most destructive stage.

Further Reading

Deck, Josef, *Differentiation of Iris Marking,* Ettlingen, Germany, 1983. This illustrated and photographed diagnostic manual for advanced students contains information on treatment, genetic disposition and principles of pathology. Each organ zone is fully described.

_____ , *Principles of Iris Diagnosis,* Institute Fund Research, Portland, Oreg., 1985. Color photographs help to explain the concepts of iris diagnosis. This authority is considered to be an expert in the field of iridology.

Farida, Sharan, *Iridology,* Thorson's, London, 1989. This book provides clear explanations and illustrations of iris diagnosis.

Jensen, Bernard, D.C., N.D., *The Science and Practice of Iridology,* Vol. 1, BiWorld Publications, Inc., Provo, Utah, 1952. The textbook of iridology, written by America's foremost authority, is a comprehensive book that provides graphic illustrations and detailed explanations of this diagnostic science.

_____ , *Iridology: Science and Practice in Healing Arts,* Vol. II, B. Jensen, Escondido, Calif., 1982. This 600-page book, which took the author 10 years to write, is considered to be the definitive text of iridology. It includes over 1,200 color plates personally chosen by the author along with charts and illustrations. Plastic overlays for the eye picture and reference every organ as reflexively seen in the iris.

_____ , *What Is Iridology?* B. Jensen, Escondido, Calif., 1984. This is an introduction to iridology and its relation to nutrition. The basic principles of healing, energy and history of this system are discussed. Color photographs of eye fiber structures are included.

J

Jin Shin Acutouch^{SM} a system that includes self-help and treatments for others by touching points on the body to stimulate the flow of QI throughout the MERIDIANS. It is an amalgamation of many Oriental systems including JIN SHIN JYUTSU, the FIVE ELEMENT THEORY, Taoist philosophy and YOGA. This system is also comprised of forms of MEDITATION, BREATH THERAPY and principles of TAI CHI combined with psychological awareness, nutrition, vitamins and herbs to create a complete healing system.

The name translates to "compassionate spirit penetrating through touch." It is a derivative of Jin Shin Jyutsu, an ancient healing system, which was rediscovered by Jiro Murai in Japan in the early 1900s and brought to America by Mary Burmeister, his pupil, in the 1950s. Jin Shin Acutouch uses the same 26 energy centers, or **keys** in specific patterns of touch. When two energy centers are simultaneously touched, the energy flows between them, promoting healing.

Jin Shin Acutouch was developed in 1978 by Barbara Clark. Clark suffered from chronic asthma, which left her with only a 35 percent lung capacity and an eight-year dependency on steroids. She looked into alternative healing methods to help her and received her first Jin Shin Jyutsu treatment in 1977. That initial treatment cleared her lungs for two hours before the wheezing began again—her first relief in years. Weekly sessions strengthened her body and helped Clark reduce, and eventually give up, most of her medications and doubled her lung capacity.

She began studying Jin Shin Jyutsu, TUI-NA, Taoist healing and philosophy and other martial arts concerned with physical or energy movements. Putting it all together, along with her knowledge of nutrition and vitamins, Clark created Jin Shin Acutouch.

When two specific points on the body are touched and held for one to five minutes, the energy of the hands activates the energy flow.

The hands act as "jumper cables," recharging the energy system. Daily self-help routines can be used to maintain good health or to help in the healing process.

Jin Shin Acutouch can be performed almost anywhere. When it is performed by a facilitator, the recipient lies on her back, dressed in loosely fitting clothes. Shoes and jewelry should be removed. Sessions last for 60 to 90 minutes.

The meridians of Jin Shin Acutouch operate on the same theory as ACUPUNCTURE except the patterns and directions may be different, especially the diagonal meridians. The main central flow pattern is the source for all other flows (meridians). The points along this main flow are primarily concerned with well-being. The major vertical pattern balances each side of the body and the organ meridians. The minor diagonal pattern harmonizes the flow between the right and left sides and upper and lower body.

As the energy circulates throughout the meridians, the recipient may experience calmness, peace and a more balanced state of health.

Further Reading
Clark, Barbara, *Jin Shin Acutouch: The Tai Chi of Healing Arts,* Clark Publications, San Diego, Calif., 1987. This book clearly explains all the various systems that combine to make up Jin Shin Acutouch.

Jin Shin Do®* Bodymind Acupressure™ translates to mean "the way of the compassionate spirit," or as "body/spirit way," is an integrated body/mind system that combines Japanese ACUPRESSURE, the psychological theories of Wilhelm Reich and Carl Jung, Taoist philosophy, breathing techniques, and verbal body focusing to release emotional and physical tensions. It honors the unity of the body/mind, which permits a return to one's inner nature and emphasizes personal growth.

---

*"Jin Shin Do" is a registered trademark owned by Iona Marsaa Teeguarden and used with permission.

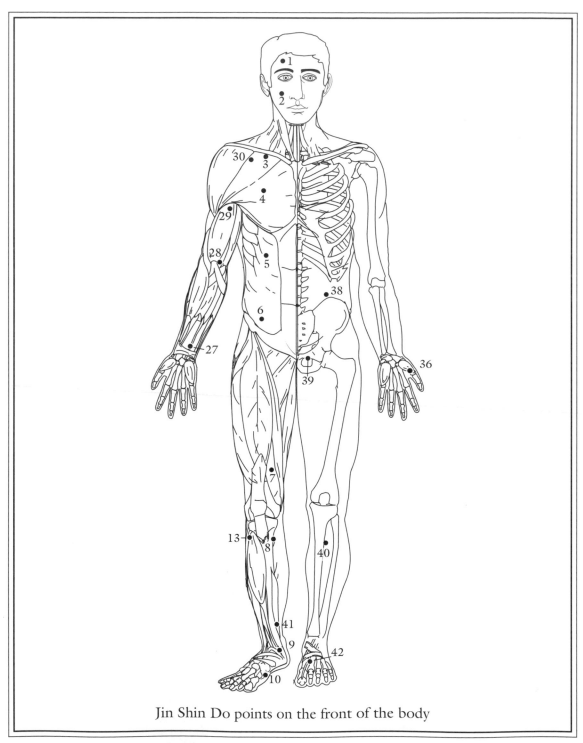

Jin Shin Do points on the front of the body

The integrated acupressure system of Jin Shin Do uses a 45-point system to release emotional and physical tensions and offer deep relaxation. Each point is held for an average of one to two minutes, using a unique finger pressure technique.

It was developed by Iona Marsaa Teeguarden, M.T., M.A., L.M.F.C.C., after nearly two decades of bodywork study and experience in the United States, Canada and Europe.

Jin Shin Do can be used to help many physical ailments such as headaches, insomnia and backaches and to reduce daily tensions and emotional stresses. It is a deeply relaxing system, which balances the body's energy.

This bodywork can be self-administered using the 30-point system, a color-coded chart and **release recipes,** which provide fast relief for many common symptoms. Professional training provides information on 45 main Jin Shin Do points plus a couple hundred additional release points, the traditional energy channels, the Chinese FIVE ELEMENT THEORY and the psychotherapy theories of Reich's **armoring** and Jung's **individuation.**

This acupressure system is the only one to emphasize the "strange flows" of the ACUPUNCTURE MERIDIAN system.[1] The Chinese consider these extraordinary channels to be reservoirs of the body's essence and don't use them as often as they do the regular channels, but Jin Shin Do recognizes them as the body's self-regulating mechanisms. They are a network of energy channels that connects with and monitors the energy flow of the 12 organ meridians, collects and releases energy throughout the meridian system and transports QI energy (life's vital energy) all over the body.[2] Jin Shin Do also uses **acu-points** along the strange flows, as well as along the organ meridians, to help balance *qi* energy. Acu-points, like acupuncture points, are concentrated points of energy, which conduct *qi* energy along the meridians.

A **local point** is held while one or more **distal points** are pressed. The distal point stimulation helps to expedite the release of tension.

The finger pressure techniques of Jin Shi Do are unique to this system. It is firm but gentle pressure on the acu-points, carefully avoiding extremes of touch, which are neither too light nor too aggressive.

Contacting the acu-point is a primary concern. This involves accurate point location and the optimum angle of pressure. On YIN areas, such as the chest or abdomen, the weight of the practitioner's arm should sink into the point. In YANG areas, which are thicker and more muscular, such as the back, the practitioner can lean into the body, producing stronger pressure. The acu-point pressure should not create resistance. The practitioner's fingers curl into the client's body for maximum pressure with minimum discomfort. *Teh qi,* or connecting with the *qi,* is achieved by getting into or under the tension. Locating the exact point at the optimum angle can melt the tension within seconds.[3]

Jin Shin Do considers emotions as positive forces that guide individuals through life and lead to self-awareness. All too often, however, these emotions are suppressed and their free expression is blocked. Unavailable emotions eventually become physical tensions, locked in specific parts of the body. Jin Shin Do seeks to unlock these tensions and reestablish a free flow of feelings. The yin meridians relate to actual emotions, while the yang meridians relate to our attitudes about emotions.

Wilhelm Reich believed that the life force, which he called **orgone energy,** flowed within vertical pathways. He also theorized that specific emotions are stored in particular body parts. For instance, the chest might hold feelings of joy and/or sadness, or the diaphragm might control anger or aggressiveness.

Unexpressed or blocked feelings are physicalized by tensions in muscle groups, called **segments.** Chronic problems, or armoring of the body, develop when free expression is withheld over a long period of time. Jin Shin Do recognizes the body/mind connection established by Reichian theories.

The Five Element Theory, which explains that the meridians relate to specific emotional energy and expression, is also incorporated into Jin Shin Do.

In each session, which lasts 60 to 90 minutes,

the client lies fully clothed on his back, removing only his shoes. The practitioner observes the client and then takes his PULSES. The practitioner palpates his body to assess where the tensions are and then begins the point work on the area(s) that require attention. Each point is held an average of one to two minutes, although, in some cases where tension is chronic, the point can be held as long as five minutes.

Channeling meditations help the practitioner channel *qi* energy and keep her own body relaxed. The trance state can also uncover any hidden talents, unexplored potential and resources, which could make the session more effective.

The Jin Shin Do Foundation was founded in 1982 to provide advanced training, to promote the growth of Jin Shin Do, to offer a network and resource center for authorized teachers and to furnish information to the public and professionals about the system.

Notes

[1] Porter, Arnold, "The Two Eyes of Jin Shin Do," *Heartwood: Journal of Experience, Expressions and Odyssey,* September/October 1988. Vol. vii, No. 4, p. 1. "Strange flows" have also been translated as "extraordinary meridians," "odd conduits" or "psychic (occult) channels."

[2] The 12 organ, or regular meridians are: bladder, gall bladder, liver, lung, large intestine, small intestine, kidney, heart, heart constrictor (pericardium), stomach, spleen and triple warmer (triple heater).

[3] Teeguarden, Iona Marsaa, "Jin Shin Do Is Acupressure," *The Acupressure News,* Vol. 11, 1994. Jin Shin Do Foundation, Palo Alto, Calif.

Further Readings

Teeguarden, Iona Marsaa, M.A., M.T., L.M.F.C.C., *The Acupressure Way of Health: Jin Shin Do®*, Japan Publications, Tokyo and New York, 1978. Teeguarden's first book describes the theory, philosophy and practice of Jin Shin Do. This illustrated book also instructs the reader in self-help techniques.

———, *Fundamentals of Self-Acupressure,* Jin Shin Do® Foundation, Felton, Calif., 1989. This booklet provides easy-to-follow self-acupressure sessions for common problems and general stress reduction. Illustrations and photographs make this a clear guide.

———, *The Joy of Feeling: Bodymind Acupressure,* Japan Publications, Tokyo and New York, 1987. This compre-

hensive, illustrated book explains the integration of Eastern acupressure and Taoism with Western psychological theories to create the unique bodywork system of Jin Shin Do.

———, *A Complete Guide to Acupressure,* Japan Publications, Tokyo and New York, 1995. Teeguarden's latest book discusses the theory of acupressure and the basics of emotional programming. Detailed chapters on many common ailments offer a variety of acu-point combinations for their relief.

Jin Shin Jyutsu® an energy-balancing art that facilitates the release of physical tensions, which may cause disease, by unblocking the energy pathways. *Jin* (man of knowing and compassion), *shin* (creator) *jyutsu* (art) translate as "art of the creator through man of knowing and compassion." Jin Shin Jyutsu harmonizes body/mind/spirit and is considered to be an art by its practitioners, rather than a technique. An art is a skillful creative process, whereas a technique is a mechanical application.

This ancient art was brought to the United States by Mary Burmeister who learned it in Japan from her teacher, Master Jiro Murai. Murai, who was raised in a family of medical professionals, was stricken in his 20s by an illness considered terminal. Since traditional medicine offered no hope for his condition, he decided to spend his remaining days at his family's mountain cabin. He instructed his family to leave him at the cabin for seven days and to come for him on the eighth to see the outcome. For those seven days, Murai meditated upon the sages he had learned about and practiced the hand poses that he had observed them using (known as *mudras* in India and *ijur* in Japan). With each passing day, Murai experienced his body becoming colder and colder. Then, on the seventh day, it was as if fire coursed through his body, and Murai felt that he was ready to die. Yet to his surprise, his body began cooling and when he regained normal body temperature, he found that he was cured. He prayed to God and gave thanks for his healing and dedicated the rest of his life to the study and research of Jin Shin Jyutsu.

A Jin Shin Jyutsu session lasts for approximately one hour. To receive a session, the client lies fully clothed, face up, on a padded surface or massage table. The Jin Shin Jyutsu practitioner utilizes a **flow** to harmonize energy pathways. A flow is a sequence in which hands are placed along the various **safety energy locks,** which are located along these pathways. When any of these 26 safety energy locks become locked or tense, they can serve as friendly reminders that we need to get ourselves back into harmony. In holding the safety energy locks, tensions are released as the circulation of energy flows freely.

Hand pressure may vary in Jin Shin Jyutsu and pressure is not necessary for the release of tensions along the energy pathways. Rather, the hands are used as "jumper cables" through which flow is limitless universal energy, which is the true harmonizer. Further, Jin Shin Jyutsu can be used as a powerful self-help tool. For example, each finger can be held for a few minutes or until a quiet rhythmic pulsation is felt, indicating the harmonizing of the energy flow.

Each finger is associated with a specific emotion or attitude as well as its share of the many functions throughout the body. Specifically, the thumb is held to harmonize worry; the index finger is held to harmonize fear; the middle finger is held to harmonize anger; the ring finger is held to harmonize sadness; and the little finger is held to harmonize pretense or trying to (making an attempt).

Further Reading

All books are written by Mary Burmeister and can be obtained at the Jin Shin Jyutsu Center in Scottsdale, Arizona, in person or by mail.

Self-Help Book 1: Getting to Know (help) Myself: Art of Living. This book contains basic daily tension releases, a history of Jin Shin Jyutsu and an introduction to the application of the universal life energy.

Self-Help Book 2: Mankind's "Safety" Energy Locks and Keys. This book locates and explains the 26 safety energy locks. Self-help routines are provided.

Self-Help Book 3: Fun with Fingers and Toes. The third book explores "jumper cable" energy, the relationship between fingers and toes and simple finger postures, which harmonize the total being.

Fun with Happy Hand. This is an illustrated guide for children, which introduces them to Jin Shin Jyutsu.

Johrei® a form of Japanese spiritual healing, which manifests through the focusing of divine light. Johrei (*jo* means "purify" and *rei* means "spirit") initiates a natural purifying process, which promotes inner spiritual balance and eases physical, mental and emotional distress. Repeated over a period of time, this system purifies the spiritual body, allowing it to become more radiant and encouraging one's divine nature to unfold. Johrei is a system used to relieve stress and promote healing.

Practitioners of Johrei believe that suffering, as well as health, is a reflection of the spiritual condition. A clouded spiritual condition will manifest in some form of disease, conflict or poverty. On the other hand, a bright spiritual condition will produce health, peace and prosperity.

As spiritual awareness and understanding begin to unfold, the consciousness expands, positively affecting all aspects of our being. Gradually, with Johrei, people become self-realized as to their mission in life: to help others become happy. The spiritual condition becomes brighter, which allows people to return to the natural state of true health.

During a session, which lasts about 20 minutes, a channeler sits in front of, or behind, a seated participant with a raised, cupped hand, meditating to receive energy. The participant closes her eyes and relaxes until she, too, experiences the flow of energy.

The Johrei Fellowship is an international association of individuals from many countries, cultures and faiths, joined together in a common spiritual practice. The Fellowship has, as its underlying principle, the belief that through the practice of truth, virtue and beauty in our daily lives, we can transform the three major sufferings of humanity: disease, conflict and poverty, into a state of health, peace and prosperity. The ultimate vision of the Fellowship is the manifestation of a true paradise on earth. All members of the Fellowship are trained to give Johrei and membership is open to all. There is never a charge for Johrei.

Mokichi Okada, also known as Meishu-sama, the Japanese philosopher, poet, artist, teacher, businessman and visionary, founded the movement in 1935. Through a series of divine revelations, Meishu-sama became aware of God's plan for the new age and of major world changes that would occur before its coming. He realized that Johrei could help humanity make the necessary change in consciousness to promote this transition.

He taught three basic activities: to give service to others, to appreciate beauty and art and to care for one's physical health and the environment. Three main activities of the Fellowship work toward these goals: Johrei, the spiritual aspect; *sangetsu* **flower arranging** ("moon over mountain") to present the hidden beauty in the flowers rather than imposing one's will on them and the arrangement; and, natural farming, which employs no synthetic chemicals in the growing of the food.

K

kahuna bodywork (see LOMILOMI) also called Hawaiian bodywork or Hawaiian temple bodywork.

ki See CHI.

ki-shiatsu a therapeutic Oriental bodywork synthesized from CHINESE MEDICINE, MACROBIOTIC MEDICINE and MACROBIOTIC SHIATSU. It is based on the ancient principle that each person is an integral part of nature. The main focus of ki-shiatsu is to free blocked, stagnated energy, or *ki* (CHI) for optimum health and to strengthen any weaknesses between the body/mind.

Ki-shiatsu was developed in the 1970s by Susan Krieger over two decades of personal and professional experience in the Oriental healing arts. Her work and studies have taken her throughout the United States, Europe and Asia. Krieger is a certified shiatsu practitioner and instructor, vice president of the American Oriental Bodywork Therapy Association (A.O.B.T.A.), a founding member of the International Macrobiotic Shiatsu Society, producer of the Ki-Shiatsu Instructional Video, a macrocounselor and lecturer.

The recipient of ki-shiatsu is given a calm, personal space in which to partake of, and participate in, the treatment. The *ki* of the environment and the healing focus of the practitioner are vital to, and are reflected in, the work.

Practitioners use their fingers, thumbs, hands, arms, elbows and (barefoot) feet to apply a varying amount of noninvasive touch pressure and techniques along the MERIDIANS, energy pathways, and TSUBOS, specific points of energy on the meridians. Yogalike movements, stretches and corrective exercises are incorporated in the treatment. When the *ki* has been released and is flowing smoothly, organs and body systems heal naturally.

Each session starts with assessments of the recipient's condition, which are based on the *do,* or way, of visual, verbal and touch techniques. The FIVE ELEMENTS-Transformations are used as an evaluation and treatment tool along with PULSE READING, facial diagnosis, posture analysis, personal history of the individual's nutritional habits and state of physical and emotional health.

The ki-shiatsu practitioner guides and supports all those who are dealing with health issues and complaints on many levels. Ki-shiatsu has been used to relieve tension, enhance postsurgical recuperation, for general health improvement, as a preventive to avoid injury or pain and to clear unexpressed emotions while addressing the recipient's physical, emotional and spiritual health.

This system also teaches individuals ways to help themselves with self-shiatsu massage, corrective exercises and QIGONG, dietary and lifestyle recommendations, breathing exercises and home remedies, such as external compresses and medicinal plant foods.

kidney meridian a YIN meridian whose element is water and sense organ is the ear. It controls the spirit and *qi* energy to the body, providing resistance against mental stress by controlling hormonal secretions. It also produces bone marrow and brain tissue. This meridian helps to detoxify and purify the blood.

Traditionally, the right kidney is called the **gate of life** where prenatal *qi* originated.

The kidney meridian flows bilaterally from the bottom of the feet, up the body to the clavicles (collarbones). There are 27 ACUPUNCTURE points along this energy pathway.

kinesiology the science of mechanics and principles of human movement. Structural kinesiology is involved with the study of muscles as they are involved in movement. Principles of kinesiology, when applied to muscles and physical development, have increased muscular strength and improved physical performance.

Structural kinesiologists can analyze any exercise or sport and recognize which muscle groups are primarily being used, developed or rehabilitated. Understanding physical laws of gravity, leverage, motion and balance are also vital factors in analyzing movement.

The Council of Kinesiology, the national association, was founded in 1968.

kripalu bodywork based on the principles of kripalu yoga, known as meditation in motion. This system emphasizes the integration of body/mind/spirit through awareness, deep relaxation and a meditative focus on physical sensation. It also seeks to release the emotional and mental obstacles held in the body through a system of sensitive touch.

The kripalu bodywork training grounds the practitioner in the basic techniques of bodywork that release and minimize tension, such as SWEDISH MASSAGE, TRIGGER POINT WORK and ENERGY BALANCING. One of the distinguishing characteristics of kripalu bodywork is that it encourages practitioners to maintain a daily spiritual practice of yoga or meditation and to bring their spiritual awareness and level of spiritual practice into the massage room. Using the heightened awareness gained from her spiritual practice, the bodyworker creates a massage experience that is spiritually profound for both practitioner and recipient.

The goal of kripalu bodywork is to stimulate *prana,* life force energy that lives in each of us, and to expand consciousness. In a kripalu bodywork session, the bodyworker guides the client through the range of physical sensations or emotional releases that may arise. Through these releases, the bodyworker stimulates the *prana* in the recipient's body, facilitating an experience of deep relaxation and integration between body/mind/spirit. To help the client maintain the balance after the massage, the bodyworker may recommend yoga *asanas* (postures) or breathing exercises for the client to practice at home.

Kripalu bodywork emphasizes the importance of creating a massage experience that is rewarding and fulfilling for both giver and recipient. To support both the client and the bodyworker in remaining present and aware of their bodies and breath, both are encouraged to breathe consciously during the massage experience.

Kripalu bodywork is taught at the Kripalu Center for Yoga and Health in the Berkshire Mountains of Lenox, Massachusetts. Named after the yoga master Swami Shri Kripalvanandaj, this nonprofit center was founded on the belief that all humanity belongs to one family and that the divine lives within each of us. Also an intentional spiritual community, the 300 resident volunteers follow the tenets of *vairagya,* simplicity, *brahmacharya,* celibacy outside of marriage, and *tapascharya,* willful spiritual discipline.

Kriya Massage™ places emphasis on the practitioner's intuitive abilities while performing the massage. It is defined as spontaneous energy movement, and the practitioner flows with this movement during the session. Kriya Massage combines universal, life-affirming energy with classical massage techniques to form a continuous dance. The **universal four forces,** centripetal, centrifugal, gravity and electromagnetic forces, are incorporated into the massage to create an individually designed treatment.

Kriya Massage was developed by Kamala Renner in 1970 as part of her ALCHEMICAL SYNERGY work.

The strokes used in Kriya Massage are a combination of ENERGY WORK, SWEDISH MASSAGE, NEUROMUSCULAR THERAPY, and SOMATO-EMOTIONAL RELEASE. The experience of Kriya Massage is often described as "stepping out of time and space" in order to take inventory of one's life.[1] The subconscious is allowed to readjust preprogrammed attitudes. Kriya Massage's healing quality takes place when these outdated attitudes are transformed into beliefs that are appropriate for the present, which can be as beneficial to the practitioner as it is to the client.

Note
[1] Kamala Renner interview, April 1994.

Kurashova massage See RUSSIAN MASSAGE.

L

Laban movement analysis a system which defines, analyzes and promotes greater awareness of all movement. The participant also learns to understand and improve upon his physical expressivity. This work can be applied to general movement such as simple gestures to more complex movements often found in performance.

Rudolf Laban (1879–1958) was born in Austro-Hungary. He was a dancer, choreographer and teacher. The system he developed incorporates three primary components of movement: the body, spatial awareness and the purpose or intent of the movement. These theories can be applied whenever movement is used for communication and expression, including dance, theater, psychology, physical therapy, bodywork, fitness, sports training and nonverbal communication.

large intestine meridian, according to CHINESE MEDICINE, is a YANG meridian whose element is metal. It helps the function of the lungs. The detoxification, secretions and excretions of the body are influenced by this meridian. It also helps in the elimination of stagnated *qi* energy. The large intestine flows bilaterally down the body from the lower eyelids to the second toes. There are 20 ACUPUNCTURE points along this meridian.

laying on of hands a healing technique in which the provider allows the universal healing energy to flow through her hands into the energy field of the recipient. This rebalanced energy flow can relieve energy blockages, which may be responsible for physical, emotional, mental or spiritual disorders.

Laying on of hands, as in all energetic healing systems, is based on the theory that the physical body is surrounded by a subtle energy, or AURA, and emotional body. It is believed that traumas

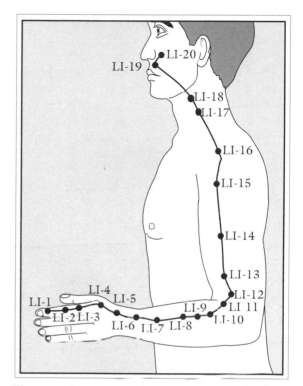

The yang large intestine meridian is involved in the function of the lungs, water metabolism, secretions and excretions. It flows bilaterally down each arm, starting from the second fingers to the side of the nostrils.

and pain can be stored within this energy biofield. The process of healing rebalances the energies within the body by focusing on the expression of the misalignment, correcting it and repairing the appropriate layer of the energy field.

Laying on of hands is practiced in many traditional cultures throughout the work, such as the espiritistas, the psychic surgeons and healers of the Philippines, usually coupled with a spiritual component.

Paintings discovered on the walls of caves in the Pyrenees, dating back 15,000 years, depict healing by touch. Medieval church carvings demonstrated laying on of hands as a healing technique. The "king's touch," as it was called, was used in England and France.

The belief is that touch restores balance and harmony to the energy bio-field, subsequently healing the recipient on all levels. The provider passes her hands over the body of the recipient, feeling for energy imbalances. These imbalances are manifested by skin temperature extremes of heat or cold, muscle tightness or pulsations. The provider touches those areas of tension, which acts as a conduit to boost the recipient's innate healing abilities.

Laying on of hands can also be self-administered.

light therapy, or radiation therapy, for healing purposes is generally limited to the use of INFRARED RAYS and ULTRAVIOLET RAYS.

Further Reading
Liberman, Jacob, *Light Medicine of the Future,* Bear & Co., Santa Fe, N.Mex., 1993. Liberman addresses the holism of a person—body/mind/spirit in a nonintrusive way. This book describes the use of light as a healing technique for cancer, PMS, sexual dysfunction, immune system disorders and learning disabilities.

liver meridian a YIN meridian in CHINESE MEDICINE whose element is wood and sense organ is the eye. It stores and distributes nutrients and energy for physical activity. It also cultivates resistance against disease and stores, analyzes and detoxifies the blood in order to maintain physical stamina.

The liver meridian, which has 14 ACUPUNCTURE points, flows bilaterally up the body from the big toes to the intercostal (between the ribs) space between the sixth and seventh ribs, just distal to the breasts.

lomi ka'ala hoku See LOMILOMI.

lomilomi originally known as **lomi ka'ala hoku,** "massage journey to the stars," is an ancient Hawaiian massage system, with many different styles, passed down from one generation to the next. Native Hawaiians believed that all nature is replete with the same energy or spirit, which they called **aloha 'aina.** It described their oneness with nature, filled with compassion and unconditional love.

The **kahuna lomi,** (*ka* translates to "keeper" and *huna* means "secret") massage masters or experts and shamanic leaders, communicated with the spirits of the body in the same way nature was addressed, respectfully and reverently. The kahuna lomi accepted the belief, passed down from ancient times, that each body part has its own consciousness, which contributed to the makeup of the larger consciousness of a person. Injury or illness was considered a problem in the life of the ailing body part. The malady often had emotional and/or psychological implications as well.

During a ritualistic dance-massage, the kahuna would enter into an altered state, which permitted him to communicate with the sick body part and ask it for cooperation in its own healing.

Originally performed as a rite of passage for adolescents, lomi ka'ala hoku was used to align and clear the spiritual and physical bodies of the children, enabling them to assume adult responsibilities. Visions of their purpose in life were commonplace during these sessions and the *mana,* or life energy, to carry out their life's work. Two to six kahuna lomi would perform the ritual, which lasted unceasingly from 10 hours to 10 days, depending on the child's status in the community. Two to six kahuna drummers and chanters accompanied the healers. It was believed that their incantations, coupled with the bodywork and *mana* flowing through the kahunas, caused the cells of the child to vibrate at higher frequencies, making it possible for the child to connect with *akasha,* universal knowledge.

The genetic vibrations experienced by the adolescent were expected to be felt by other members of the family, healing and uplifting them as well.

Babies were lomied in tide pools using hands and the soft, inner aspect of the arms, the way lomi ka'ala hoku is performed. Children who misbehaved were massaged to clear the disruptive energy, while the parents and family addressed that which was not in harmony with themselves.

This sacred healing art was handed down from kahuna to student in an unbroken chain for a millennium. This system was kept secret until the late 1970s when Abraham Kawai'i began to share the knowledge with the West. Modern use of lomi has not veered very far from its ancestral roots. No longer an exclusive ritual for adolescents, it is still used as a rite of passage to mark milestones in a person's life.

The massage can also be a physical therapy or a vehicle for the release of emotions, traumas, tension, stress and blocked energy. It is used to revive the body, to move blood and lymph, release muscle spasms and facilitate waste product removal from muscle and connective tissue. The concepts of unconditional love, grace, beauty and spirituality are inherent in lomi.

Currently, Abraham Kawai'i, the kahuna who passed down this lineage of lomi ka'ala hoku, is a teacher of this form. Harriette Sakuma is another teacher who does healings and has worked with this particular system for many years.

Another recognized form of Hawaiian bodywork is lomilomi. The healer most associated with lomilomi today is Aunty (a term of affection and respect) Margaret K. Machado (1916–) who has been practicing and teaching this ancient tradition for over 50 years. She calls lomilomi "the loving touch—a connection between heart, hands and soul with the source of all life."[1]

The most distinctive movement of traditional lomilomi is a kneading motion done toward the heart, using either thumbs, palms or forearms. However, a full range of massage strokes, EFFLEURAGE, PETRISSAGE, FRICTION, VIBRATION, PERCUSSION and kneading are also used. Special attention is paid to the *na'au,* the lower abdomen (see HARA), which is the center of all emotion and power, according to ancient Hawaiian philosophy.

In lomi ka'ala hoku, draping is a tool of the treatment. The recipient, lying on a massage table, can be draped to enhance the nurturing aspect of the treatment or the sheet can be used shamanically at the end of the session to cleanse and align the energy. Unscented oil is used as an energy transmitter.

Music is still an integral part of the session, which can last anywhere from two hours to all day. Trance-inducing drumming may begin a treatment, followed by more lyrical music, ending with ethereal sounds. Depending upon how an individual integrates the work, all Hawaiian music may be used.

The practitioner, in constant dance motion with the rhythm of the music, pulls energy from the universe (heaven and earth). She will look at the geomancy of the individual's body and will try to "raise the valleys" and "lower the hills," open the joints and lengthen the muscles and structure. The movement is choreographed in the moment, as the unique spirit and need of each person's body ultimately guides the session. The practitioner receives the healing as the energy pours through her. The movement is a dance of the spirit and soul of the recipient.

Strokes of an elongating nature are used to expand the body. The practitioner may rotate the joints, lift, cradle, hug and even turn the passive recipient. Before receiving the treatment, individuals are advised to fast or refrain from eating for up to four hours in order to expand their awareness of feelings and the intent of the sessions.

Ever conscious of working with nature, the practitioner will predominantly use the soft part of the forearms coupled with the dance to create the long, gliding strokes intrinsic to lomi ka'ala hoku. She may also use fingertips, hands, knuckles and elbows. In ancient times, a shamanic carved stick was used for deeper pressure and release. Each level of tissue can be treated, from the skin level to the bone level, using the mind and *mana* in conjunction with the pressure of the touch. The light work at skin level deals with more recent issues and the mind (relax the skin, relax the mind), while deeper and/or older traumas are found on deeper tissue levels.

It is a good idea to drink lots of water afterward, to continue the cleansing process. One usually feels the benefits on all levels for a period of time after the session.

Note
[1] Bogardus, Stephen, "Aunty Margaret Revisited," *Massage and Healing Arts Magazine,* Vol. 1, Issue 6, 1986, p. 30.

LooyenWork™ a painless approach to deep tissue therapy, which works with the CONNECTIVE TISSUE and FASCIAL components of the body to produce dramatic changes in posture. It is a combination of several restructuring systems, such as ROLFING, POSTURAL INTEGRATION, FELDENKRAIS, and ASTON-PATTERNING.

Ted Looyen, founder of LooyenWork, was born in Holland and received his education in Australia. In 1973, he sustained a serious back injury, which prompted him to become a bodyworker. His injury was most successfully treated by the deep tissue work of Rolfing, yet he did not believe that the pain involved was necessary to produce structural changes.

After many years of study and research, he developed his system in 1985, which provided all the benefits of deep tissue work without eliciting the pain. Looyen felt that causing such discomfort would be a repetition of the trauma, which initially created the problems. He believed in a process of gentle, slow release.

LooyenWork considers each person's individuality and his **core issue,** or the effects of emotional, physical and/or psychological traumas. Once the practitioner has determined the core issue, a treatment program is planned, addressing each physical problem as it arises.

The fingertip pressure of the practitioner is penetrating yet gentle. The practitioner works to release adhesions (fibers that stick together, forming nodules or "knots") of the connective tissue, stretch contracted muscles and separate tendons.

In addition to helping restructure the client's body, LooyenWork is also a way of working that protects the practitioner against injury.

lung meridian, according to CHINESE MEDICINE, is a YIN meridian whose element is metal and sense organ is the nose. The lung meridian also dominates the skin, especially the pores and body hair. (The hair of the head is governed by the KIDNEY meridian.) The lung meridian is involved with the intake of CHI energy and air. This energy is essential to help the body build resistance against external intrusions.

The lung meridian balances the water passages and eliminates stagnant *chi* energy through exhalation. It spreads vital fluids throughout the body.

The lung meridian flows bilaterally from the upper chest to the thumbs. There are 11 ACUPUNCTURE points along this energy pathway.

lymphatic drainage massage also known as manual lymph drainage or Dr. Vodder's Manual Lymph Drainage®, is a CONNECTIVE TISSUE massage technique, which accelerates the movement of lymphatic fluid (see LYMPHATIC SYSTEM), reduces **edema** (a condition in which the tissues of the body contain an excessive amount of fluid) and decongests all lymphatic pathways from the affected limb to the confluence of lymphatic and blood systems in the neck.

The lymphatic drainage massage was developed by Dr. Emil Vodder and his wife, Astrid, in 1932. These two Danish massage therapists were practicing in Cannes, on the French Riviera. Most of their clients were English vacationers who were recovering from chronic colds, due to the weather in England. Most had swollen lymph nodes in their necks. Although the prevailing attitude was to avoid massaging the lymphatic system directly, the Vodders recognized the need to stimulate lymph flow. Their results were successful and their client's colds finally got better.

For the next several years, they worked on developing the technique known as Dr. Vodder's Manual Lymph Drainage, expanding its applications and teaching throughout Europe. This system enhances immune system function and toxin removal, reduces edema (coupled with compression bandaging and exercise), increases tissue metabolism, improves nutrition to the tissues, promotes eliminative functions, establishes fluid balance in the tissues, reduces pain and induces deep relaxation.

Lymphatic drainage massage has made it possible for many people suffering from lymphedema and other conditions of obstructed lymph pathways to have relief. Lymphedema is the consequence of an insufficiency of the lymph vessel system, which may be caused by the surgical removal of the lymph nodes or radiation therapy. In cases of swollen extremities, the therapist uses manual lymph drainage to shunt the excess fluid to those areas where the lymph vessels are healthy and can reabsorb the fluid. The treatments must be frequent, anywhere from twice daily for serious lymphedemas to two to three times a week, with sessions lasting anywhere from 30 minutes to one hour. It is based on promoting the movement of lymph through gentle massage.

Lymphedema can create major medical complications: swelling of the limb or other affected body part that worsens over time, heaviness and limitation of movement, repeated episodes of infection, skin thickening, limited activities and the need for constant medical supervision.[1]

Lymphedema is either **primary** or **secondary**. Primary cases are caused without any obvious reason. They may be present at birth (lymphedema congenital), occur later in life (lymphedema praecox) or after the age of 35 (lymphedema tarda). It is more common in women than men and usually occurs in the lower extremities.

Secondary lymphedema is caused by injury, scarring or excision of lymph nodes, radiation therapy, traumas or infections to the lymph system. It is estimated that there are over 2,000,000 cases of secondary lymphedema in the United States, most commonly as a result of aggressive cancer therapies. In Third World countries, parasites are responsible for the obstruction of the lymphatics.[2]

The massage is always performed following the course of lymph flow, toward the heart. There are five basic techniques of lymphatic drainage massage: **stationary circles, pumping, scooping, rotary** and **thumb circle movements.**

Using manual lymphatic drainage massage helps to maintain adequate tissue oxygen and accelerates the removal of metabolic byproducts. Since inappropriately applied pressure can lead to tissue oxygen deprivation, correct pressure is an important consideration. The amount of pressure necessary to deflate lymph vessels is low, as little as 20-40 Hg pressure (one-tenth of a pound).[3]

The lymphatic system is responsible for keeping the connective tissue surrounding the cells of the body free from excess water, proteins, bacteria, viruses, inorganic materials such as dust and dyes, destroyed cells resulting from surgery or trauma, red blood cells, and other dead cells. Dr. Vodder called these materials the **lymph obligatory load** (L.O.L.). They make up approximately 10 percent of the fluid delivered to the connective tissue by the arterial capillaries as well as other debris that has found its way into the tissue. Because these molecules are all rather large, it is the "obligation" of the lymphatic system to remove these substances. The remaining 90 percent of the fluid, which consists of small molecular substances such as salts, sugars, water and gases, are removed by the capillaries of the venous system.[4]

The therapist uses precise, gentle, rhythmic strokes. The pumping action of the massage causes small capillaries to open and close, enhancing reabsorption of lymph from the tissues back into the lymph vessels and allowing the materials of the lymph obligatory load from the surrounding tissues to make their way by diffusion into the lymph vessels.

As a secondary effect, manual lymph drainage also stimulates the venous capillaries to reabsorb more materials, especially excess water (edema), from the tissue spaces. Healthy lymphatic and venous systems do this automatically.

For those people who have healthy lymph vessels but have sustained an injury, undergone surgery or are experiencing chronic inflammation, manual lymph drainage is beneficial. It helps by speeding up removal of the lymph obligatory load substances thereby allowing healthy fluids to move into the affected area and promoting healing.

Manual lymph drainage works consistently with the body's physiology. In addition to speeding up the removal of the lymph obligatory load, this system may stimulate the immune system to combat pathological conditions such as chronic inflammations. The repetitive and soothing movements stimulate pain-inhibitory reflexes, which may temporarily reduce pain. These movements also lower the activity of the sympathetic nervous system, permitting the client to experience deep relaxation. The effects of stress can be reduced and the body's self-healing mechanisms may be enhanced.

Remedial exercises are usually prescribed for each client. Exercise activates each muscle group and joints of the affected limb, resulting in increasing lymph flow. Compression bandaging, proper diet, hygiene and daily precautions are also important considerations.

Lymph massage is contraindicated in cases of active cancer, major heart trouble, recent thrombosis, phlebitis, acute inflammation related to infection or other severe conditions without medical approval.

Recognition of the value of manual lymph drainage has spread throughout Europe where it is practiced widely in hospitals and clinics. In Germany, it is the third most prescribed physical therapy.[5] It was formally introduced in North America in 1982 and is now being taught and practiced widely in the United States, Canada and Mexico.

Therapists of Dr. Vodder's Manual Lymph Drainage system must complete four weeks of training and pass an internationally recognized examination through the Dr. Vodder School of Walchsee, Austria, before receiving certification. Currently, there are approximately 250 certified Vodder therapists in the United States and Canada. Many other therapists are trained in lymphatic massage through other schools.

Notes

[1] Lymphedema Services, P.C., "Complete Decongestive Physiotherapy: An Innovative and Logical Approach to Lymphedema," Lymphedema Services, N.Y., 1991, p. 6.

[2] Ibid., pp. 2–3.

[3] Elden, Harry R., Ph.D., "In Class: Massage and Lymphatics—A Question of Pressure and Domain," *Massage Magazine,* Issue 16, October/November 1988, pp. 40–42. Millimeter mercury pressure is the quantitative measurement of touch pressure.

[4] Wyrick, Dana, "European Manual Lymph Drainage," Body Therapy, Dallas, Tex, October/November 1994, p. 2.

[5] Ibid., p. 2.

Further Reading

Kurz, Ingrid, *Introduction to Dr. Vodder's Manual Lymphatic Drainage,* Vol. 2, Therapy I, Karl F. Haug Publications, Heidelberg, Germany, 1986. This illustrated text provides the scientific basis and theoretical explanation of the action of Manual Lymphatic Drainage.

———— , *Introduction to Dr. Vodder's Manual Lymphatic Drainage,* Vol. 3, Therapy II, Karl F. Haug, Publications, Heidelberg, Germany, 1990. The therapeutic application and spectrum of diseases, including the contraindications of the massage and precautionary measures, are included in this text.

Wittlinger, Hildegard, *Introduction to Dr. Vodder's Manual Lymphatic Drainage,* Vol. 1, Basic Course. Karl F. Haug, Publishers, Heidelberg, Germany, 1986. This illustrated guide explains the basic course of this lymphatic massage system.

lymphatic system the body's drainage system composed of **lymph, lymph nodes, lymph vessels** and **lymph glands** such as the spleen, thymus gland and tonsils. The lymph system drains protein-containing fluid from the tissue spaces back into the cardiovascular system, filters the blood, transports fats from the digestive tract to the blood, produces blood cells (lymphocytes) and helps protect against disease and infection.[1]

Lymph is a clear, viscid fluid that is a by-product of tissue circulation and metabolism. It carries white blood cells and some red blood cells and is contained in the lymph vessels. It is slowly propelled through the lymph system by inter-vessel contractions, surrounding muscle contractions, intestinal movements, respiration and proper massage.

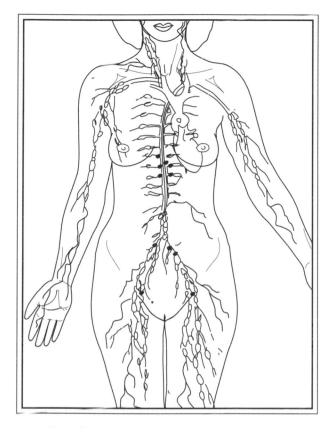

Lymph vessels, which are anatomically similar to veins, have numerous valves and hundreds of nodes that filter the lymph. Lymph is propelled toward the great veins in the neck, where it combines with blood on its way to the heart.

Lymph flows up the body, against gravity, in the same direction as venous blood flow.

There are over 600 lymph nodes, oval or bean-shaped structures, which are the system's filtering centers, scattered throughout the body. They are typically arranged in two sets: **superficial** and **deep.** Each node contains millions of lymphocytes (a type of white blood cell that fights infection) and can produce 10,000 to 100,000 different types of specially sensitized lymphocytes. During a serious illness, 2,000 specialized antibodies can be manufactured per second.[2]

Lymph circulates through a network of lymphatic vessels. These structure are anatomically similar to veins, contain numerous valves and nodes and are delicate and thin. Some lymph vessel walls are so thin that lymph is visible. The vessels carry the lymph from tissue spaces to lymph nodes and empty the processed fluid, about two quarts per day, back into the bloodstream. There are more lymph vessels and blood veins in the human body, but they are smaller in size.

There are several lymphoid organs, which are only related to this system in terms of their immune functions. The spleen is the largest lymph organ. It forms blood cells, filters harmful particles from the blood, stores iron for the manufacture of hemoglobin,[3] stores blood, manufactures bilirubin[4] and supplies antibodies to fight bacteria and parasites. The thymus gland is located in the upper thoracic cavity. About half of the **T cells,** lymphocytes that are responsible for cellular immunity, migrate to the thymus gland where they are processed. In some way, the thymus confers **immunologic competence** to these specialized T cells.[5] The tonsils, located in the pharynx, manufacture lymphocytes. When an infection is present in the body, the lymph nodes swell as lymphocytes multiply to defeat the illness.

Notes
[1] Tortora, Gerald J., and Anagnostakos, Nicholas P., *Principles of Anatomy and Physiology,* Harper & Row, N.Y., 1981, pp. 9, 524.
[2] Calvert, Robert, "Lymphatics: The Body's Drainage System," *Massage and Bodywork* Magazine, Vol. 1, Issue 5, 1986, p. 27.
[3] Hemoglobin is contained within red blood cells and is the pigment that unites with the oxygen and is carried to the tissues of the body.
[4] Bilirubin is a bile pigment derived from hemoglobin during the normal and pathological breakdown of red blood cells.
[5] Tortora, Gerald J., and Anagnostakos, Nicholas P., *Principles of Anatomy and Physiology,* Harper & Row, N.Y., 1981, p. 545.

M

macrobiotic medicine promotes a lifestyle based on the use of natural, native foods and proper cooking methods, SHIATSU or other forms of Oriental bodywork, exercises and breathing techniques to treat illnesses and maintain health.

As interpreted from ancient Greece, macrobiotics is the way of achieving longevity and happiness according to the principles of nature. In modern-day terms, this system offers a way to reach the universal dream of mankind—world peace.[1]

At the turn of the 20th century, George Ohsawa (1893–1966), who had cured himself of tuberculosis using this natural diet and coined the term macrobiotics (*macro* means "great" or "large" and *bios* means "life"), revitalized these theories. He lectured all over the world on the benefits of leading a lifestyle based on nature's laws. He arrived in the United States in 1959.

Ohsawa outlined several basic principles that explain macrobiotic theories: health is the natural condition of all human beings while illness is unnatural, or a sign of being out of balance with nature; health or sickness are not achieved accidentally; sickness is a direct result of a poor lifestyle; food is an important key in determining sickness and health; and seasonal foods that are locally grown are best to promote and maintain health.[2]

Food is a major factor in a person's health. People are advised to eat only when hungry, to eat only natural, whole foods according to the season and climate, consume a low-fat, high-fiber, high complex carbohydrate and low-protein diet, chew food well and eat only up to 80 percent of capacity. Foods, therefore, can become a person's medicine.

Macrobiotic medicine also recommends: adequate sleep, daily exercise, moderate sexual activity, medicinal food preparations, an attitude of appreciation for one's life, developing a positive acknowledgment and relationship with others, respecting the environment and the world at large and bodywork to provide a healthy lifestyle, respectful of nature's laws.

Notes
1 Kushi, Michio, *The Book of Macrobiotics,* Japan Publications, Inc., Tokyo, 1977. On book cover.
2 Yamamoto, Shizuko, and McCarthy, Patrick, *The Shiatsu Handbook,* Turning Point Publications, Eureka, Calif., 1986, p. 21.

Further Reading
Jack, Alex, *Let Food Be Thy Medicine,* One Peaceful World Becket, Mass., 1991. 185 scientific and medical reports demonstrate the importance of a grain-based, natural foods diet.

Kushi, Michio, *The Macrobiotic Way: The Complete Macrobiotic Diet and Exercise Book,* Avery Publishing Group, Inc., Wayne, N.J., 1985. Written by the foremost authority on macrobiotics, this book provides information about the healing properties in foods and illustrates exercises to maximize health.

———, *Standard Macrobiotic Diet,* One Peaceful World Press, Becket, Mass., 1996. This introductory guide to the macrobiotic way of eating includes recommendations for different climates, basic recipes and lifestyle suggestions.

———, *The Teachings of Michio Kushi,* One Peaceful World, Becket, Mass. The lectures of Michio Kushi included in this book cover various topics, such as the I Ching, diagnosis and physiognomy, war and peace, and what is happiness?

Ohsawa, George, *Art of Peace,* George Ohsawa Macrobiotic Foundation, Oroville, Calif., rev. ed., 1990. The principles of judo and akido are used to explain the nature of happiness, justice, freedom and world peace.

———, *Philosophy of Oriental Medicine,* George Ohsawa Macrobiotic Foundation, Oroville, Calif., 1960. A classic in macrobiotic writings, this book provides information about the macrobiotic lifestyle.

macrobiotic shiatsu supports a natural lifestyle and heightened instincts for improving health. It was founded by SHIATSU expert Shizuko Yamamoto and is based on George Ohsawa's (the originator of macrobiotics) philosophy that each individual is an integral part of nature.

Treatment involves noninvasive touch and pressure using hand and barefoot techniques combined with stretches to facilitate the flow of

QI, life's vital energy, and to strengthen the body/mind. Dietary guidance, medicinal plant foods, breathing techniques and home remedies are emphasized. Corrective exercises, postural rebalancing, palm healing, self-shiatsu and QI-GONG are also included in macrobiotic shiatsu.

Further Reading

Yamamoto, Shizuko, *Barefoot Shiatsu,* Japan Publications, Inc., Tokyo and New York, 1979. A respected text on shiatsu, including hand and foot techniques. The relationship between internal organs and fascial diagnosis is detailed.

Yamamoto, Shizuko and McCarthy, Patrick, *The Shiatsu Handbook,* Turning Point Publications, Eureka, Calif., 1986. This guide to shiatsu also includes an illustrated chapter on treating common problems.

———— , *Whole Health Shiatsu,* Japan Publications, Inc., Tokyo and New York, 1993. The system of macrobiotic shiatsu is explained and illustrated in this book, written by the originator of the technique.

magnetic field work   See ELECTROMAGNETICS.

magnetic therapy   also called biomagnetics, utilizes specially constructed magnets for therapeutic purposes. The magnets stimulate the body's natural forces to promote healing by increasing blood circulation and subsequent oxygen to a specific area. This therapy should not be confused with the harmful electromagnetic field generated by electrical appliances and high tension wires.

One of the earliest references to magnets was made by Aristotle, approximately 350 B.C., when he spoke of their therapeutic powers. First century B.C. Chinese physicians recorded the effects of the earth's magnetic field on health.

In the late 18th century, Dr. Franz Mesmer, a Viennese doctor, believed that magnetic forces flowed throughout the body affecting health. He used iron rods, along with soothing words and gestures, to realign the "magnetic fluids" in his patients. Although the results of his experiments were not taken seriously by his peers, he did pave the way in the understanding of the power of suggestion and HYPNOTISM, or being "mesmerized."

During the 1950s, European and Japanese doctors used magnets to relieve pain and to treat many symptoms that had failed to response to conventional treatments.

There are two types of magnets used today. The **ferrite magnet** is small and hard and is placed inside mattress pads and pillows so people may benefit from the magnetic force throughout the night. It is also placed inside joint supports and jewelry. The other magnet is a flat, flexible, rubberlike pad that is placed directly on the injury or the site of pain.

Blood flow to an area is stimulated as magnetic waves pass through the tissues. The magnetic polarity, which is created, dilates blood vessels and increases blood flow to specific areas. The magnets also promote a relaxation of musculoskeletal pain and tension.

Magnetic therapy has been used to treat sprains, broken bones, skin lesions and burns and joint diseases such as arthritis.

Dr. Richard Markoll of Melville, New York, has had success in treating osteoarthritis with biomagnetic therapy.[1] His treatment has prompted new cartilage growth to replace the worndown cartilage. A machine with a pulsating magnetic field is placed six inches above the affected area for 30 minutes, 18 times, for a five-week period. This therapy claims to be 80 percent effective.[2]

Most people wear the magnets for at least 48 hours before feeling any change. If there is no difference in their physical condition, the magnet is repositioned elsewhere on the body.

Magnetic therapy is generally contraindicated for people with pacemakers and automatic internal defibrillators. It is never applied to a fresh wound, acute sprain or hematoma within the first 24 hours.

Notes

[1] Eighty percent of all arthritis is osteoarthritis. This is a degenerative condition of bones and joints.

[2] Swirksky, Joan, "Magnetic Therapy to Relieve Arthritis Pain," *New York Times,* January 17, 1993. This therapy transmits less than 1 percent of the power used in the diagnostic MRI.

makko-ho exercises   are postures designed to stretch and stimulate the 12 regular MERIDIAN channels. These pathways carry vital life energy, or QI, and relate to specific organs and physiological functions.

Each exercise affects a YIN and its YANG meridian counterpart. When practiced daily, these exercises provide flexibility to the joints, increase elasticity of the muscles and free obstructed energy within the pathways.

The yin HEART/yang SMALL INTESTINE stretch begins in a seated position, knees bent outward, feet touching at the soles. On the exhalation, bring your head to your toes and apply simultaneous pressure to the knees with the elbows. Breathing is normal and the pose should be held for several seconds. It is the pressure on the knees that stretches these arm meridians.

The yin LUNG/yang LARGE INTESTINE meridians are also found in the arms. While standing, clasp your hands behind your back and bend forward at the waist. Touch your head to your knees and stretch your arms overhead.

The final pair of arm meridians are the yin HEART CONSTRICTOR (pericardium)/yang TRIPLE WARMER. Sit in a full lotus or cross-legged position and place your hands on opposite knees. Bend forward on the exhalation, bringing your head to the floor. Breathe normally. On the next movement, reverse hand positions.

The yin KIDNEY/yang BLADDER meridians are found in the legs. Stand straight and inhale. On the exhalation, bend forward and bring your head to your knees. Hold this pose for a minute or so breathing normally.

The yin SPLEEN/yang STOMACH are also found in the lower extremities. To stretch these meridians, kneel on your knees and bend back as far as you can until you are lying on the floor. This stretch can also be performed leaning back on your elbows. The stretch should be felt in the front of the thighs.

The yin LIVER/yang GALL BLADDER meridian stretches are performed seated on the floor. Spread your legs and inhale. On the exhalation, bring your head to one knee, keeping the leg as straight as possible. Breathe normally. Reverse legs.

Each stretch can be performed for one or two minutes, bringing the entire sequence to approximately a 10 to 15-minute exercise session.

massage   See SWEDISH MASSAGE.

Massage Body Mechanics^{SM} or Constitutional Body Mechanics^{SM}, is a dynamic means of transmitting force and energy from the therapist to client, making use of the greater reservoir of power in the therapist's lower torso. In Massage Body Mechanics, the upper body acts as a flexible conduit of energy from the hands through the upper torso to the lower abdomen. Forces are then sent through the legs to the bottom of the feet.

The benefits of this system allow the therapist to remain free from harmful stresses in the upper torso, enhancing the fluidity of the massage. It incorporates the basic tenets of TAI CHI and particularly Zen HARA development. It is also grounded in classical physics, particularly in terms of the application of vectors of force and the center of gravity.

The wrist, shoulder and neck muscles usually build up most of the stress during a massage treatment. In order to unload this tension, and avoid injury, Massage Body Mechanics instructs its practitioners to **set the *chi* muscle.** This region includes the urogenital diaphragm, the pelvic diaphragm, anal sphincter and pubococcygeus muscle. By way of historical perspective, this zone is known from antiquity in Taoist practices, *zazen* (sitting) meditation and *akido*.

To isolate the *chi* muscle, simply squeeze the muscles posterior to the sexual organ (the perineum) without tightening the gluteal muscles. During the inhalation, the abdomen will expand. On the exhalation, the abdomen slightly contracts. During this phase of the breath, squeeze the *chi* muscle. The sacrum will extend forward slightly and the entire spine will straighten. As the *chi* muscle contracts, the center of gravity lowers, dropping the stress from the upper torso.

To enhance the transmission of force through the body to the feet, it is important for the therapist to determine his **optimum posture** or

line of force. This is the posture that allows for the maximum amount of force with the least amount of stress. Reducing the curve of the lower back and bending the knees, the **zero gravity posture,** helps to absorb the pressure from the upper body and bring it down to the lower body.

Massage Body Mechanics has proven to be effective in helping massage therapists and other bodyworkers work deeply and efficiently without injury.

McMillan massage technique laid the groundwork for many innovative uses of the five basic SWEDISH MASSAGE strokes and variations of them, particularly in medical applications.

Mary McMillan, a nurse in Liverpool, England, prior to World War I, was an associate of Sir Robert Jones, a lead orthopedic surgeon who was a proponent of massage for the treatment of fractures.[1]

McMillan was brought to Walter Reed Army Hospital in the United States and served as chief aide and instructor of special war emergency courses in 1918 in the newly established reconstruction department. From 1921 to 1925, she was director of physiotherapy at Harvard Medical School, Cambridge, Massachusetts.

She defined massage as "the manipulation of soft tissues or as movements done upon the body."[2] She prescribed dry massage, preferring lubrications only in cases of excessive scarring, weakened patients or after the long use of splints or casts. She required her students to use both hands with equal strength and dexterity. Two-handed contact was always maintained in her system, and the pressure of the strokes was toward the heart, distal to proximal. She suggested draping patients to keep them warm and a length of time no longer than 50 minutes in which to provide a full-body massage. Pillows were placed under the knees with patients in a supine position and under the abdomen in a prone position for added comfort.

Her EFFLEURAGE strokes were either light or deep, molding the hand to the body part and pressing upward, toward the heart; alternate hand stroking, particularly on large surfaces such as the back or thigh; simultaneous stroking; and one-handed stroking. PETRISSAGE consisted of one- or two-handed kneading, using the flat palm or fingers and thumb; two-fingered petrissage for small surfaces, using the forefinger and thumb; and alternate one-hand wringing of muscles.

FRICTION was used primarily around bony prominences and articulations. Circular pressure was put on the underlying tissues. The benefits provide enhanced absorption of intercellular fluid, greater flexibility and mobility to the joint and breaking down of adhesions (muscle fibers that stick together). She advised using effleurage after friction to increase circulation, thereby promoting reabsorption of the by-products of inflammation. Fingertips, thumbs or thener eminences (thick pad below the thumb) are used in friction. Running frictions are used to calm inflamed nerves, such as in the case of sciatica.[3]

Her TAPOTEMENT techniques included **hacking, clapping, tapping** and **beating.** Hacking is performed with the ulnar surface of the opened hand in rapid succession. Clapping uses cupped hands and tapping employs the fingertips. Beating in a percussion that uses the ulnar surface of closed hands. VIBRATION is performed using the whole hand or fingers.

The first stroke of the massage is always effleurage, followed in order by petrissage, friction, tapotement and vibration.

Notes
[1] Tappan, Francis M., *Healing Massage Techniques*, Reston Publications, N.Y., p. 8. This idea, developed in France in 1880 by Just Marie Marcell in Lucas-Championniere, theorized that soft tissue involvement should be considered along with bone integrity during treatment of a fracture.
[2] Ibid., p. 196.
[3] Ibid., p. 200. Sciatica is an inflammation of the sciatic nerve, which runs down the back of the legs.

mechanotherapy See RANGE OF MOTION.

medical massage the application of any combination of the SWEDISH MASSAGE THERAPY strokes to treat medically diagnosed physical conditions. EFFLEURAGE, PETRISSAGE, FRICTION, VIBRATION and TAPOTEMENT each produce a different effect on the body, which helps in the treatment of illnesses and injuries. Medical massage is usually a half-hour treatment applied to an affected area. It is used to treat conditions of most major physiological systems, such as skeletal, nervous, circulatory, digestive and muscular as well as a powerful rehabilitative procedure.

Effleurage, which has a direct effect on the circulatory system, increases blood and lymph flow. This assisted circulation may counteract the early stages of inflammation by retarding the buildup of blood corpuscles and accumulated fluid at the injured area, such as in the case of sprains. Increased circulation promotes tissue nutrition and waste product removal. When the stroke is applied distally to the injured site, effleurage will drain excess fluid buildup, thereby reducing pain and permitting other manipulations to be performed on the inflamed tissues.

Petrissage is particularly valuable in promoting increased nutrition, elevated cellular activities and containing atrophy (muscle shrinkage). The alternate movements of petrissage assist in the reabsorption of LYMPH and restoration of a fresh blood supply to nourish the tissues.

Friction is very important in treating muscle spasms and joint disorders. The cross-fiber action of friction breaks down muscle adhesions (sticking together) and inflammatory products. At the articulations, friction prevents joint stiffness by promoting elasticity, flexibility and increased RANGE OF MOTION.

Tapotement, or percussion, a locally applied stroke, increases nerve irritability and is effective in arousing languid motor or sensory nerves. Tapotement for a short amount of time, less than 10 seconds, causes contraction to the underlying tissue and blood vessels, so it can be used as a means to remove blood from a region. A longer duration will expand the blood vessels, thereby flushing an area with blood. It will also sedate excited nerves and relax muscle spasms.

Vibration, the last massage stroke, stimulates glandular activity, circulation and the nerve plexi.

Medical massage is contraindicated in the presence of tumors, with a fever, on the site of open skin lesions, herpes lesions or contagious skin conditions (e.g., poison ivy) or directly on top of varicose veins. Local massage should be avoided in the abdominal region in cases of gastric or duodenal ulcers or hypertension.

medical orgone therapy a form of body-work, sometimes coupled with psychotherapy, used to free the body of its **armoring** (muscular holding and tension brought on by repressed feelings and emotions from early infancy and childhood) and restore the natural flow of the body's energy.

Dr. Wilhelm Reich (1879–1957), an Austrian psychoanalyst, was a student of Dr. Sigmund Freud. Reich was the first to discover that feelings and emotions are reflected in the posture, attitude and behavior of a person. His therapeutic approach employed both character analytic, verbal techniques as well as direct work on the body's musculature. It employs breathing to bring to the surface repressed emotions and these are then encouraged expressions. Rage, fear, sadness and longing are released in controlled sessions. Reich's work was originally for the treatment of neurotic and psychotic illnesses, but has been modified by many bodywork practitioners. They found the connection between spastic musculature and repressed emotions to be true, and this has influenced bodywork and added a dimension that differentiates it from the purely physical approach. Dr. Reich is considered to be the father of body-oriented therapies.

Reich held that the biological basis of emotions and sexuality exists as a specific energy, which he named **orgone energy.** He derived the name from the term organism and orgasm. He created an **orgone box,** which was designed to accumulate this energy for therapeutic purposes. The orgone accumulator was used to increase the individual's biologic charge and to help his patients overcome disease.

He held that emotions could be trapped in the body in the form of muscular contractions, or armor. The contraction serves to block the perception of painful feelings, but, in so doing, pleasurable sensations are also avoided. Reich's goal was to relieve repressed emotions and feelings by dissolving the armor, allowing the free flow of orgone energy to be restored.

Dr. Reich's advocacy of and lectures on sexuality forced him to move from city to city in Europe. He came to the United States in 1939 and accepted a position at the New School for Social Research in New York City. In that year, he founded the Orgone Institute in New York.

Reich was never arrested for fraud, but a federal injunction was ordered prohibiting interstate shipments of orgone accumulators. Reich failed to obey the injunction and was found in violation by a federal court. He refused to defend his scientific discoveries in a court of law and was imprisoned for failure to obey the injunction. He died in 1957, just two days before his parole hearing. None of his scientific claims were ever disproved by objective, controlled studies.

In his therapy, Reich employed varying methods to break down physical and emotional armoring. Deep breathing was used to build up an energetic charge, which facilitated emotional release. It was often used in concert with deep pressure work, applied to those areas of the body that were spastic and held tension.

Reich encouraged gagging to relieve the spasticity held in the diaphragm. Stamping, kicking, limb shaking and other expressive movements encouraged expression, as was shouting out with full expression.

Inhibited respiration was a significant source of armoring. To release this tension, the Reichian therapist may sometimes push down on the client's chest during exhalation. This is always done cautiously to avoid injury.

A session of Reichian work includes character analytic work to point up attitudes and behaviors that are defensive or maladaptive. When the client is ready for biophysical work, he or she is asked to disrobe to a bathing suit or underwear. This is done to better observe areas of muscular armoring or rigidity and allow direct work without the encumbrances of clothing. Deep breathing brings about repressed emotions and long-buried feelings and full expression of them is encouraged. When feelings surface, the therapist allows them to continue. If they don't surface, the therapist will sometimes work deeply into those muscle groups she believes are holding, or obstructing, free expression. This method of direct work on the armored muscles relieves armoring, slowing and over time, and the work proceeds in a systematic fashion from head to pelvis.

There are only a few dozen Reichian therapists who are truly medical orgone therapists in the United States. The American College of Orgonomy, in Princeton, New Jersey, trains and certifies therapists. Requirements for training include personal restructuring and medical licensure with board certification in psychiatry or internal medicine.

Further Reading

Bean, Orson, *Me and the Orgone*, St. Martin's Press, N.Y., 1971. This book describes an individual's personal experience in medical orgone therapy.

Boadella, David, *Wilhelm Reich: The Evolution of His Work*, Dell Publications, N.Y., 1975. This heavily researched book is a biography of the man, his life and his work.

Reich, Wilhelm, Dr., *Selected Writings: An Introduction to Orgonomy*, Farrar, Straus & Giroux, N.Y., 1973. Dr. Reich explains his energetic theories and discusses his scientific discoveries.

Totton, Nick and Edmonson, Em, *Reichian Growth Work*, Prism Press, Bridport, England, 1988. This book presents Reich's principles in the light of bodywork as practiced by nonphysicians.

The Wilhelm Reich Foundation, *Orgone Accumulator—It's Scientific and Medical Use*, Reich Foundation, Princeton, N.J., 1951. This manual describes the theories and use of Dr. Reich's invention.

meditation   an ancient self-help practice that quiets and trains the mind, as it helps an individual realize his inner nature and attain spiritual enlightenment. It is beneficial in relieving anxiety and in achieving a deeper understanding of life.

Meditation has been practiced for centuries, in the East more than in the West.[1] Shamanistic rituals included meditations for finding guidance from the spirits. Japanese Buddhists developed Zen meditation, a form that is still familiar and widely practiced.

Different forms of meditation vary only in their focus. In the Oriental ritual, meditation emphasizes mental control and may use mantras, mandalas or chants to achieve the meditative state. Freeing the mind and keeping it open to all thoughts is another type of meditation that helps to provide insights into particular problems.

Other forms, such as YOGA, are based on the idea of body control (rather than mind control) to integrate the body/mind, while still other forms encourage deliberate relaxation and release of muscular tension.

Meditation, in all its variations, generally requires certain procedures for achieving total relaxation. First, the environment should be isolated and free from distraction. The space should be quiet and comfortable. Concentration on a specific point, object, sound or word helps to focus attention. Meditation requires a passive attitude—an individual does not "do" or cause the meditative state to happen.

The individual should sit in a comfortable position, free of restrictive clothing. Finally, meditation takes practice to reach deeper levels of relaxation and insight.

To begin, 20 minutes of meditation a day is suggested. Mastery of the practice can take several years, and deep concentration is not achieved with each session.

Meditation practices are varied. Transcendental meditation was popularized in the 1960s by Maharishi Mahesh Yogi. This form of meditation is an adaptation of an ancient Indian system in which a secret mantra is repeated. Enlightenment and world peace are the ultimate goals of this practice.

Vipassana (insight) meditation is the moment-to-moment investigation of the body/mind through calm and focused awareness. It originated in the Theravada tradition of the teachings of Buddha. Insight meditation is a way of seeing clearly the totality of one's being and experience. Growth in clarity brings insight into the nature of who we are and increased peace in our lives.

Regardless of the form it takes, meditation offers many physiological and psychological benefits. This self-help technique eases tension, lowers blood pressure, decreases the level of lactic acid in the blood, lowers heart rate and can reverse the harmful effects of stress, promoting a much calmer, controlled lifestyle.

Note
[1] In 1875, the Theosophical Society was founded in the United States by Helena Petrovna Blavatsky and Annie Besant. This organization introduced Eastern meditation practices and philosophies to the West.

Further Reading
Fontana, David, Dr., *The Meditator's Handbook: A Comprehensive Guide to Eastern and Western Meditation Techniques,* Element, Rockport, Mass., 1992. This book is an easy-to-follow guide on various meditation techniques, their backgrounds and practices.

Mennell massage technique a form of MEDICAL MASSAGE that uses a slow rhythm and light pressure. Healthy tissue is massaged first, leading up to the area of injury. The length of time depends upon the pathology, and herbally blended oils are often prescribed. Support is placed under the knees with the patient in a supine position and under the legs and chest in a prone position. Elevation of the limbs was used to promote greater LYMPHATIC drainage.

James B. Mennell was a medical officer and massage lecturer at the Training School of St. Thomas's Hospital in London, England, from 1912 to 1935. He was a strong proponent of the use of massage and worked to interest the medical community of its values.

He classified the movements as: **stroking,** subdivided into superficial and deep, and **com-**

pression, including kneading, FRICTIONS, pressures, PETRISSAGE, TAPOTEMENT and VIBRATION. He stated that the patient must be completely relaxed, since any tension would be counterproductive. The direction of his deep strokes is toward the heart in proximal to distal segments, promoting lymphatic drainage. He called that the "removal of the cork from the bottle."[1] His system was the first to use this approach.

Superficial stroking is done slowly and lightly with the practitioner maintaining two-handed contact at all times. The direction of the stroke is optional and constant, relying upon the client's response. Deep effleurage is also done at a slow pace, following the rate of blood and lymph flow.

Kneading is performed in a gentle, circular manner using open hands working in opposite directions. The pressure is deepest at the onset of the stroke and gradually lightens. Petrissage is an alternate pick up of muscle between the fingers and thumbs of both hands. Frictions, as he called the stroke, can be done circularly or transversely to long muscle fibers.

Tapotement consists of hacking, using the ulnar surface of the open hands striking soft blows, clapping, which uses cupped palms, and beating, using a half-closed fist on either the ulnar or palmar side. Beating is the most vigorous of the percussive strokes.

Mennell preferred mechanical vibrators to the practitioner's techniques, saying that proficiency in this stroke is difficult to achieve even thought a shaking stroke could provide a firm vibration.[2]

Notes
[1] Tappen, Francis M., *Healing Massage Techniques,* Reston Publications, N.Y., 1980, p. 207.
[2] Ibid., p. 212.

mentastics® See TRAGER®.

meridians a complex network of pathways that circulates QI (life's vital energy), blood (*hseuh*) and essence (jing) throughout the body. Meridians are an integral part of the concepts of

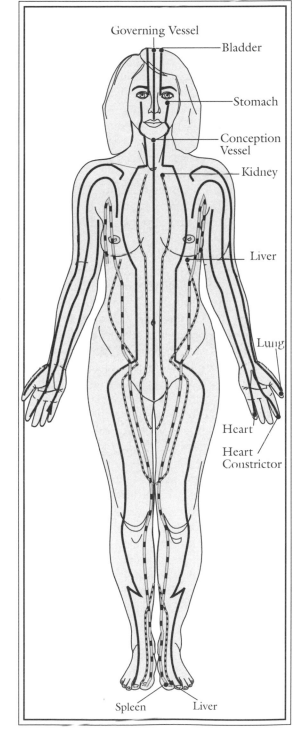

The 14 regular meridians run up and down the front, side and back of the body. This front view shows yang leg and yin arm energy pathways.

CHINESE MEDICINE, ACUPUNCTURE and other related Oriental therapies. Treatment points along the meridians are the acupuncture points.

The meridians relate to the organs (*zang-fu*) interiorly and extend over the body exteriorly, linking tissues and organs. The meridians run longitudinally and internally within the body. The **collaterals,** which are branches of the meridians, run transversely and superficially from the meridians. Together, they are called *jingluo* (meridians and collaterals).

This system includes 12 regular meridians, 8 **extra** meridians, 15 collaterals, 12 **divergent** meridians, 12 **muscle** regions and 12 **cutaneous** regions.

The meridians and collateral channels are distributed internally and externally throughout the body. They function to transport *qi* and blood, which nourishes the internal organs, skin, muscles, tendons and bones. HOMEOSTASIS, or balanced, normal function, is ensured when energy flows freely through all the pathways.

The theory of meridians and collaterals was developed by the ancient Chinese, probably in relation to their keen observation of disease symptoms, the transmission of needling sensations, TUI-NA (Chinese remedial massage), breathing exercises called *daoy* and anatomical knowledge.

The 12 regular channels are made up of three YIN[1] hand meridians: LUNG, HEART CONSTRICTOR (pericardium) and HEART; three YANG meridians: LARGE INTESTINE, TRIPLE HEATER and SMALL INTESTINE; three yin foot meridians: SPLEEN, LIVER and KIDNEY; and three yang foot meridians: STOMACH, GALL BLADDER and BLADDER. They are called regular meridians because they are the major trunks of the entire system. These regular channels are bilateral, running up and down the right and left sides of the body.

The eight extra meridians include the GOVERNING VESSEL, which runs up the midline of the back and governs all the yang meridians. The CONCEPTION VESSEL runs up the midline of the abdomen and controls all the yin meridians.[2]

Chong meridian, "the sea of the twelve primary meridians," regulates the flow of *qi* and blood within the 12 regular meridians. *Dai* meridian, "girdle," binds all the meridians at the waist. *Qiao,* "heel," starts at either aspect of the ankle and controls motion regulation of the lower limbs. *Yangqiao* and *yinqiao* are representative of the yang and yin lower extremity meridians. *Wei* denotes connection and network, so the *yangwie* meridian connects and networks the exterior yang meridians of the entire body, while the *yinwei* affects the yin meridians in the same manner. They regulate the flow of *qi* in the yin/yang meridians and help maintain the coordination and equilibrium between the yin/yang meridians. They both strengthen and connect the internally/externally related meridians.

The divergent meridians govern the inside of the body without having specific organ points. The collaterals control the body surface and each of them has a *luo* (connecting) point used to treat certain diseases.

Connected with their own relating regular meridians are the 12 muscle regions and 12 cutaneous regions of the regular channels. The muscle regions are deeply distributed under the skin, while the cutaneous regions are much more superficially located. The muscle regions are the vessels that distribute *qi* and blood of the 12 regular channels to nourish the muscles and connect all the bones and joints of the body. The cutaneous regions refer to the place where *qi* and blood of the meridians become superficial. These regions have 12 distinct areas of the body's surface within the system of the 12 regular channels. They provide the initial protective function to the body, since they are the most superficial.

This intricate network of meridians and collaterals functions closely with the body's tissues and organs. They transport *qi* and blood, regulate yin and yang, resist external pathogens and reflect symptoms and signs of disease, transmit needling sensations and regulate deficiency and excess conditions.[3]

Notes

[1] Yin and yang are counterparts of each other and the balance between them is considered to produce optimum health. Yin energy flows upward, from earth to heaven. Yang flows downward, from heaven to earth. Yin meridians are mainly found on the medial aspect of the limbs, while the yang meridians are on the lateral aspect.

[2] The 12 regular channels plus the governing vessel and conception vessel make up the 14 meridians.

[3] Xinnong, Cheng, ed., *Chinese Acupuncture and Moxibustion,* Foreign Language Press, Beijing, 1987, p. 278. Deficiency and excess are the two principles that categorize the strength of the antipathogenic *qi.* Hyperactivity of pathogenic factors causes an excess condition, while the consumption of *qi* results in deficiency. These two categories are part of the **eight principle patterns,** which describes the patterns of disharmony. The description is made up of four pairs of opposites: yin/yang, interior/exterior, deficiency/excess, and cold/hot.

Further Reading

Bensoussan, Allan, *The Vital Meridian,* Churchill Livingstone, N.Y., 1991. This book clearly describes the functions of the meridians.

Denmei, Shudo, Brown, Stephen, trans., *Introduction to Meridian Therapy,* Eastland Press, Seattle, 1983. Each meridian is carefully described and treatments are provided for common ailments.

Di Ling, *Acupuncture Meridian Theory and Acupuncture Points,* China Books and Periodicals, San Francisco, 1992. This detailed book provides historical information about meridian therapy and acupuncture.

Ellis, Andrew, Wiseman, Nigel, and Boss, Ken, *Fundamentals of Chinese Acupuncture,* Paradigm Books, Brookline, Mass., 1986. A concise text on the theory of Oriental medicine and detailed analysis of the meridian system.

Lade, Arnie, *Acupuncture Points: Images and Functions,* Eastland Press, Seattle, 1989. A detailed description of the meridians and the acupuncture points are illustrated in this book.

Worsely, J.R., *Traditional Chinese Acupuncture, Vols. I–II,* College of Traditional Acupuncture, London, England, 1990. This text clearly explains the theories of Chinese medicine, the meridians, acupuncture, moxibustion and massage.

meridian therapy   See SHIATSU.

misalignment   See SUBLUXATION.

MotherMassage^{SM}   a hands-on system specifically designed to treat the discomforts of pregnancy and maintain optimum health for the expectant woman, from her nine months of pregnancy, through labor and postpartum, to the nursing period. This massage system is a combination of various techniques, including SWEDISH MASSAGE, REFLEXOLOGY and SHIATSU.

Centuries before technology provided us with sonograms and fetal monitors, birthing women and their caregivers considered massage to be a vital part of prenatal and postpartum care. While a woman is pregnant, the demands placed on her body are great and dramatically ever-changing. MotherMassage is a safe, nurturing and effective way to reduce many of the adverse results of stress and the accompanying discomforts.

There is a lot of literature and scientific data that validates the prodigious, beneficial effects of massage. One of its most powerful accomplishments is stress reduction. During pregnancy, stress and anxiety can cause blood catecholamine levels to increase, potentially interfering with the work of oxytocin and other labor-promoting hormones.[1] These compounds traverse the placenta and can affect the developing fetus.

MotherMassage can counteract the deleterious effects of stress and promote the secretion of endorphins, the "feel good" compound. These, too, traverse the placenta. Therefore, what the expectant mother feels, whether it is good or bad, creates biochemical reactions, which can be passed on to the developing fetus.

MotherMassage was created in 1980 by massage therapist, teacher and author Elaine Stillerman of New York City. Her extensive research into tribal societies' birthing practices and traditional massage techniques led her to develop a system that contributes to an easy, empowered and confident experience for the pregnant, laboring and postpartum woman.

Stillerman believes that a woman should not have to define her pregnancy by its aches and pains. MotherMassage treatments provide general relaxation as well as relief from some of the most common discomforts of pregnancy: abdominal pressure; allergies and sinus congestion;

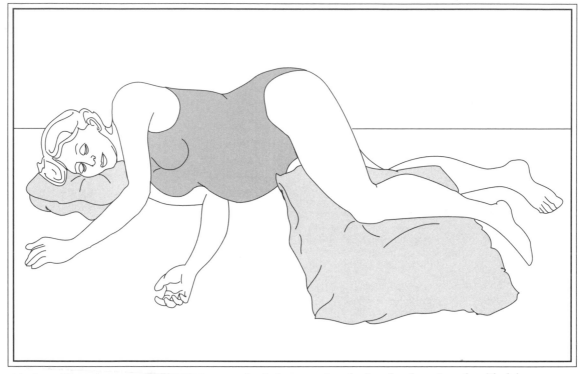

Placing pillows between the expectant mother's knees and under her head, makes the side-lying posture of MotherMassage very comfortable.

anemia; backaches; breast soreness; carpal tunnel syndrome; charley horse and leg cramps; constipation, heartburn and gas; edema (swelling); fatigue; headaches; hemorrhoids; insomnia; morning sickness and nausea;[2] sciatica; sore nipples and varicose veins.[3]

Emotionally, self-esteem and a better body image can also be promoted with MotherMassage.

During pregnancy, the stimulation of glandular secretions from massage and specific shiatsu point pressures can stabilize hormone levels, rendering their side effects less severe. Leg massage, particularly light EFFLEURAGE, can control varicose veins by draining the legs and reducing edema. An increase in blood and LYMPH circulation (due to massage's enhanced effect on the circulatory system) brings greater nutrition to all tissues of the body and speedier waste removal. This includes enhanced circulation to the placenta.

Red blood cells, which may line the walls of the blood vessels instead of circulating, are reintroduced into the bloodstream by massage's mechanical pressure. This raises the red blood cell count and hemoglobin, which is of particular importance to those women who might develop anemia.

Muscle strain, pressure on weight-bearing joints, myofascial (see FASCIA) discomfort and fatigue may be relieved through Mother-Massage.[4]

In preparation for labor, MotherMassage promotes the use of Kegel exercises (the contraction/relaxation of the pubococcygeal muscles) and self-administered perineal massage. This technique promotes flexibility and elasticity to the sensitive region between the anus and the vagina and may eliminate the need for an episiotomy, a surgical incision to avoid "tearing" the perineum during the second stage of labor. Perineal massage also helps the woman identify the muscles she will use for pushing and to recognize some of the same physical sensations she will experience when the baby's head crowns.

MotherMassage provides specific points that may help to stimulate or speed up labor, while promoting calmness and relaxation. Ligaments, tendons and joints enjoy greater flexibility. Back labor can be relieved with MotherMassage back massage.

MotherMassage promotes a greater kinesthetic sense to the pregnant or laboring woman. In addition to this heightened physical awareness, women report feeling more confident and in control of their body. During this emotional time, studies have shown that touch reduces C-section rates and shortens labor.[5,6]

The postpartum recovery period, considered to be the six weeks after the birth, is a physically and emotionally demanding period of adjustment. MotherMassage can help realign the pelvis and possibly avoid pregnancy-related back pain. Uterine involution, or the return of the uterus to its prepregnant condition, can be expedited by a clockwise, circular PETRISSAGE, performed every four hours. The MotherMassage full-body treatment offers relief for general soreness and fatigue and promotes rapid healing. In addition, postpartum blues, which affect almost two-thirds of postpartum women, is minimized with a general, relaxing treatment.

Medicated births and postpartum stress can sabotage milk letdown. Specific points and massage techniques can promote the release of prolactin and other lactation-inducing hormones. Breast massage, usually self-administered, can ease breast engorgement or soreness.

The treatment is given in a chair, with the pregnant woman comfortably leaning on pillows placed on a table, or on a massage table, lying on her side, with pillows or cushions placed under her head and knees. She is unclothed, but draped in a sheet and towel. Half her body is massaged on one side, then she slowly turns over for the other half. The treatment, done with lubrication, lasts one hour, and special attention is paid to those areas of greatest discomfort.

MotherMassage is designed for professional massage therapists, childbirth educators and nurse midwives to use with their pregnant clients. A simpler variation of the technique is offered to the expectant woman or couple, to help them share the entire experience together.

Notes

1. Stillerman, Elaine, L.M.T., *MotherMassage: A Handbook for Relieving the Discomforts of Pregnancy*, Dell Publications, N.Y., 1992., p. xix. Catecholamines are compounds responsible for the "fight or flight" response to stress.
2. General massage is contraindicated when a client is nauseous or vomiting. However, when the symptoms subside, specific shiatsu points can relieve the severity of the symptoms.
3. Massage directly on varicose veins is contraindicated. The congestion in the legs can be reduced, however, through Swedish massage techniques that do not compromise the weakened vessels.
4. Stillerman, Elaine, L.M.T., *MotherMassage: A Handbook for Relieving the Discomforts of Pregnancy*, Dell Publications, N.Y., 1992, pp. 1–2.
5. Sobel, David S., M.D., M.P.H., "Childbirth: Emotional Support in Labor Reduces C-Sections and Shortens Labor," *Mental Medicine Update*, Center for Health Sciences, Los Altos, Calif., 1993, p. 7. Of the 204 patients at the Jefferson Davis Hospital in Houston, Texas in the control group who did not receive massage, 18 percent had C-sections. Of the 212 patients who had labor support, such as massage and emotional support, only 8 percent had C-sections, a reduction of 56 percent. In addition, the use of epidural anesthesia was reduced by 85 percent and labor averaged two hours shorter. There were also fewer neonatal complications from the group that received massage.
6. Op. cit., pp. 85–86. *The Journal of Nurse-Midwifery*, Vol. 31, from Stillerman, Elaine, L.M.T., *MotherMassage*, No. 6, November/December 1986, pp. 270–276. Reported in a study on touch during labor, women overwhelmingly felt greater confidence and an ability to cope when someone held or touched them.

Further Reading

Stillerman, Elaine, L.M.T., *MotherMassage: A Handbook for Relieving the Discomforts of Pregnancy*, Dell Publications, N.Y., 1992. This illustrated book, written for the expectant couple, carefully explains the beneficial effects of massage during pregnancy. The first part of the book explains the massage strokes that are involved and then applies them to the relief of over 20 common complaints of pregnancy. A full-body massage is also provided for general stress reduction. Labor preparation, labor massage, postpartum massage and nursing care are detailed. A chapter on infant massage is also included and is easy to follow. Stillerman includes quick reference charts on reflexology and shiatsu points, as well as herbal remedies.

moxibustion, also called igni-acupuncture, is an ancient healing method, possibly dating back as far as the Stone Age, which developed along with ACUPUNCTURE. Instead of using needles for the treatments, ignited herbs are usually placed on the back, on or just above acupuncture points. It is generally believed that moxibustion was more commonly used in damper climates, like Japan, where internal warming was a desired effect. The charts for moxibustion indicate treatment points, which are slightly different from acupuncture points, although the latter are commonly used.

The herb used in moxibustion are old, dried moxa leaves, also called mugwort (Artemisia vulgaris). The herb is ground into a fine powder and the coarse residue is removed. This "moxa wool" has properties that make it suitable for therapeutic purposes: it is deeply warming, can unblock energy obstructions within the MERIDIANS and promotes improved organ function.

The moxa wool may be shaped into a cone or rolled into a cigarette shape, which is wrapped in paper and sealed at both ends. The moxa stick is used more frequently in current moxibustion treatments.

Moxibustion is administered topically in two manners: **scarring** and **nonscarring.** In the former, the cone is placed directly on the skin until it is completely burned. It is replaced with several more cones on the same point. This technique is rarely performed any longer.

The nonscarring method burns the cone until the patient can no longer tolerate the heat. It is then rapidly removed and several more cones are added and removed until the area becomes red.

Indirect moxibustion is performed by placing a thin slice of garlic, ginger or salt on the point and putting a lit moxa cone on top. Each barrier is used for different purposes: the garlic for pulmonary disorders and ginger for arthritis. The salt is poured into the navel, covered with a slice of ginger and topped with a moxa cone. This is used for emergency cases such as coma or diarrhea.

The moxa stick is placed about $\frac{1}{4}$ inch above the acupuncture point and is held there by the practitioner until the area becomes pink, about 5 to 10 minutes.

Moxibustion may also be used to conduct heat into an acupuncture needle. The deep tissues benefit from the point stimulation and the additional penetrating heat.

Further Reading
Auteroche, B., et al., *Acupuncture and Moxibustion: A Guide to Clinical Practice,* Churchill Livingstone, N.Y., 1992. This easy-to-use book offers a detailed analysis of the use of acupuncture and moxibustion.
Baek, Sung, *Classical Moxibustion Skills in Contemporary Clinical Practice,* Blue Poppy Press, Boulder, Colo., 1990. This text provides an historical perspective of moxibustion and offers clinical treatments for specific ailments.
Feit, Richard and Zmiewski, Paul, *Acumoxa Therapy: Reference and Study Guide,* Paradigm Books, Brookline, Mass., 1990. This book explains the history and use of moxibustion in a clear, concise way. Detailed treatment points are provided.

mud baths, packs and wraps See BODY WRAPS.

muscle energy work a direct, soft tissue approach for normalizing joint movement through human structure. It is an evaluation and diagnostic system that may eliminate somatic dysfunction, which often inhibits an individual's RANGE OF MOTION.

The corrections occur through gentle, cooperative interaction between the provider and the participant. This system is based on the theory that once the primary dysfunction is eradicated, the body's self-correcting mechanism will be facilitated.

Isometric, positional and contraction methods, respiratory and active exercises are used to identify and release restricted joints. Once these articulations are released, the mobility and function of the related soft tissue structures also increases.

Muscle energy technique focuses on the fundamental aspects of spinal motion on segmented and group levels. The assessment and treatment of the cervical (neck), thoracic (upper back), thoracolumbar (midback) and lumbar (lower back) segments of the axial skeleton[1] are addressed along with the dysfunctions of the sacroiliac.[2]

Notes

[1] The axial skeleton is composed of 7 cervical, 12 thoracic, 5 lumbar spinal bones called vertebrae and the sacrum and coccyx at the base of the spine.

[2] The sacroiliac joint is a suture joint, one with small but important movement, between the sacrum and the iliac bones of the pelvis.

muscle testing See KINESIOLOGY.

music therapy the use of music to rehabilitate and maintain a person's physical and mental health. Individuals can actively participate by playing instruments or be involved by listening to music.

Moods and attitudes, as well as physiological functions, such as respiration and heartbeat, can be affected by music. The most relaxing music seems to mimic the pulse rate of 70 to 80 beats per minute.[1]

Music therapists use music and therapy to offer a creative treatment medium. Musical modalities combined with psychodynamic, behavioral and biomedical approaches, help clients of all ages and varying disabilities to reach their therapeutic goals.

As early as the sixth century B.C., Pythagoras, a Greek philosopher and mathematician (c. 582–500 B.C.) recognized the healing value of music. He believed that music and diet were the primary means of purifying the body and soul and maintaining health.[2]

Today, music therapists bring their skills to hospitals, outpatient clinics, day care treatment centers, senior centers, correctional facilities, schools, halfway houses and nursing homes. In hospitals, both the doctors and patients reap the benefits of music therapy. Linda Rodgers, a clinical social worker and daughter of the composer Richard Rodgers, has created a set of tapes containing "anxiolytic" music, or music composed exclusively to reduce stress and anxiety and promote rapid healing.[3] Rodgers claims that the tapes, which have neither recognizable melodies nor distinctive rhythms, override the noises of surgical procedures and can affect the patients subliminally even if they are under anesthesia. Instead of the noises, patients hear synthesized music and Rodgers's reassuring voice proffering messages of calmness.

Surgeons also agree with a study published in the Journal of the American Medical Association that concluded that surgeons performed better when working to the music they like. The study showed that the 50 doctors studied had lower blood pressure and pulse rates.[4]

On an energetic level, music is purported to balance the CHAKRAS, the AURIC FIELD and consciousness (see TONING). Each of the seven chakras (vortices of energy) vibrate at specific frequencies or the same as related notes. If a chakra is not vibrating at its usual rate, the complementary note will restore the balance.

Music therapists have been able to overcome many barriers, whether physical, mental or emotional, through music.

Notes

[1] Reader's Digest, *Family Guide to Natural Medicine,* Pleasantville, N.Y., 1993, p. 139.

[2] Kastener, Mark, L.Ac., *Alternative Healing,* Halcyon Publications, La Mesa, Calif., 1993, pp. 163–164.

[3] Miller, Leslie, "Reassuring Music to Have Surgery By," *USA Today,* September 6, 1994, p. 6D.

[4] Lawson, Carol, "Doo-wop, Doo-wop, Scalpel, Scalpel," *New York Times,* October 5, 1994, p. C1.

myofascial release® a mild and gentle hands-on form of stretching that evaluates and treats the FASCIAL system.

This system concentrates on treating the fascia, a tough CONNECTIVE TISSUE, which spreads throughout the body in a three-dimensional network from head to toe, without interruption. Fascia is made of two types of fiber: **collagenous** and **elastic.** Collagenous fibers, whose main component is collagen, are tough and have little stretchability. Elastic fibers, composed chiefly of elastin, are stretchable. Fascia, which is denser in some areas than others, surrounds and infuses with tissues and organs of the body, including nerves, vessels, muscles and bones, down to the cellular level.[1]

Anatomically, fascia is divided into three layers. The first layer, the **superficial layer,** lies directly below the dermis (skin) and contains fat, nerve endings and blood vessels. The second layer is referred to as a **potential space.** This portion of fascia may increase in size with extra tissue fluid or edema. The third layer is the **deep layer.** Muscle groups are enveloped by fascia separating one muscle group from the next. Free movement is made possible by the lubrication of fluid between the fibers of one muscle past another.[2]

Any malfunction in this pervasive network, due to trauma, bad posture or inflammation, can create a tightening of the fascia, resulting in abnormal pressure on all the structures it covers. This can produce pain or dysfunction throughout the body, sometimes with unusual side effects and unrelated symptoms. Many people suffer with fascial problems that go unrecognized because advanced technological diagnostic tests do not reveal the condition of the fascial network.

The role of fascia in the body is varied. At the cellular level, fascia creates the tissue spaces and plays an important role in support, protection, separation, cellular respiration, elimination, metabolism and fluid and LYMPHATIC flow.[3] In addition, fascia is involved in the body's postural balance, motion, circulation and nervous system.[4]

This connective tissue acts as a shock absorber throughout the body, is a major area of inflammatory processes, will often change prior to chronic tissue congestion and fluids and infections often travel along fascial planes. Dysfunctions in these tissues, therefore, can have far-reaching effects.

Myofascial release offers evaluation and treatment of the entire fascial structure. Therapists are taught to assess the system through visual analysis of the human frame three-dimensionally in space, by palpating tissue textures and by observing the symmetry and quality of the CRANIOSACRAL rhythm.

Once the facial restrictions have been determined, the therapist applies gentle pressure into the direction of the restriction. Initially, the elastic component of the fascia releases, eventually followed by the collagenous component. The therapist follows the motion of the tissue, barrier after barrier, until release is felt.

Hand placement should be comfortable for both the therapist and the client. Each hand, or finger(s), is placed proximal to the attachments of the muscles being stretched. The pressure is adequate enough to stretch the superficial skin, fascia and underlying muscle(s) in the direction of the muscle fibers. The position is held until the soft tissue is felt to relax. The stretch is repeated, taking up additional slack produced by the release. This process is repeated until no further stretch is possible and both muscle and related soft tissues are fully elongated and relaxed. Another evaluation is taken by the therapist for any additional restrictions that may still be present.

Myofascial release was developed by John F. Barnes, P.T. Born in Philadelphia, Pennsylvania, Barnes studied PHYSICAL THERAPY and received his license in 1960. He had sustained a serious back injury from weight lifting when he was 17 years old and was reinjured years later when he stepped into a gopher's hole. After the first injury, he had back surgery, which fused his lumbar (lower) spine, yet the later accident started him on a program of self-help. Almost without realizing it, Barnes had started developing the myofascial release technique by working on himself.

He believed that a much older form of myofascial release had been practiced for centuries in Europe. Barnes realized that trauma or inflammation causes the body to lose fluid content, resulting in a solidifying of body tissues. He also maintains that the fascia may be the physical medium for ACUPUNCTURE'S MERIDIAN system.

John F. Barnes is an international lecturer, author and president and director of the Myofascial Release Treatment Centers and Seminars in Paoli (suburban Philadelphia), Pennsylvania, and Sedona, Arizona.

Myofascial release relieves fascial restrictions all over the body, promoting strength, flexibility, full RANGE OF MOTION, aligned posture and fluid movement. Myofascial release treats chronic problems and reduces pain throughout the body and aids in neurological dysfunction and rehabilitation.

Notes
1. Barnes, John F., P.T., "Myofascial Release—An Introduction for the Patient," *Physical Therapy Forum*, October 3, 1988, p. 1.
2. Manheim, Carol J., M.Sc., P.T., and Lavett, Diane K., Ph.D., *The Myofascial Release Manual*, Slack, Inc., Thorofare, N.J., 1989, pp. 3–4.
3. Barnes, John F., P.T., "Myofascial Release," *Physical Therapy Forum*, September 16, 1987, p. 2.
4. Ibid., p. 2. The central nervous system is surrounded by fascial tissue, which connects to the inside of the skull, the foramen magnum, and the second sacral region.

Further Reading
Barnes, John F., P.T., *Myofascial Release,* Rehabilitation Services, Inc., Paoli, Pa., 1990. This book explains evaluation and treatment techniques with clear illustrations. Over 15 different authorities contribute their experiences with myofascial release.

Cantu, Robert I, P.T., M.T.C., and Grodin, Alan J., P.T., M.T.C., *Myofascial Manipulation: Theory and Clinical Application,* Aspen Publication, Gaithersburg, Md., 1992. This illustrated and photographed text discusses the history of myofascial manipulation, the physiology of this important connective tissue and provides treatment techniques.

Manheim, Carol J., M.Sc., P.T., and Lavett, Diane K., Ph.D., *The Myofascial Release Manual,* Slack, Inc., Thorofare, N.J., 1989. This text describes the different strokes of myofascial release in a clear form. Photographs elucidate the various techniques.

myotherapy® See BONNIE PRUDDEN MYOTHERAPY®.

N

Naprapathy™ from the Czechoslovakian word *napravit,* "to correct," and the Greek word *pathos,* "suffering." A hands-on healing system that focuses on manipulating the soft tissues of the body (muscles, tendons, ligaments and fascia) to relieve tension and promote fluidity in motion. Practitioners believe that any assault to these tissues, either through trauma, injury or stress, can interfere with the normal functioning of the nervous and circulatory systems. Exercise, dietary and nutritional recommendations are also part of the care, since naprapaths believe that the chemistry of the body must be, like the soft tissues, in balance.

Naprapathy was developed by Dr. Oakly Smith, a chiropractor and medical student in 1905. These two disciplines have much in common, although chiropractors focus on structural alignment through osseous (bony) adjustment, while naprapaths concentrate on soft and CONNECTIVE TISSUE manipulations.

In 1905, Dr. Smith founded the Chicago College of Naprapathy, which is now called the Chicago National College of Naprapathy. Currently, naprapaths can be trained in Chicago, School of Naprapathy in Sweden or in Spain. In Chicago, graduates of the four-year program receive a Doctor of Naprapathy (D.N.) and are licensed to practice naprapathic medicine. At the present, Illinois and Ohio are the only states to grant licenses to doctors who work with connective tissue.

Naprapaths use hand palpation and an acute sense of touch to evaluate the soft tissues. Once a painful, contracted, or restricted area has been located, the practitioner performs gentle manipulative movements called **directos** to gently stretch the tissues.

Sessions usually last 30 minutes. Some naprapaths do "mono treatments," concentrating on only one problem area, although whole body treatments can be done for corrective and preventive purposes.

Naprapathy has been used to treat neuromusculoskeletal pain. However, it may be used to treat many physical problems that involve restricted mobility, scar tissue problems, pain syndromes, obstructed nerve supply, LYMPHATIC drainage and circulation.

neural organization technique a noninvasive technique that corrects structural faults in the body, which may create disorganization within the nervous system. Neural organization allows the body to function in a subtle, synchronous manner.

The body has self-regulatory "switches" that can be turned on with outside intervention. Neural organization technique was developed in 1979 by Dr. Carl A. Ferreri, a chiropractor with extensive knowledge of ACUPUNCTURE and APPLIED KINESIOLOGY. He recognized that there is an orderly neurological priority system and developed neural organization technique to intervene in reorganizing normal function to the body.

A central circuit (nerve) system, organized in the brain and controlled primarily by the nervous system, controls the body's major physiological functions, such as circulation, hormone secretion, digestion, excretion and learning. Signals from the body, as well as exogenous factors, come through receptors on the body into these circuits, which then transmit information to the brain. In the brain, these messages are organized and then redirected back to the body to affect change in a particular body part.

Many health problems develop when improper signals, from either environmental, chemical, physical or emotional sources, cause a breakdown in the circuitry. This results in a disorganization in a particular system, often causing an inappropriate physiologic reaction.

This system uses digital pressure found in the MERIDIAN system of acupuncture and other points on the LYMPHATIC SYSTEM in an organized manner to switch on these regulatory points.

Precise pressure and location can help reconnect the circuits.

Neural organization technique has been used to treat scoliosis (abnormal curvature of the spine), multiple sclerosis, Down's Syndrome, cerebral palsy, allergies, dyslexia and other learning disabilities. A pilot study examining the application of neural organization technique on children with learning disabilities was published in *Concern,* a British children's journal. All children showed significant improvements in intellectual functioning and in the 10 skills that were tested. Every child improved in at least two skill areas with some improving in as much as six. Almost 7 percent of the children showed improvements in full scale I.Q. tests, with gains from 4 to 14 percent.[1]

An individual's success depends on the stage or progression of his or her particular condition.

Note

[1] Kitay, Annalee, Dr., "Neural Organization Technique—Treatment for Learning Disabilities," *Relevant Times,* March/April 1993, p. 18.

NeuroCellular Repatterning™ a holographic, somatic and psychotherapy process that uses affirmations of love and forgiveness as its basic modality. This system purports that all disease and emotional or physical breakdowns are brought on by dysfunctional behavior patterns. According to this system, the disease does not have to be diagnosed or named. All that is required is knowing what created it, then release it with love and forgiveness.

Practitioners, or teachers, of NeuroCellular Repatterning instruct people to love themselves and receive love in order to make the shift to the conscious mind, rather than permitting the ego and subconscious mind to rule, to promote permanent healing. In order for any therapy to be effective, the participant must get in touch with his feeling self. Healing is governed by the law of love.

NeuroCellular Repatterning locates all fears on the left side of the body and anger on the right. Rejection is deposited along the spine as well as within 60 specific locations, each relating to a particular emotional dysfunction. When a person is sick, the cellular structure breaks down at that site because it can no longer process or absorb nutrients. In this system, the cellular memory of emotional rejection, lack of love or any negative emotion is erased. This helps the affected body parts recover their original function and rebuild healthy, new cells.

With NeuroCellular Repatterning, the core issue, or cause, of the illness is uncovered. At the same time, the negative subconscious mind-set is released. On a physical level, the cellular memory is released, permitting the tissues to return to their healthy function.

Sessions of NeuroCellular Repatterning are one hour and 15 minutes long. Participants are clothed and no special preparations are required. ACUPUNCTURE points, which relate to the incident in question, are located and pressed. Momentary discomfort may be experienced at these sensitive sites, but once the details of the illness are explored and forgiven, the pain will disappear. The affirmations communicate the changes that are expected to take place. The release of the trauma may be registered on a BIOFEEDBACK instrument, which substantiates the individual's subconscious response.

It is actually the individual who permits himself to release his negative programming. The practitioner acts as a facilitator who conjoins with the client to let the change happen.

NeuroCellular Repatterning was developed in 1978 by psychologist Arthur Martin. He began his healing career as an intern psychologist in the 1970s as well as studying many forms of alternative therapies. His own physical problems, a deteriorating spine, led him to study alternatives to allopathic medicine. He learned that the body stores cellular memories, which often cause numerous physical/emotional/spiritual dysfunction. He recognized that suppressed emotions from his childhood were causing his physical problems. His technique can remove harmful patterns from the neurological system and replace them with revitalized cells and restored health.

Further Reading
Books by Arthur Martin are available from the Wellness Institute for Personal Transformation, Penryn, California: Martin, Arthur, *Recovering Your Lost Self,* Personal Transformation Press, Penryn, Calif., 1996. *Your Body Is Talking, Are You Listening?* 1996. *Being a Spiritual Being in a Physical Body,* 1994 and *The Doorway to Self-Empowerment,* 1996. Personal Transformation Press, Penryn, Calif.

neuro-linguistic programming®

neuro-linguistic programming® an educational and psychological approach to changing behavioral patterns, thoughts, feelings and perceptions in oneself and in communication with others. It provides the tools to heighten and direct consciousness, to develop the internal world, to enhance communication effectiveness and to increase the knowledge and understanding of oneself and others.

The neuro-linguistic programming model of human communication and personal evolution is based upon the concept that **how** our minds work, **how we** think is precisely knowable, that our perceptual, cognitive and behavioral patterns can be understood and used to positively affect our emotions, thoughts, physiology, sense of self, success, relationships and the future. By influencing internal dialogues that create behavioral patterns, neuro-linguistic programming offers more response choices.

Based on the theories of John Grinder, neuro-linguistic programming follows six principles and presuppositions: the meaning of your communication is the response you get, independent of the intention; there is a positive intention beneath every behavior; failure is feedback; the map is not the territory; people make the best choices available to them; and everyone has the resources needed to accomplish what they really want.[1]

Note
[1] New York Training Institute brochure, 1995, p. 4.

Further Reading
Bandler, Richard and Grinder, John, *Frogs into Princes,* Real People, Newark, Calif., 1979. This book is made up of transcripts from introductory neuro-linguistic programming workshops.

Dilts, Robert, Grinder, John, Bandler, Richard, and DeLozier, Judith, *Neuro-Linguistic Programming: Vol. 1—The Study of the Structure of Subjective Experience,* META, Capitola, Calif., 1980. This book compiles findings of anchoring, elicitation and polarity strategies of neuro-linguistic programming.
Dilts, Robert, *Roots of Neuro-Linguistic Programming,* META Publications, Capitola, Calif., 1983. This book offers a concise presentation of the theories of this system, including sensory experience, chunking, coding, patterning, etc.
Grinder, John, and Bandler, Richard, *Neuro-Linguistic Programming and the Structure of Hypnosis,* Real People, Calif., 1981. This sequel to *Frogs into Princes* explains the use of hypnotic patterning in changing your life.
Linden, Anné and Spaulding, Murray, *The Enneagram and NLP,* Metamorphous Press, Portland, Oreg., 1994. The Enneagram personality typing system is integrated with the transformational techniques of NLP to form a methodology for therapy and a systematic approach for personal evolution.
O'Conner, John, and Seymour, John, *Introducing Neuro-Linguistic Programming,* Aquarian/Thorson's, San Francisco, 1993. This concise book explains the theories of neuro-linguistic programming.

neuromuscular reprogramming

neuromuscular reprogramming also called Conscious Bodywork®, an integrated MASSAGE THERAPY that addresses structural problems at the mechanical, emotional and energetic levels. It incorporates massage, MUSCLE TESTING, conscious attention and advanced techniques to assess and correct coordination dysfunctions affecting joint mobility, RANGE OF MOTION, strength and comfort of joints and muscles.

Conscious BodyWork® accelerates recovery from injuries and helps athletes to optimize their performance. It enables people experiencing the daily wear and tear of life and aging to regain physical capabilities they may have lost. This system blends well with other massage and bodywork modalities, providing the missing ingredient of detailed and thorough neuromuscular reprogramming. It is noninvasive and achieves quick results when dealing with chronic tension and muscle spasms.

Conscious BodyWork uses neuromuscular reprogramming to engage the motor control center of the brain in a kinesthetic conversation to correct the dysfunctional postural and movement patterns that contribute to pain, aging and degeneration in muscles and joints. It also addresses the emotional and energetic components of physical tensions that prevent full recovery from injury or trauma to the body.

When the body experiences shock or trauma, or damage to the tissues, there is a concurrent disruption of the reflex motor patterns governing coordinated movement in those areas. After the tissue damage has healed, these patterns of compensation and protection still exist, even if rehabilitative exercises are performed. Conscious BodyWork addresses the source of these patterns, facilitating full recovery.

Conscious BodyWork neuromuscular reprogramming enhances body awareness by improving the clarity of sensory feedback. It recognizes conscious attention and intention as powerful agents of change in the body, tools that enable the client to fully participate in his or her own healing and realignment process.

Focusing conscious attention and intention, while engaging the sensory feedback system via neuromuscular reprogramming, elicits an intelligent, organized response from the motor coordination center. Newly integrated signals are relayed through the nervous system into the muscles. As a result, posture and movement patterns are quickly changed and pain is alleviated. Clients often experience an improved sensory relationship with their body, heightened body consciousness and new freedom of movement.

Neuromuscular reprogramming was developed by the renowned massage practitioner Jocelyn Olivier. She is the founder and director of Alive and Well! Institute of Conscious Body-Work in San Anselmo, California, and has dedicated her life to the development of this system. Neuromuscular reprogramming is taught only through Alive and Well! Institute of Conscious BodyWork, Inc. Practitioners receive 560 hours of comprehensive, hands-on training, including massage, anatomy, kinesiology, lymphatic, deep tissue, neuromuscular reprogramming, educational and specialized kinesiology, emotional/ energetic balancing techniques and several other relevant modalities.

neuromuscular therapy   See SOMA NEUROMUS-CULAR INTEGRATION.

nuad bo-rarn   See THAI MASSAGE.

O

occupational therapy a type of PHYSICAL THERAPY that helps an individual correct or compensate for a loss of function and to promote independent daily living skills.

Activities are selected to offer neuromuscular, sensory, perceptual, cognitive and/or social skills training. The activity, or the "doing," is the medium that provides individuals with successful functional experiences, in spite of any physical limitations or debilitating diseases.

Many common activities, designed to achieve functional goals, may include creative projects such as gardening, arts and crafts, drawing and painting.

Occupational therapy was first suggested by Dr. J.G. Spurzheim in his book, *Observation on the Deranged Manifestations of the Mind* (Boston, Mass., 1833). The idea was developed by George Combe of Edinburgh, Scotland, a lawyer and phrenologist who popularized the ideas of occupational therapy.[1]

Note

[1] Law, Donald, *A Guide to Alternative Medicine,* Dolphin Books, Garden City, N.Y., 1976, p. 160. Phrenologists believe that the mind operates the body through the brain and links unhealthy mental activity with specific illnesses. Phrenology was founded by Dr. F.J. Gall (1756–1828) and Dr. J. G. Spurzheim.

Further Reading

Border, Bette, Ph.D., *Psychopathology and Function: A Guide for Occupational Therapy,* Slack, Inc., Thorofare, N.J., 1994. This text presents the psychiatric diagnostic system used in the mental health field and explores the role of the occupational therapist.

Lewis, Sandra Cutler, *Elder Care in Occupational Therapy,* Slack, Inc., Thorofare, N.J., 1994. A comprehensive review of the aging process and practical guide for educators and therapists specializing in elder care.

McColl, MaryAnn, Ph.D., Law, Mary C., Ph.D., and Stewart, Debra, B.S., *Theoretical Basis of Occupational Therapy,* Slack, Inc., Thorofare, N.J., 1993. This book references 691 articles relevant to the development of occupational therapy.

Ohashiastu® a method of bodywork that elevates traditional Japanese SHIATSU to a more complete experience of self-development and healing, available to provider and recipient alike. It was developed by the shiatsu master and teacher Wataru Ohashi after years of practicing, teaching and observing human nature. It incorporates psychological and spiritual dimensions to shiatsu, Zen philosophy, movement, exercises and MEDITATIONS to balance the energy of the body/mind/spirit.

Wataru Ohashi was born near Hiroshima, Japan, in 1944. He had a weak constitution as an infant, which made him vulnerable to illness. His strength was restored as a young child by the healing techniques that became central to his teachings.

He came to the United States in 1970 and founded his school, The Ohashi Institute in New York City, in 1974, dedicating himself to the teaching and practice of the Eastern concept of health for 20th century men and women.

To traditional shiatsu, in which pressure is applied to points along the ACUPUNCTURE MERIDIANS, **tsubos,** to relieve pain, tension, fatigue and other symptoms, Ohashiatsu introduces psychological and spiritual components. Rather than focusing on specific points, this system emphasizes sensing and working with the overall flow of energy throughout the body. The quality of a session depends on the provider's technical skill and the empathy, or connection, established between provider and recipient. The qualities of empathy, compassion and reverence are central to Ohashiatsu courses and sessions.

The study and practice of Ohashiatsu helps develop a sensitivity to and an awareness of KI energy, life's vital force. This system seeks to facilitate the flow of *ki* energy throughout the body to achieve a state of balance and harmony. The balanced state promotes and maintains the health and well-being of the body/mind/spirit.

In a typical session, the recipient, dressed in comfortable clothing, lies on the padded floor while the provider moves around him, stretching his body, repositioning limbs and applying firm but gentle pressure to stimulate and balance energy and to induce a peaceful state of well-being.

There are five principles in the Ohashiatsu system. The first, **don't press, just be there,** directs the provider to communicate from her center and to "listen" for the tsubo to draw her in to the exact spot and depth. **Use both hands,** is the second principle. The **mother** hand is always stationary, while the **son** hand moves. Both hands provide support to the recipient. The third principle, **be continuous,** relies upon a continuity of movement in order to keep the *ki* energy constant. Ohashiatsu movement is a way of harmonizing with the flow of the universe.

Be natural, the fourth principle, suggests that the provider should maintain a clear mind, be honest, comfortable and intuitive. The final principle, **be reverent to life,** infers a respect to self, partner, others and the universe.

There are twelve locations in the United States and Europe where Ohashiatsu is taught and the Institute's motto is "Touch for Peace."

Further Reading

Ohashi, Wataru, *Do-It-Yourself Shiatsu,* E. P. Dutton, N.Y., 1976. This clearly illustrated and photographed book explains the principles of Ohashiatsu and provides easy-to-follow techniques for the relief of many symptoms.

———, *Reading the Body: Ohashi's Book of Oriental Diagnosis,* Penguin/Arkana, N.Y., 1991. This book clearly explains how the body can provide all the clues about inner health or illness.

———, *The Big Book of Relaxation,* The Relaxation Company, Emeryville, Calif., 1994. This book describes Ohashiatsu techniques for achieving relaxation.

Okazaki Restorative Massage^{SM}, also called Long Life Massage^{SM}, is a massage based on the ancient Japanese tradition of *seifukujitsu,* or "restoration arts," popularized by Professor Henry S. Okazaki. Historically, martial arts schools in Japan trained their students in fighting skills as well as healing techniques. *Seigotsu* (bone-setting), *kuatsu* (resuscitation techniques) and *seifukujitsu* survived within the realm of jujitsu and judo schools. The most skilled practitioners were usually the most advanced martial artists who practiced their techniques in the dojos, the studios of martial arts. *Seigotsu* practitioners are still seen at judo tournaments in Japan, although *seifuku* practitioners have become rare.

In 1924, Professor Okazaki traveled to Japan to study martial and healing arts required to develop his system of jujitsu. Later, he settled in Hawaii where he learned about the island's ancient healing ritual LOMILOMI. He also studied ancient Oriental massage techniques from which he drew a variety of strokes: pressing, kneading, rubbing, pinching, pulling, rocking, scraping, rotating, jerking, etc.

His system emphasizes the projection of internal energy (KI) to perform the techniques correctly and makes liberal use of deep elbow work. His treatments include joint manipulations to increase flexibility and improve circulation.

He passed his massage techniques on to his jujitsu students and sometimes to health practitioners. In 1958, the American Judo and Jujitsu Federation was incorporated as an educational public benefit organization. In 1983, the first publicly offered class of Okazaki Seifukujitsu Therapy^{SM} was held in Sacramento, California. There are currently over 250 certified Okazaki Restorative Massage technicians in the United States. Okazaki's son, Hachiro, and grandson, Keith, continue to operate Professor Okazaki's massage studio in Honolulu.

Ortho-Bionomy™ a gentle, noninvasive, OSTEOPATHICALLY based reeducation process, which seeks self-correction and balance by accentuating the existing physical condition. The concept of self-healing and the innate wisdom of the body is fundamental to Ortho-Bionomy. By placing the body in its **preferred position,** the position which is most comfortable, and moving it the way it wants to go, the body's healing reflexes are initiated, relaxing muscles and freeing the body of its stresses and tensions.

Ortho-Bionomy was developed by British osteopath Dr. Arthur Lincoln Pauls, D.O. Dr.

Pauls was a black belt in judo and felt that the forceful adjustment techniques he learned in school were contradictory to the movement he had mastered in the martial arts. He began teaching his work in the United States in 1976 and has spread his teachings throughout Europe.

Pauls read an article by the American osteopath Dr. Lawrence Jones called "Spontaneous Release by Positioning," which described how muscular release would occur spontaneously when patients were comfortably, specifically positioned, or put into the position the body was trying to attain. Placing the body in its preferred position stimulates the proprioceptive nervous system (the sense of self-experience) to recognize healthy patterns. This movement triggers a release of the old pattern as the body rebounds to self-correct. Pauls agreed with this concept and developed a system that achieved release and relaxation painlessly and quickly.

He called his system Ortho (correct) Bionomy (the science of the laws of life). This system is designed to teach people how to be more at ease in their bodies and to accomplish the most by expending the least amount of energy. The gentle touch of the practitioner, basic movements and discussions attempt to help the client discover new patterns of balance. The practitioner acts as an observer who facilitates the way as the body heals itself. The Ortho-Bionomy practitioners uses movement and gentle compression to find positions of comfort, which permit the body to change stress and pain patterns.

Ortho-Bionomy has been used to treat arthritis, whiplash, muscle pain and spasms, repeated movement syndrome (repetition of the same movement creates musculoskeletal problems) and imbalanced posture. This system has been effective in increasing joint RANGE OF MOTION, relaxation, circulation and reduction of physical stress and emotional tensions.

Ortho-Bionomy has been incorporated by many bodyworkers, such as massage and physical therapists, chiropractors, osteopaths and naturopaths in their work.

osteopathic medicine a branch of medicine that emphasizes the unity of all body systems. Disturbances in one system, including the musculoskeletal, can alter the function of other systems.

Doctors of osteopathic medicine (D.O.s) observe the Hippocratic philosophy of patient-centered, holistic care and take the osteopathic oath. D.O.s believe that medicine must be more than an attempt to repair or remove the byproducts of disease and are concerned with returning a patient to a state of optimum physical, emotional and mental health.

Osteopathic medicine emphasizes that the musculoskeletal system is central to health. This system, comprised of bones, muscles, tendons, tissue, nerves and the spinal column, makes up almost 60 percent of the body's mass.[1] It works with all other organs and can reflect many internal illnesses.

Osteopathic medicine recognizes the body's own ability to heal. The goal of achieving a high level of efficiency in patient health and function includes preventive medicine, nutritional advice, appropriate exercise and following a healthy lifestyle.

Doctors of osteopathic medicine use all of the recognized medical procedures and technologies for prevention, diagnosis and treatment of disease, such as drugs, radiation and surgery, but they also may use palpation and manipulation of the spinal column as well as other bodywork modalities. Osteopathic physicians may do residencies and specialize in all areas of medicine, such as surgery, psychiatry and radiology.

Manipulation offers an additional dimension to the D.O.s diagnostic and therapeutic arsenal. Palpation provides information about soft tissue changes or structural asymmetries. Corrective manipulations, or **adjustments,** relieve dysfunctions or joint restrictions.

There are a number of manipulation procedures used by osteopathic physicians to treat somatic dysfunctions. In addition to palpation and manipulation, the doctor may employ MYO-FASCIAL RELEASE, CRANIALSACRAL THERAPY, LYM-

PHATIC TECHNIQUE, STRAIN-COUNTERSTRAIN, thrust technique or muscle energy technique.

Myofascial release concentrates on releasing the fascial network, directing dysfunctional tissues along a path of least resistance until free movement is achieved.

Craniosacral technique employs gentle, non-invasive manipulations to treat the craniosacral system, which runs from the covering of the inside of the skull (the dura), down the inside of the spine to the sacrum.

Lymphatic technique is designed to promote circulation of the lymphatic fluids and can be used to treat upper and lower respiratory infections.

Strain-counterstrain identifies TRIGGER POINTS, hypersensitive areas on the muscle and myofascia, and then moves the patient's body or limbs away from the restricted motion toward the position of greatest comfort.

The thrust technique is a form of manipulation that utilizes the physician's high velocity/low amplitude thrust to restore specific joint motion. This technique resets neural reflexes and establishes a fuller joint RANGE OF MOTION. The procedure reduces and/or nullifies the physical signs of somatic dysfunction: tissue changes, asymmetry, tenderness and restricted range of motion.[2]

Muscle energy technique directs the patient to use his muscles from a precise position, and in a specific direction, against the physician-applied counterforce. Muscle energy technique restores motion, decreases tissue changes and modifies the asymmetry of somatic dysfunction.[3]

Osteopathic medicine was founded in 1874 by Dr. Andrew Taylor Still on the Missouri frontier. Dissatisfied with the medical practices of his time, he developed a philosophy of medicine based on body unity, focusing on the musculoskeletal system.

He identified palpation and the human touch as vital to gaining patient trust and confidence and as a means of providing effective medical care. He stressed manipulation over the more commonly accepted practices of the 19th century, which were rudimentary drugs and surgical procedures.

Dr. Still began to teach his four sons the art of manipulation in 1887 and founded the American School of Osteopathy in Kirksville, Missouri, in 1892.

Modern osteopathic physicians have the same practice rights as medical doctors (allopathic physicians) throughout the United States and treat patients in both osteopathic and allopathic hospitals and clinics.

Notes

1 American Academy of Osteopathy, "Osteopathic Medicine: A Distinctive Branch of Mainstream Medicine," American Academy of Osteopathy, Indianapolis, Ind., p. 1.
2 Ibid., p. 4.
3 Ibid., p. 4.

Further Reading

Northup, George W., D.O., F.A.A.O., *Osteopathic Medicine: An American Reformation*, American Osteopathic Association, Chicago, Ill., 1987. This book provides an overview of osteopathic medicine, its history and theories.

———, *Osteopathic Research: Growth and Development*, American Osteopathic Association, Chicago, Ill., 1987. This book traces the development of osteopathic medicine to the present. Recognition is given to the study of the nature and effect of somatic dysfunction as well as basic scientific research done under the auspices of the osteopathic profession.

P

PNF stretches (proprioceptive neuromuscular facilitation) is a physical therapy method developed to rehabilitate patients by using a unique stretching technique. The idea behind PNF stretches is to cause the injured muscles to accomplish specific goals by "tricking" the proprioceptors within the soft tissue.

Proprioceptors are nerve mechanisms, which help an individual identify the physical activities and position of muscles, tendons and joints. This sense provides information of the degree of muscular contraction and the amount of tension in the tendons. With this sense, which is also called the kinesthetic sense, we can recognize the location and rate of movement of body parts in relation to others and estimate how much muscle strength is required to perform a specific task.

PNF stretching, based on contraction/relaxation, was initially developed during the 1940s and 1950s to rehabilitate patients with paralysis. CRAC, the acronym which describes the technique stands for contract/relax/antagonist/contract. A client fully extends an arm, for example, and the therapist holds that stretch while the client tries to contract the arm. Since the muscle tenses during this process, upon release, it can stretch or extend even further.

The application for PNF has reached beyond rehabilitation. During the 1980s, it was adopted by athletes to increase performance and enhance flexibility and strength.

Further Reading

McAtee, Robert E., *Facilitated Stretching: PNF Stretching Made Easy,* Human Kinetics Publications, Champaign, Ill., 1993. This photographed book explains the history and theory of PNF stretching and its application in rehabilitation as well as performance enhancement.

Parma Training Program™ a system that facilitates the removal of blocks, obstacles, hindrances and limitations, which prevent the vital life force from its fullest expression within the mind/body system. It is an integration of several disciplines designed to restore harmony and balance to the mind/body/spirit of an individual.

It is a combination of SHIATSU, HOSHINO THERAPY, TRIGGER POINT, NEUROMUSCULAR THERAPY and Eastern energetic work.

Parma work includes pressure point release and myofascial (the connective tissue sheath that enfolds muscles) spreading. It also includes breath awareness work, relaxation imagery and therapeutic stretches.

This system was developed by Vincent Parmentola, R.M.T., C.S.P., of Boca Raton, Florida. His 15 year and rather eclectic background, which involves MASSAGE THERAPY, SOMA THERAPY and CRANIALSACRAL THERAPY in addition to those methods listed above, combined to create the unique blend of Parma.

Parma **Symmetry** is based on the 10-step procedure for structural alignment. The first three sessions, "Setting the Stage," is defined as a complete unit. It establishes a foundation for the facilitator and the partner (Parmentola refers to his clients as partners). Session one begins the process of head and shoulder alignment while expanding the rib cage. Session two is a "grounding" experience as the partner develops a physical connectedness to the earth. Session three lengthens and balances the shoulder/pelvis axis. These sessions form an independent segment of Parma Symmetry.

Sessions four through seven focus on freeing the pelvis and attaining maximum length of the **coreline,** an imaginary track that runs the length of the body from the feet to the head. These four sessions are central to the entire construct of the 10-session format. **Corecenter** is accessed and the proper body mechanics training is emphasized.

The final three sessions consist of organizing and balancing the structure so that **dynamic symmetry** results. The upper/lower and the front/back aspects demonstrate greater integration and harmony in expression and function. "Becoming friends with gravity" makes life flow with greater ease and comfort as the transformed body moves with greater efficiency through the gravitational field.

past life regression a psychotherapy process that retraces former lives in the hopes of resolving obstacles and problems in this life. It assists in understanding and changing unhealthy behavior patterns and focuses on the individual's life purpose. Past life regression may be used as a tool for transformation within the fields of integrative medicine and psychology.

Although many ancient cultures have recognized reincarnation, there are no religious overtones in past life regression nor do people necessarily have to believe in reincarnation for the regression to be effective.

Hypnosis or guided meditations are the most popular ways of accessing the unconscious mind to reveal past traumas. Reliving an incident may explain current behavior patterns or physical problems and provides closure to the incident.

Adults and children alike can partake of this system without harm. Children seem to be particularly easy subjects, since they are so close to their previous life.

Past life regression has been accepted in the United States and Europe for about 25 years, with a modest following. The Association for Past Life Research and Therapies, in Riverside, California, provides information and referrals on past life regression.

Further Reading

Chaplin, Annabel, *The Bright Light of Death*. This book provides the author's personal account of her work with people whose problems are directly related to the influence of deceased relatives or close friends.

Netherton, Sandy and Amodeo, John, *Past Lives Therapy*, William Morrow & Co., N.Y., 1978. This informative book provides a general overview of the history and explanation of past life regression.

Schlotterbeck, Karl, *Living Your Past Lives*, Ballantine Books, N.Y., 1987. The psychology of past life regression is explained in this text.

Weiss, Brian L., M.D., *Many Lives, Many Masters*, Simon & Schuster, N.Y., 1988. This book details a case history of a young woman who suffered from many anxieties. Under hypnosis, she recalled several incidents of dying, which explained and finally relieved her problems.

pericardium See HEART CONSTRICTOR MERIDIAN.

Pesso Boyden system psychomotor an innovative method of psychotherapy or emotional reeducation, originally designed by dance educators Albert and Diane Boyden Pesso in 1961, to heighten the skills of dance students and performers.

Formerly called psychomotor, this method emphasizes bodily movement, especially action by the client and appropriate interaction by others whose roles are typically played by members of a therapy group. Through the years, Pesso Boyden system psychomotor has evolved into a coherent system that fits well with both psychodynamic and cognitive-behavioral, as well as neurobiological models of therapy.

Assured of the therapist's respectful understanding and acceptance, the client may speak about thoughts and feelings as they occur and how that affects what is being sensed in the body. The emotion felt by the client is named by the therapist as if by a **witness figure** and is linked to its context. Any **inner voice** that the client seems to be following is identified and made external. For instance, the client chooses someone from the group to role-play **the voice of shame,** indicating what the voice should say. This very often mimics parental wording. The client can then relive the experience where needs were not adequately met. In this case, however, it is reexperienced in a place of support and security.

New, more ideal parents (or other important figures) can role-play past events where the client's feelings and needs were denied. This new experience can be taken in by both mind and body as an alternative and can be corrective to the client's literal past history, enabling positive patterns of behavior and self-awareness.

petrissage, also called kneading, is the second stroke in SWEDISH MASSAGE. Petrissage lifts the

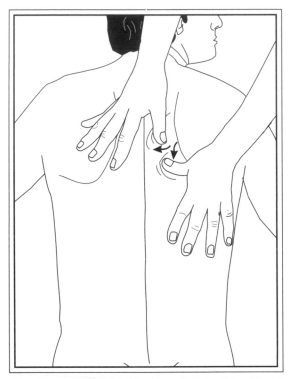

Circular petrissage to the scapula (shoulder blade) is applied in a centrifugal direction, with the pressure away from the center. Petrissage lifts the skin from underlying structures. Light work affects the tissues directly below the movement, while deep work penetrates into the muscle fibers.

skin from underlying structures and can be either superficial or deep. The pressure of the stroke is applied in a centrifugal (away from the center) direction and can be applied in several different ways: with the palmar surface of one or both hands for larger areas or circularly with fingertips or thumbs for more detailed work. Other forms of petrissage include **fulling, rolling, wringing, chucking** and **pick up.**

Fulling is a type of petrissage where the skin is compressed between the thumbs and the first fingers. It is a pinching movement, which acts upon the skin and the loose, underlying tissues. The skin is released at the point of greatest strain to ensure the maximum effect of emptying and refilling blood and lymph vessels. Fulling is an alternative hand movement.

Rolling is a back and forth movement where the tissues are compressed against underlying structures. The fingers are straight and held closely together. The movement is rapid, about 200 to 400 strokes per minute, and works from the proximal aspect of the limb (the region closest to the body) to the distal end (the region farthest away from the body). The pressure exerted during rolling can be strong.

Wringing is performed by grasping a limb with both hands close together and moving simultaneously in opposite directions.

Chucking is a petrissage where a limb is supported by one hand while the other hand firmly grasps the fleshy portion and drags it up and down. Movements are made two to six times at each part of the limb. Chucking helps to stretch contracted muscles and acts upon the blood vessels and nerves.

Pick up is performed as the skin is lifted between both thumbs and fingers. The hands alternately lift and twist the tissue, bringing blood to the surface. The hands are held close and there is always skin in one hand as the movement progresses. Pick up is beneficial to maintain muscle tone and to contain atrophy (shrinkage).

The rate of kneading is generally 30 to 90 strokes per minute, except where noted. Petrissage acts upon the deep vessels, accelerates venous and lymph circulation and brings arterial blood to the body part being treated. As a result of its effects on circulation, nutrition is promoted and weak muscles are stimulated.

Superficial petrissage affects tissues directly below the movement, while deep work penetrates into the muscle fibers. Petrissage improves the functional activity of the skin and increases general glandular activity. The absorption of inflammatory exudate (accumulated fluid) is enhanced. Kneading to the colon improves the tone of the intestinal walls and promotes peristaltic activity (the wavelike motion of the intestines during excretion).

Cellular respiration is increased and the exchange of gases is increased. Petrissage produces a great amount of heat to the body.

Thérèse Pfrimmer Method of Deep Muscle Therapy® a refined, deeply penetrating system of corrective treatment specifically designed to aid in the restoration of damaged muscles and SOFT TISSUE throughout the whole body. By employing a specialized series of cross-tissue movements, the trained Pfrimmer Deep Muscle therapist can concentrate on all the layers of muscles that have become depleted of their normal, and essential, blood and LYMPHATIC flow. This precise therapy helps restore the circulation to the tissues along with its natural healing properties.

Pfrimmer, a massage therapist and physiotherapist in Ontario, Canada, was stricken with paralysis to her lower extremities in 1946. Her condition was diagnosed as incurable, yet she believed otherwise. This prognosis prompted her to work on herself and led to the discovery of her technique and the reversal of her paralysis. Until her death in 1980, 34 years later, Pfrimmer did extensive research on muscles and trained others in her technique.

While she was ill, she started to manipulate her legs and found them to be extremely painful. She recognized that healthy muscles should not register pain to the touch. As she worked deeply into her leg muscles, she discovered that she was growing stronger each day. Evidently, the muscles were acutely involved in the paralysis, more so than the nerves. She was determined to work on other crippling conditions to see if her technique could also help others.

Pfrimmer's second subject, Ethel Brown, was completely paralyzed. She could only move her eyes and lips, but could not speak. She was discolored, edemous (full of fluid), had a strong mephitic odor coming from her body and had been brought to the hospital to die.

The first treatment Pfrimmer gave her lasted four hours. During this introductory session, the stench was so nauseating that Pfrimmer had to leave the room many times to vomit. The deep treatments were identical to those she had performed upon her own paralyzed legs.

By the third treatment, Brown was running a fever, indicating that her body was functioning, and feebly spoke for the first time in several months. In March 1948, five months after their initial encounter, Ethel Brown was sitting up in bed and was able to exercise slightly.

That same year, Pfrimmer received her massage license. Throughout her research and experimentation, she learned that, although paralysis might be present, the muscles were not alienated from the brain, and when the circulation to the limbs was restored and they were released from their adherent factors, muscles could begin to function again.[1]

From 1946 to 1949, Pfrimmer worked without pay as she continued to develop her theories. To support herself, she took a job as a night cook at a local restaurant. This proved to be serendipitous. While cutting up a side of beef, she came across a tough section of meat, which felt similar to the way muscle fibers of paralytic conditions feel. She understood that her deep muscle therapy restored circulation to unhealthy muscle cells, permitting them to function again. Her observation convinced her that the answers to crippling conditions were in the muscles.[2]

Pfrimmer Deep Muscle Therapy establishes a foundation for corrective massage into which other, specific trouble-shooting techniques can be incorporated.[3] It is a preventive as well as restorative therapy. It is designed to cause corrective changes to damaged or adherent muscles and the adjacent soft tissues. The resulting improved circulation on a cellular level, improves and restores the damaged muscles and any soft tissues that may be impaired by poor circulation, as well as the total body health of an individual.

Where muscles become "dry," Pfrimmer Deep Muscle Therapy promotes lymphatic fluid flow. Since those adherent and fibrous muscle conditions that exist within the layers of muscles are released, this system actually corrects damaged muscles and soft tissues. In order to be effective, the pressure of the treatment takes place at the discomfort level, as much as the client can tolerate.

These back and forth, specialized cross-fiber movements have been successful in the treatment of amyotrophic lateral sclerosis (ALS), a progressive muscular atrophy (Lou Gehrig's disease), arthritis, carpal tunnel syndrome, cerebral palsy, digestive distress, headaches, joint and muscle pain, multiple sclerosis and muscular dystrophy, occupational injuries, paralysis, Parkinson's disease, poor circulation, sciatica, sports injuries, tendinitis, trauma and whiplash.

The professional course is a two-week intensive program, totaling 80 hours. Offered at the Alexandria School of Scientific Therapeutics in Alexandria, Indiana and the Pennsylvania School of Muscle Therapy, Wayne, Pennsylvania, it is suitable for advanced massage therapists, physical therapists, doctors, nurses and chiropractors.

Notes
1 Pfrimmer, Thérèse C., *Muscles: Your Invisible Bonds,* Blythe Printing, Blythe, Ontario, Canada, 1970, p. 10.
2 Ibid., p. 11.
3 Mixing Pfrimmer Deep Muscle Therapy with Swedish massage, for example, would nullify the corrective system of Pfrimmer. Swedish massage, a relaxing system, enhances circulation to the heart, while Pfrimmer Deep Muscle Therapy is used primarily for corrective purposes. Only those systems that work in concert with Pfrimmer's precepts can be combined with this precise technique.

Further Reading
Pfrimmer, Thérèse C., *Muscles: Your Invisible Bonds,* Blythe Printing, Blythe, Ontario, Canada, 1970. Written by the developer of the system, this easy-to-read book gives the background of Pfrimmer Deep Muscle Therapy and its application in the treatment of many conditions.

Phoenix Rising yoga therapy an integrated system of supporting and holding the body in positions based on classic HATHA YOGA postures, called *asanas,* while using verbal dialogue techniques to create conscious awareness. This hands-on yet noninvasive work allows for the release of both physical and emotional ten-

sions as well as those belief systems that have been holding them in place for so long.

Phoenix Rising yoga therapy is based on the idea that unresolved emotional experiences are stored in the body/mind and are often hidden from conscious awareness. The body's innate freedom is inhibited and, over time, the body begins to "wear" the postures reflected by those beliefs. These postures can create deep-seated tension.

Hatha yoga was developed approximately 6,000 years ago by Indian masters to unblock the flow of life force energy, called PRANA. Physically, each asana releases patterns of holding as well as having a metaphysical signature relating to emotions. For example, a posture of willingness, when held long enough, will eventually yield to surrender. A posture of positive affirmation, such as one of self-confidence, will grow stronger. Phoenix Rising yoga therapy also includes techniques of humanistic psychology to create a system available to anyone who is committed to personal growth.

This system was created by Michael Lee, M.A., who began his professional life in education in the outback of Australia. He became a lecturer at the Administrative College of Papua, New Guinea. Eventually, he found himself working for the South Australian government, designing and implementing a human relations and organizational effectiveness program. In 1978, while teaching at college in Adelaide, Lee was introduced to yoga. Deeply inspired, he brought new programs, such as metaphysical sciences, to the college curriculum.

His growing desire to develop aspects of body/mind therapy brought him to the United States and the KRIPALU Center for Yoga and Health in Lenox, Massachusetts, in 1984. His work continued to evolve, resulting in the development of Phoenix Rising yoga therapy in 1986. Training is currently offered across the United States, Canada and Europe.

Lee believes that discomfort is a "call for transformation."[1] It affords an individual an opportunity for the spirit to explore these fears that caused the discomfort, and then go beyond it. Lee thinks of yoga as a way to confront the entire self through the body.

Personal transformations are possible during the session as the practitioner supports and moves the client's body, permitting deeply held tensions to be explored, released and integrated. Further supporting this process are the dialogue methods specially created to stimulate internal awareness, especially those that frame and construct behavior. These dialogue techniques are not used until the clients feel comfortable with the physical scope of yoga therapy. As a completion for the dialogue technique, clients are led through a GUIDED MEDITATION, which invites them to connect with the innate sense of knowing that underlies all cognitive experience. Client-generated affirmations, which are linked to the body, close each session with a reinforced healing power and self-awareness.

The training to become a Phoenix Rising yoga therapy practitioner consists of three levels. Levels one and two are each four-day residential programs, while level three is a six-month, non-residential internship-practicum.

Note
1 Ruch, Meredith Gould, Ph.D., "Release Your Body's Healing Wisdom," *Changes,* June 1993, p. 34.

physical deep muscle therapy See DEEP TISSUE MASSAGE.

physical therapy a specialized rehabilitative healing science designed to relieve pain, restore function and movement and prevent injury. People seek help from licensed physical therapists, for specific reasons, with a doctor's prescription.

Physical therapists are an important part of the rehabilitation and preventive health care team. They are involved in the recovery of cardiac, pulmonary, medical, surgical and orthopedic patients. There are also specialized therapists who are highly trained to work in burn units of hospitals and with developmentally delayed infants and children.

Early Chinese and Roman societies used physical methods, such as massage, HYDROTHERAPY and heat treatment, for many ailments. During the Dark Ages, Middle Eastern physicians discovered the value of exercise in the treatment of injuries. Massage was recognized by European doctors during the mid-19th century, as a valuable tool for health.

Physical therapy, as we know it today, began during World War I when the United States needed health professionals to rehabilitate the wounded. The Surgeon General's Office formed the Division of Special Hospitals and Physical Reconstruction, employing about 2,000 "reconstruction aides," as the physical therapists were then called. Practicing in hospitals and later in veterans' hospitals, these reconstruction aides used hydrotherapy, ELECTROTHERAPY, mechanotherapy (RANGE OF MOTION), muscle reeducation, active exercises, indoor and outdoor games and passive exercises in the form of massage to help restore the wounded.[1]

Women formed the first professional association, in 1921, called the American Physical Therapy Association which had 274 chapter members. By the end of the 1930s, men were admitted and membership grew to almost 1,000.[2]

With the advent of World War II and the nationwide polio epidemic during the 1940s and 1950s, the demand for these trained professionals was great. The membership in the organization increased to 8,000 members.

In the 1960s, the APTA membership reached almost 15,000 with 52 education programs nationwide. Currently, more than 62,000 physical therapists, physical therapist assistants and students are represented by the association, located in Alexandria, Virginia. One hundred and thirty-one institutions offer physical therapy education programs and 135 offer physical therapist assistant education programs in the United States.[3]

Modern physical therapists employ a number of modalities in the evaluation and treatment of physical problems. Initially, an evaluation or assessment is made to attain information about the condition or dysfunction. A personal history is taken, which may include the medical history, occupation, daily activities, history of medications and explanation of the injury and its accompanying pain pattern.

The physical therapist palpates, or feels, the area for moisture, swelling, temperature, mobility, limitations and muscle spasms.

Routine tests are generally performed to determine muscle strength, range of motion and sensation. All of this information is gathered to develop a specialized treatment program. This program is usually based on the principles of pain reduction, neurological rehabilitation, increased range of motion and increased strength.[4]

Many different treatment therapies may be combined to reach the therapy goals. For the relief of pain, the physical therapist may employ heat therapy and cold treatments, such as ice or hot packs, ULTRASOUND, and hydrotherapy, a hands-on system of joint and soft tissue mobilization, such as massage and/or exercise. Electrical stimulation is used when muscles are immobilized or extremely weak. An automatic contraction helps increase muscle strength.[5]

Neurological rehabilitation helps the patient coordinate basic movements used in daily life. Patients who are suffering from strokes, head injuries, spinal cord traumas, birth defects or neurological disorders generally receive this form of treatment. Neuromuscular reeducation helps the body to learn basic movements again. If the muscles have contracted abnormally due to the physical condition, specific tone reduction exercises and positioning may be used.

Exercises are an integral part of recovery. They strengthen the muscles, restore balance and promote self-care. Stretching exercises can help elongate muscle tissue and are often used to prevent back injuries and athletic injuries.

Treatments usually last 20 to 30 minutes, two to three times a week, as needed. A licensed profession in each state, many physical therapists work in hospitals, although the majority of them work in private physical therapy offices, sports facilities, rehabilitation centers or health centers.

Notes
[1] American Physical Therapy Association: A Historical Perspective, Alexandria, Va., no date.
[2] Ibid.
[3] Ibid.
[4] Krames Communication, ''Physical Therapy,'' Daly City, Calif., 1984, p. 5.
[5] Ibid., pp. 5–6.

Further Reading
American Physical Therapy Association, ''A Future in Physical Therapy,'' Alexandria, Va., 1995. This booklet provides an overview of physical therapy for the patient as well as potential student.
Matthew, Jane, M.P.H., P.T., *Practice Issues in Physical Therapy,* Slack, Inc., Thorofare, N.J., 1994. This education resource analyzes current and future physical therapy practice patterns. It provides operational information about setting up a practice. The author is a past president of the American Physical Therapy Association.

The Pilates® Method a full-body exercise system, which emphasizes body alignment and correct breathing. The abdomen, lower back and buttocks are used as a power center, which enables free movement of the rest of the body.

A series of controlled exercises and specialized equipment create variable resistance for muscular exertion. The Pilates Method excludes the use of weights, although resistance is provided by springs and the client's own body weight, jumping and running.

An exercise called running can be done, however, lying down with feet placed against an adjustable bar. The primary focus is on balance of the entire neuromusculoskeletal system. The main apparatus is called the **reformer.** It is a bedlike platform with a carriage that slides along tracks. The carriage may be moved by pushing against a bar or pulling leather straps with the arms or legs. Exercises may be done from reclining, sitting, kneeling, standing or piking positions. Other equipment pieces are the **Cadillac** (a bedlike platform surrounded by a metal frame, which includes a push-through bar, trapeze bar and leg straps), **barrel** (a rounded structure, which strengthens the legs and spine), the **chair,** the **tower** (a vertical frame housing adjustable spring tension) and the **mat** (upon which a repertoire of abdominal and spine exercises, which focus on controlled breathing, may be performed).

This system was developed by physical culturist Joseph Pilates (1880–1967). Growing up in Germany, he sought ways to strengthen his frail body, which helped to create his lifelong interest in physical culture.

While living in England during World War I, Pilates became a nurse. His experiments with resistance using springs attached to a hospital bed proved to strengthen his immobilized patients. These discoveries led him to design the mat exercises and the **universal reformer,** which enhanced his mat exercise program and became the foundation of The Pilates Method. In 1926, Pilates emigrated to the United States and introduced his exercise system.

Some of the first people to use this system were dancers, such as Martha Graham and George Balanchine. It is now widely used by physical therapists and orthopedists who employ it as an adjunct to the rehabilitation of their patients.

Pilates called his work "contrology," meaning that the body must be controlled and trained through the mind. He believed that corrective exercise begins with education and total conditioning. He preferred more precise moves to, what he considered to be, mindless repetition. The movements of more than 500 specifically designed exercises on the five main pieces of equipment are purposely concentrated. As the mind is directed through the movements, a greater awareness takes place.

Pilates sessions, which are tailored to each individual, are usually done on a one-to-one basis or in closely supervised, small groups with a certified teacher. The certification process by the Pilates Studio has some of the highest standards in the country for exercise instruction, with over 600 hours of apprenticeship required to become a certified Pilates instructor.

The Pilates Method is available to all people, regardless of age or level of physical fitness, who want to improve their strength and flexibility without increasing muscle bulk. This system facilitates muscle harmony and balance. People who consistently use it report that they walk and sit straighter, are more graceful, sleep better and develop firmer, sleeker, more powerful muscles.

pointing therapy a special PHYSICAL THERAPY that treats certain illnesses and symptoms by activating ACUPUNCTURE points or **stimulant lines** (similar to the MERIDIAN system) with specific hand pressure techniques. These techniques include **pointing, pressing, pinching, clapping** or **knocking.** This system is part of the heritage of CHINESE MEDICINE, which holds that pointing therapy can promote vital energy (QI) and blood circulation, thereby enhancing healing.

The chief method of treatment is the placement of one or two fingers directly on a specific acupuncture point or stimulant line. Its name is derived from this form of treatment. Pointing skill emerges from the ancient Chinese martial arts that were used not only for self-defense, but also for treating disease. Pointing therapy has been used to treat common illnesses as well as those that are difficult to treat, such as polio, cerebral paralysis and herniated disks (intervertebral disks). No special instruments are required for pointing therapy and it produces no adverse side effects.

The acupuncture points and stimulant lines of pointing therapy are directly connected to the energetic system.[1] If the function of the points or pathways is obstructed, disease will occur. Pointing therapy promotes channel and organ function by increasing vital energy and blood circulation, restoring the balance between YIN and YANG, supporting healthy energy, clearing channels and expelling pathogenic factors. In

Western terms, pointing therapy may regulate the function of the nervous system, improve local circulation and metabolism and assist in the healing of diseased tissue.

Pointing therapy is indicated in numerous conditions, such as paralytic diseases, nerve injuries, extremity pain syndromes, headaches, impotence, myopia, painful menses and temporomandibular joint disorder.

There are also certain contraindications for this system: acute diseases of the abdomen or inflammatory conditions, hypertension, heart disease or pulmonary tuberculosis, hemophilia, and severe skin diseases.

Diagnosis is made by the practitioner using the four methods of examination: observation, inquiring, listening and palpation, which includes PULSE DIAGNOSIS. Pressure of the treatment should match the client's tolerance level and treatments may be given once a day in general cases and twice daily in acute situations. The course of treatment may be 10 days for those people with mild symptoms or as long as two months for chronic cases. Treatment for paraplegia may last up to six months.[2]

This system requires strength on the part of the practitioner. There are specific types of pointing skills and preparatory exercises used to develop the craftsmanship and power needed for this work.

The hand technique of pointing is made up of three gestures. The first one is a slight flexion of the fingers with the middle finger pressed between the thumbs and the index finger. The last two fingers are tightly closed. The second pointing gesture supports slightly bent index and middle fingers on the thumb as the last two fingers are tightly closed. The third gesture brings all fingertips together. These are the most basic hand positions used to treat diseases, acupuncture points and stimulant lines.

Pressing uses the tips of the thumb, with or without the other fingers, on common points or stimulant lines. Pinching, usually applied to fingers and toes, is performed by the edge of the

practitioner's thumb or index fingernail. This method is used to stimulate the meridians.

Patting is a percussive movement done with the hands in a loosely held, tentlike position. It is used to promote circulation, dredge the channels and enhance organ function. Knocking is another percussive movement performed with all fingertips touching each other.

Pointing therapy also incorporates combinations of these hand positions in its treatments.

Notes
[1] The meridians are the pathways for vital energy (*qi*).
[2] Hui, Jia Li, and Xiang, Jia Zhao, *Pointing Therapy: A Chinese Traditional Therapeutic Skill,* Shandong Science and Technology Press, Beijing, China, 1987, p. 8.

Further Reading
Hui, Jia Li, and Xiang, Jia Zhao, *Pointing Therapy: A Chinese Traditional Therapeutic Skill,* trans. Yuan, Jiang Qi, M.D., Gao Ying, Shandong Science and Technology Press, Beijing, China, 1987. This book, translated from the Chinese, makes some unusual references. However, it does offer an explanation of pointing therapy. Clear illustrations help to clarify the explanation.

polarity therapy a health system based on the concept of the HUMAN ENERGY BIO-FIELD. The basic premise is that there is an electromagnetic energetic pattern that precedes human structure and function. The term "polarity" is used to describe the basic nature of this energy flow: cycles of expansion/contraction and attraction/repulsion. Polarity therapy was originated by Randolph Stone, D.O., D.C., N.D. (1890–1981) as a synthesis of his study of the traditional philosophies and health concepts of India and the Far East.

In polarity, health conditions are viewed as reflections of the condition of the energy biofield and therapies are designed to stimulate and balance the field for health benefit. Polarity incorporates bodywork, diet, exercise and counseling in a comprehensive physical, emotional, mental and spiritual approach to total health care.

Polarity therapy was developed by Dr. Stone in the mid-20th century. As a young physician

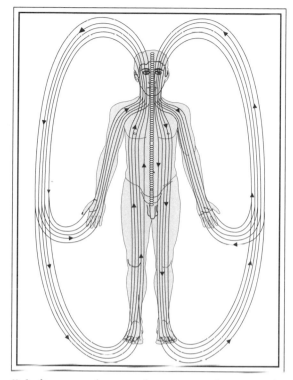

Polarity recognizes an electromagnetic, energetic pattern that precedes human structure and function. Health is viewed as a reflection of the condition of the energy bio-field and therapies are designed to stimulate and balance the field.

in the 1920s, he was shown a simple bodywork technique, which proved to be extremely valuable with patients. OSTEOPATHIC manipulations lasted longer, deeper levels of awareness were experienced and profound relaxation and healing was achieved. Fascinated by consistent results, which had no conventional anatomical explanation, he began a lifelong search for understanding of the deeper causes of health and disease. His quest led to the Oriental idea of the human energy bio-field, and to a thorough investigation of this revolutionary, yet ancient, approach to the healing arts.

Dr. Stone published his findings in the late 1940s in five books and numerous pamphlets. He chose the word "polarity" to describe the basic nature of the electromagnetic force field of the body. He taught that polarized energy currents precede physical form and are primary factors in well-being.

Dr. Stone found that the human energy bio-field is affected by touch, diet, movement and sound, attitudes, relationships and environmental factors. Polarity therapy sheds light on all these subjects; the scope of polarity practice can therefore be very broad, with implications for health professionals in many therapeutic disciplines.

Dr. Stone treated patients and conducted research at his office in Chicago for over 50 years. When he retired in 1974, his students continued development of the system, diversifying its applications across a broad spectrum of disciplines.

In the 1980s, polarity leadership was assumed by the American Polarity Therapy Association (APTA). APTA created a "Standards for Practice" to define the scope and content of polarity and organized polarity education and practitioner certification.

Modern science has described and exploited the phenomenal power of the attraction and repulsion at the heart of physical matter. The (+) quality of the proton and the (−) quality of the electron in dynamic relationship is the fundamental glue of the universe.

The significance of this electromagnetic field on the atomic or microcosmic level is also found on a macrocosmic level. Relationships of attraction and repulsion and their cycles of expansion and contraction are the primary pattern of all existence, from cellular to interplanetary.

The human body is also a collection of energetic relationships. In the polarity model, health is experienced when these systems are functioning normally. Energy flows smoothly without significant blockage or fixation on any level. Disease and pain occur when energy is blocked, fixed or imbalanced. Blockages arise primarily from trauma, self-defeating attitudes and expectations and unhealthful lifestyles. Polarity therapy deals with finding the blockages, releasing the energy to normal flow and balance and maintaining the energy bio-field in an open, flexible condition.

Polarity therapy is best known for its bodywork. The basic premise of polarity bodywork is that touch affects the human energy bio-field. Placing the hands on the body affects energy flow, with one placement stimulating and the reverse placement having a sedating effect. In the human body, the head has a positive charge, while the feet have a negative charge. The right side of the body is positive, the left side is negative.

During a polarity session, the client lies on a massage table, dressed in loose-fitting clothing. The practitioner looks for areas of tension or blockage. The manipulations of polarity are gentle and are designed to encourage the client to relax. The practitioner places both hands on two designated body areas, creating a polarity. The touch stimulates the flow of energy, and, in combination with the currents of the client, areas of blockage, pain or trauma are revitalized and released.

People receiving polarity report remarkable results. Deep relaxation, new insight into cause and patterns and a sense of calm power are often expressed. In diet, polarity espouses a vegetarian diet with periodic cleansing practices. In exercise, Dr. Stone recognized that the human energy bio-field was affected by movement, posture, sound and other self-applied therapeutic possibilities.

Polarity therapy is unique among the holistic health systems due to its comprehensive scope and a remarkable diversity of applications. While it is often found in conjunction with other healing practices, it offers a spiritual/mental/emotional/physical integration, which bridges ancient philosophy and modern science. It has proven to be effective in a wide range of health situations and continues to grow in acceptance today.

Further Reading

Beaulieu, John, *Polarity Therapy Workbook,* Biosonic Enterprises, N.Y., 1994. This work organized polarity therapy into a set of learning protocols that are quite simple to understand. It contains over 500 annotated photographs and illustrations that explain polarity therapy theory, bodywork and evaluation.

Chitty, John, and Muller, M.L., *Energy Exercises,* Polarity Press, Boulder, Colo., 1990. This book is a complete source of self-help techniques described by Dr. Randolph Stone. It contains an extensive treatment of polarity body readings, determining the condition of the energy field by the shape of the body.

Sills, Franklyn, *The Polarity Process,* Element Books, Shaftsbury, England, 1989. This is an excellent synthesis of the theory and applications of polarity therapy. It organizes the diverse concepts put forth by polarity's founder, Dr. Randolph Stone, into a sequence that is understandable for beginning readers as well as advanced students.

Stone, Randolph, *Polarity Therapy, the Collected Works: Vol. I, Vol. II,* CRCS Publishing, Sebastopol, Calif., 1986, and *Health Building: The Conscious Art of Living Well,* CRCS Publishing, Sebastopol, Calif., 1985. This three-volume set was originally published in the 1950s and considered heretical when it first appeared. At the core of these works is the revolutionary understanding of energy articulated by Dr. Stone, the systematic function of this energy and the myriad applications available. Also discussed in a large variety of spiritual and healing traditions, including reflexology, yoga, acupuncture and Auyrvedic medicine.

positional release   also called origin-insertion technique in CHIROPRACTIC, is a neuromuscular and educational technique that deals with acute and chronic pain. Positional releasepractitioners place a muscle in a supershortened position to trick the proprioceptors (a receptor stimulated by the body's own action) into releasing.

postural integration   a unique method for releasing tensions in the body/mind. It is a powerful and loving way of moving deep, blocked layers of CONNECTIVE TISSUE and releasing inhibited emotions and thoughts. It is "postural" insofar as it addresses and frees rigid postures, and it is "integration" because it helps individuals assimilate this energy and freedom into their lives.

Connective tissue, or FASCIA, is a thin, dense and elastic material that wraps around muscles and muscle groups. When tension is present, the fascia is a principal means by which physical imbalance is sustained because it tenses in response to stress. The practitioner of postural integration uses his fingers, hands and forearms to systematically release tightened and disorganized layers of fascia, allowing the contracted muscles to relax and the overstretched muscles to contract. Once muscular balance has been achieved, skeletal alignment is improved, creating flexible posture and free-flowing energy.

Deep breathing is encouraged during the bodywork to promote expression of blocked emotions and thoughts and to explore the possibility of new physical movements.

This system was developed by Jack Painter (1933–) during the 1970s. Painter holds Ph.D.s, in philosophy, literature and psychology from Emory University in Atlanta, Georgia. Many years of self-exploration in MASSAGE, ACUPUNCTURE, GESTALT THERAPY, REICHIAN THERAPY and ROLFING led to his development of postural integration.

Postural integration is given in 10 steps or phases. Each phase consists of several 75-minute sessions. During the first seven phases, called **the release** ("letting go of the old self"), the legs, pelvis, torso, arms and head are each thoroughly and deeply released. The basic emotional defense armor also dissolves during these phases. This results in softer, more consistent and malleable musculature. The body can now begin to find new proportions: wide hips may narrow, small chests may expand, torsos may lengthen, faces relax and buttocks may fill and round out. This integrated system recognizes the emotional component of physical change and, at this stage of the process, suppressed emotions and thoughts surface and may become more flexible and expressive.

The final three phases, integration ("bringing it all together"), the released parts of the person are carefully brought into harmony with one another. Two phases concentrate on fine-tuning the top and bottom of the body, while the final phase balances the left and right sides, front and back and masculine and feminine.

In the final part of the integration process, the practitioner stabilizes the breathing, facilitates the even distribution of energy and makes the client more aware of his or her emotions.

The release and integration of the self through postural integration is a powerful, redirecting experience.

Further Reading
Painter, Jack, Ph.D., *Deep Bodywork and Personal Development, Harmonizing Our Bodies, Emotions and Thoughts,* Body-Mind Books, International Center for Release and Integration, Mill Valley, Calif., 1987. A unique synthesis of deep tissues, Gestalt therapy and Reichian work. This illustrated book is full of theory and technique.
———— , *Technical Manual of Deep Wholistic Bodywork,* Body-Mind Books, International Center for Release and Integration, Mill Valley, Calif., 1987. This book presents a systematic outline for reorganizing the myofascia of the musculature.

prana the Hindu word for life's vital energy. See also CHI.

Pranic Healing℠ a new, highly effective therapy that corrects the energetic imbalances underlying physical and psychological disorders. It is the distillation of more than 20 years of research conducted in the Philippines by Choa Kok Sui, a scientist and master healer, who synthesized many of the ancient healing sciences and arts.

Pranic Healing utilizes PRANA, the vital energy, or life force, that keeps the body alive and healthy. Disease occurs when blocks in the energy system starve organs, tissues and cells of the *prana* needed to function properly. Pranic healers remove these blocks (diseased, devitalized bioplasmic matter) from the affected parts and infuse the body with fresh, bioactive *prana*. Cleansing and energizing the energy field in this way enhances the ability of the physical body to heal itself, often within a very short period of time.

Pranic Healing works primarily through the bioplasmic (etheric) body, or aura, and the CHAKRAS, which interpenetrate the physical body and extend beyond it to varying degrees in different people. The chakras are crucial in healing because each one controls and energizes specific organs and glands. They are like power stations that supply vital energy to parts of the body under their influence. After cleansing the energy system, practitioners project energy into the chakras; and the chakras transfer the healing energy to ailing parts in a biologically usable form.

Pranic healers use their hands to scan, or sense, the condition of the aura, chakras and organs. They then select precise energy vibrations, or colors, to use in healing protocols for a broad spectrum of ailments, ranging from muscle pain and fever to digestive disorders and arthritis to heart and lung problems, kidney stones and many others. It requires no physical contact and is painless.

Pranic Healing can be used as a preventative measure. There are techniques to boost the immune system and help people manage stress. Evidence also exists that working with energy can rejuvenate and revitalize the body. Pranic Healing is holistic in that it affects well-being on every plane—physical, emotional, mental and spiritual.

Pranic psychotherapy uses the principles of Pranic Healing to relieve many psychological and emotional problems such as anger and irritability, depression, obsessions/compulsions and violent or paranoid behavior. Pranic psychotherapists routinely employ several methods of shielding individuals from negative psychic influence.

Further Reading

Sui, Choa Kok, *Pranic Healing*, Samuel Weiser, Inc., York Beach, Maine, 1990. The foremost authority on Pranic Healing describes step-by-step how to heal, using this ancient healing science and art.

———— , *Pranic Psychotherapy*, Samuel Weiser, Inc., York Beach, Maine, 1993. A sequel to *Pranic Healing*, this book shows how to apply Pranic Healing techniques to prevent and alleviate psychological ailments.

pregnancy massage See BODYWORK FOR THE CHILDBEARING YEAR℠; MOTHERMASSAGE℠.

process acupressure a new psychophysical process system designed to foster psychological and spiritual development through integrative bodywork. It is a method for understanding and processing who we are and how we grow and live as integrated individuals.

Process acupressure was developed by Aminah Raheem, Ph.D., a transpersonal psychologist and diplomate of process oriented psychology. Her 30 years of research into holistic development, which included studying ACUPRESSURE, ZERO BALANCING and other body systems, transpersonal psychology and psychotherapy, and rooted in spiritual practice, led to the creation of this system. The work of the personality is profoundly interfaced with the direction of the soul.

The bodywork of process acupressure employs principles of traditional acupressure, Zero Balancing and CHAKRA ENERGY WORK to assist in understanding and strengthening the body/mind/emotion/soul of the whole person. It operates out of the knowledge of somatic energy systems—MERIDIANS and chakras—and uses significant power points to get into the body's currents. Tissues, organs and glands are addressed within the integration of these energies.

Four basic factors are used in the hands-on method to help focus and facilitate process: **touch, breath, attention** and **heart love.** Touch may include acupressure to stimulate energy flow and the Zero Balancing touch of **interface,** for accessing deeper energy currents within the body, clearly defining boundaries between client and practitioner and for maximum conservation and recharging of energy. Heart love is an attitude of compassion and unconditional respect toward the client.

A process acupressure session is performed in four phases. The beginning orients the session and opens the body's energy. The middle processes material that emerges from the body. Soul work may follow when the client is ready to go to the deepest level of consciousness and guidance. The end of the session, which includes chakra balancing and grounding, integrates and completes the work for that session.

Process acupressure incorporates various psychological modalities, including process oriented psychology developed by Dr. Arnold Mindell of Zurich, Switzerland. Dr. Mindell studied the connections between consciousness, symptoms and dreaming and developed ways of working with the whole person to return awareness, authority and will to the individual. Mindell and Raheem both claim that there is an inherent wisdom within each person that guides transformation. Process work teaches how to follow the natural development within each person.

The fundamental purpose of process acupressure is to facilitate individual, holistic growth as it occurs naturally. Attention of both practitioner and client is brought to the client's process, thus strengthening awareness and understanding of the factors underlying both symptoms and development. This consciousness is profoundly interfaced with the direction of the soul. Process acupressure teaches both client and facilitator how to respectfully follow their own unique process of knowing and growth.

Process acupressure principles can be incorporated into the framework of other bodywork or psychological approaches and can be performed with one client, several partners or self-administered.

Further Reading

Raheem, Aminah, Ph.D., *Soul Return: Integrating Body, Psyche and Spirit,* Aslan Publications, Lower Lake, Calif., 1987. The role of spirituality in psychology is discussed. Physical well-being is only part of a person's wholeness, and this book addresses the roles of love, wisdom and enlightenment in total health.

Raheem, Aminah, Ph.D., *Process Acupressure I,* Upledger Publishing, Palm Beach Gardens, Fla., 1991. This book represents the basic text for process acupressure. Accompanying illustrations demonstrate this system's points, centers and body areas as well as the chakras of the body. *Process Acupressure II* and *III,* Aminah Raheem Publications, Capitola, Calif., texts advance the work in specificity and complexity.

Bonnie Prudden Myotherapy® a system that relieves muscular pain by pressure to specific sites in the muscle tissue called **trigger points.**

Although trigger points are not completely understood, it is known that they are highly sensitive and irritable spots in the muscles and CONNECTIVE TISSUE, which contribute to pain. They can also **refer** the pain to other parts of the body. Trigger points are impregnated in the muscles throughout life by any insult or trauma to the SOFT TISSUES.

A trigger point can remain dormant in the muscle without producing sensation until an injury or the insult of repetitive motion activates it. At that point, the muscle is thrown into spasm, shortening and limiting its RANGE OF MOTION and creating a spasm-pain-spasm cycle of pain. Until the cycle is interrupted, the pain will continue, interfering with strength, flexibility, function and form.

There are two types of trigger points, according to Bonnie Prudden myotherapists: **matrix points** and **satellite points.** Matrix points are capable of referring spasm and pain to other areas of the body. Satellites, while equally painful, confine themselves to their point of origin.

Trigger points are created in a number of different ways. They may be produced initially by the birth trauma or positioning in the womb (e.g., pigeon toes). Colic is often caused by trigger points in muscles on the skull. Headaches cause pain and this pain causes almost constant crying. Swallowing air adds stomach pain, and unless the trigger points in the head, neck and face are addressed, this behavior can go on for weeks.

Accidents have the potential for creating trigger points, which may be hidden for years, only to surface when physical or emotional stress is high. It is a common phenomena for car accident victims to suffer effects from their injuries years after, when trigger points are reactivated. All too often, the original cause, the accident, has been forgotten. Thus, the resulting chronic pain becomes mysterious and treatments unhelpful. Illnesses and surgical procedures can create trigger points, as can sports injuries, work and life styles.

Trigger point therapy is effective, according to Dr. Janet Travell, who discovered her SPRAY AND STRETCH TECHNIQUE while research trigger point injection therapy, because the muscle in spasm is being denied oxygen.[1] The sensitive spot is found by palpation and then injected with procaine and saline solution. Bonnie Prudden Myotherapy substitutes the injection with finger, knuckle or elbow pressure to the sensitive trigger point. The pressure is held for five to seven seconds, the trigger point is defused and the muscle relaxes to its painless, resting state. Thus, there is no invasion. The muscle release is followed by vital corrective exercises, which hasten the recovery of strength, flexibility and coordination as well as preventing the return of pain.

The amount of pressure applied to the muscle in spasm is entirely in the hands of the person receiving the myotherapy. A scale of one to ten is used to judge the degree of pain reaction. Anything below a seven or eight is acceptable. Above nine is counterproductive. Bearing unbearable pain has the effect of causing spasms in other parts of the body under stress.

Myotherapy was developed by Bonnie Prudden (1914–), author and physical fitness expert, almost by accident. On a mountainclimbing trip with Dr. Hans Kraus, a leader in the study of trigger points, she developed a painful stiff neck, a result of an earlier fall from a horse. Dr. Kraus treated her with direct thumb pressure to a spot in the back of her neck and then used his specialty, immediate mobilization. It was discovered that applying Bonnie Prudden Myotherapy to trigger points within the first hour after injury gives the best results.

Prudden was working with Dr. Desmond Tivy, an internist, in 1976, when a patient came to her with a painfully stiff neck. As Prudden was palpating the neck muscles for trigger points, which she then circled for injection by Dr. Tivy, she pressed a little harder on a sensitive spot than we usually did. The patient snapped her head up at once, straight, free and painless.

A second patient's ailment, tennis elbow, was also relieved by pressure to sensitive points used as guidelines for elbow pain injection. The result was the same—freedom from spasm, pain and dysfunction. These successes, and all the ones since, were followed by the vitally important corrective exercises.

It is the exercise after Bonnie Prudden Myotherapy that puts future comfort and improved function into the hands of the ordinary person.

In 1979, she founded the Bonnie Prudden School for Fitness and Myotherapy, now located in Tucson, Arizona, where she offers a ninemonth program leading to certification as a Bonnie Prudden myotherapist, C.P.B.M. The course includes anatomy, myotherapy and exercises for all ages and abilities, aqua-exercise, animal myotherapy, life drawing and sculpture, business and marketing skills, student clinic and daily exercises, which lead to a fit body for each graduate.

Note
[1] Prudden, Bonnie, *Pain Erasure: The Bonnie Prudden Way,* Ballantine Books, N.Y., 1980, p. 15.

Further Reading
Prudden, Bonnie, *Pain Erasure: The Bonnie Prudden Way,* Ballantine Books, N.Y., 1980. This book offers the history and applications for Bonnie Prudden Myotherapy. Photographs demonstrate exercise techniques, while clear illustrations depict the locations of trigger points throughout the body.
———— , *Myotherapy: Bonnie Prudden's Complete Guide to Pain-Free Living,* Ballantine Books, N.Y., 1985. This book includes updated techniques from her earlier book and a "quick fix" chapter for self-help. It also includes presport and preperforming arts training, as well as Bonnie Prudden Myotherapy after acute or chronic pain.

psychic healing   See SPIRITUAL HEALING.

pulse reading   one of the methods of diagnosis in CHINESE MEDICINE. The pulses are located above the wrist where the radial artery can be felt. They are divided into three regions: *cun, guan* and *chi.*[1] The area opposite the styloid process of the radius bone (the bony eminence at the wrist, thumb side) is *guan,* the middle pulse. *Cun* is found closer to the wrist, while *chi* is found after *guan.*

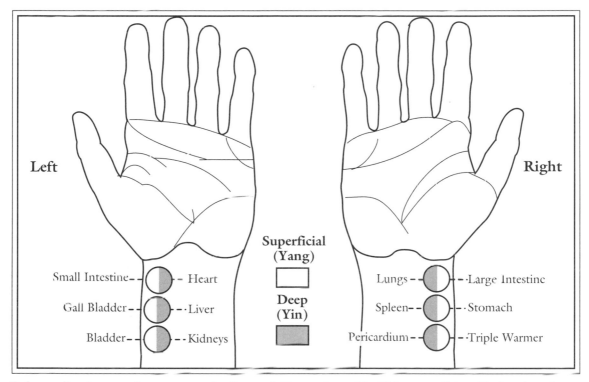

Left

Small Intestine – – Heart

Gall Bladder – – Liver

Bladder – – Kidneys

Superficial (Yang)

Deep (Yin)

Right

Lungs – – Large Intestine

Spleen – – Stomach

Pericardium – – Triple Warmer

Pulse reading is a very important evaluation and diagnostic tool in Chinese medicine. Each pulse relates to a different organ. The yang organs are felt superficially, the yin organs deep.

The pulses on each hand relate to different organs. The YANG organs are felt superficially; the YIN organs are felt deeper on the pulse. The *cun* region on the right hand corresponds to the yang LARGE INTESTINE superficially, and yin LUNG deeply. The *guan* region of the right hand indicates the condition of the yang STOMACH superficially and the yin SPLEEN deeply. Finally, the *chi* position correlations are the yang TRIPLE HEATER superficially and the yin HEART CONSTRICTOR (pericardium) or kidney yang, deeply.[2]

On the left hand, the superficial *cun* pulse is the yang SMALL INTESTINE, while the deep pulse reveals the condition of the yin HEART. The *guan* pulse corresponds to the yang GALL BLADDER and the yin LIVER. The *chi* pulse relates superficially to the yang BLADDER and deeply to the yin KIDNEY.

In feeling the pulses, the arm of the client

should be relaxed, palms facing up. The *guan* (middle) pulse is felt first with the practitioner's middle finger, followed by *cun* and *chi*, using index and ring fingers. The fingers should also be relaxed, in a gentle arcing position. The space between the fingers, and therefore the positions of the pulses, depends upon the client's size.

The pulses are palpated using three different finger pressures, superficial, middle and deep. The pulse is read and interpreted according to its depth, speed, strength, shape and rhythm.

A normal pulse is considered to be smooth, even and forceful, numbering four beats per breath. Variations may occur due to age, gender, constitution, emotional health and climate.

Abnormal pulse readings are described in a variety of ways. Chinese medicine describes at least 28 different classifications of pulses.

A **superficial** pulse indicates early illnesses of an external nature or prolonged, internal disease.

A **deep** pulse can only be palpated with heavy pressure. This indicates interior syndromes. A **slow** pulse generally means cold syndromes, while a **rapid** pulse indicates heat in the body.

A **deficient** pulse indicates QI and blood deficiency, while an **excess** pulse signifies stagnation. A **surging** pulse is broad, large and forceful and indicates excess. A **thready** pulse can signify overexertion or strain or weakness.

A **rolling** pulse means excessive fluid and phlegm in the system, while a **hesitant** pulse reading may be interpreted as blood deficiency. A pulse that is **string-taut** signifies liver-constrained **qi** and pain. A **tense** pulse represents cold, pain and the retention of food. A **soft** pulse means damp and weak disorders.

A **weak** pulse may indicate various disorders of *qi* and blood deficiency. An **irregular** pulse, with skipped beats, is a sign of *qi* or blood deficiency. A **knotted** pulse is excessive yin, cold phlegm and stagnant blood. A **regularly inter**mittent pulse is slow, with missed beats at regular intervals. This indicates declining organ *qi,* wind syndromes, pain and disorders of fear and fright.

In most cases, it is common to find a combination of two or more pulses. This is referred to as a **complicated** pulse.

Notes
[1] Xinnong, Cheng, ed., *Chinese Acupuncture and Moxibustion,* Foreign Language Press, Beijing, China, 1987, p. 268. Babies' pulses are felt with only one finger in the *guan* middle region.
[2] The kidney meridian, which is generally considered to be yin, has both yin and yang functions. The yin function controls water and heat, while the yang controls fire and cold.

Further Reading
Amber, Reuben, and Babey, Brooke, *Pulse Diagnosis: Detailed Interpretation for Eastern and Western Holistic Treatments,* Aurora Press, N.Mex., 1993. Pulse diagnosis from a cultural and historical perspective including Arabian, Aruyvedic, Chinese and Western theories and traditions.

Q

qi See CHI.

qigong, or *chi kung,* is a self-training method that combines moving, stationary and breathing exercises to achieve and maintain optimum health. It translates to "breathing exercises" or "energy skill." Its origins date back to ancient China where references were made to it in early medical texts. This venerable art, thought to be over 2,000 years old, may have been recorded during the Zhou dynasty (c. 1100–221 B.C.). It continued to develop and was greatly influenced by Indian Buddhist yoga during the Han dynasty (A.D. 25–220). *Qigong,* an important component of Chinese medicine, was widely used as a medical treatment to cure many diseases.

Chinese medicine recognizes that QI energy, or vital energy, is the foundation of all life. *Qigong* breathing exercises increase *qi* energy to build vitality and prevent illness. Currently, *qigong* is regarded as a system that builds vitality and wards off disease.

There are many variations of *qigong,* but main elements are constant in all forms: the regulation of posture, mind and breath. All these factors interact with each other to produce *qi.* Self-massage is sometimes included within the system.

The three most common qigong exercises are the **relaxation exercise,** the **strengthening exercise** and the **inward training exercise.** Exercises may be performed in standing, sitting or lying positions and movements are gentle and controlled.

Relaxation is a major benefit of *qigong* exercises, which can be performed by young and old alike. The heart rate decreases, gastrointestinal peristalsis (the wavelike movement of the bowels) is promoted and digestive juice secretion is enhanced. *Qigong* has also been effective in the treatment of high blood pressure, constipation and ulcers.

Further Reading

China Sports Magazine, *The Wonder of Qigong,* Wayfarer Publications, Los Angeles, 1985. This illustrated guide describes the history of *qigong* along with exercises to enhance internal energy, reduce stress and increase productivity.

Connor, Danny, *Qigong: Chinese Movement and Meditation for Health,* Samuel Weiser, York Beach, Maine, 1992. This easy-to-follow book describes the history of *qigong,* the origin of *qi* energy and employs photographs to demonstrate the exercises.

Jwing-Ming, Yang, Dr., *Chi Kung: Health and Martial Arts,* Yang's Martial Arts Association, Jamaica Plain, Mass., 1985. This photographed and illustrated book provides information on the history and principles of *chi kung.* Included in this text are massage and exercise techniques as well as Chinese poetry.

Kit, Wong Kiew, *The Art of Chi Kung: Making the Most of Your Vital Energy,* Element, Rockport, Mass., 1993. This illustrated book provides exercise for health and longevity, martial arts training and mind-expanding exercises.

Shih, Tzu Kuo, *Qi Gong Therapy,* Station Hill Press, Barrytown, N.Y., 1994. This book provides a detailed history of *qigong,* the three main methods and aspects of *qigong* according to Chinese medical principles

R

The Radiance Technique® a seven-level, ancient science that employs the vibration of universal energy for energy-balancing purposes. It is a gentle, noninvasive energy technique that activates, amplifies, directs and balances the universal life force within any individual and within any person or living energy with whom that individual may wish to share this energy.

The Radiance Technique®, or TRT℠ also known as Real Reiki®, The Official Reiki Program®, and The Authentic Reiki®, is promoted by The Radiance Technique Association International, Inc. Its founder and first president was Barbara Ray, Ph.D., the world's foremost authority on TRT. Dr. Ray writes that this technique is effective for the prevention of disease and energy imbalances on all levels of being and can be used in conjunction with any other sources for restoring vital energy and promoting health. She was taught the full seven degrees by Hawaiian Hawayo Takata (c. 1900–1980), the then grand master of this system, in 1979. Dr. Ray is the only person to hold the keys to all seven degrees of this system.

The complete system of The Radiance Technique is made up of universal symbols, which are components of the **attunement** processes that distinguish each of the seven degrees.

The first degree teaches students to share the universal energy force through their hands with themselves, others, animals and plants using hands-on positions. Students are taught, in seminars, 12 suggested hands-on positions. Radiant energy accessed at this level can be used on a daily basis. There is also a four-part attunement process, which allows for the expansion of the student's access to universal life force energy. This attunement process is activated by the instructor with each student. A full session of The Radiance Technique consists of the hands-on application of the 12 positions on the body, beginning at the top of the head, for as long as desired. Five minutes per position is a good beginning.

The second degree student begins to learn the symbols of the inner language of this vibrational science and the process of directing energy beyond time and space, or distance directing. These skills promote personal unfolding and expansion and can be used to help others. The second degree student also learns how to focus more on the emotional/mental levels and on more serious disorders.

The third degree involves another attunement process and is divided into three aspects. The first two aspects can be studied for the individual's interest in personal growth and enlightenment. The third aspects is a teacher certification process as well as a level of study for personal growth and enlightenment.

The fourth degree was made available in 1985. Since then, the fifth degree, the sixth degree and the seventh degree have been opened for study. Dr. Ray is permitting a naturally slow evolution of The Radiance Technique.

Further Reading
Ray, Barbara, Ph.D., *The "Reiki" Factor in The Radiance Technique*, Radiance Association, St. Petersburg, Fla., 1983. Part I of this book explains the history and science of universal energy in The Radiance Technique. Part II provides The Radiance Technique for self-help and the helping of others.

radionics the science of diagnosing and treating diseases using radionic instruments. These sensitive instruments can sense vibrations in the human body and sometimes generate vibrations for the purpose of treatment.

The basis for this theory is the belief that all animate or inanimate matter emits specific frequencies. In the human body, each organ and system vibrate at their own particular rate. Diseases also have a unique vibratory pattern, which can be registered.

Radionics was pioneered by Dr. Albert

Abrams (1863–1924), a prominent San Francisco neurologist and dean of clinical medicine at Stanford University Medical School, Palo Alto, California. Abrams believed that since diseased tissue could be measured by instrumentation, it could also be treated as a vibratory deviation. He initially developed a variable resistance box to measure diseased tissue. Years later, he created the "Abrams Generator," which treated diseases by neutralizing abnormal emanations.

Radionics had some supporters who were eventually frustrated in their attempts to gain recognition from their medical colleagues. Today, in the United States, radionics has not received the approval of the American Medical Association, although it does enjoy a modest acceptance in England.

Further Reading

Tansley, David, *Radionic Healing: Is it for You?,* Element Books, Shaftesbury, England, 1988. Explains radionics, how it works and how it is used for diagnostic and treatment purposes.

Tansley, David, *Radionics and the Subtle Anatomy of Man,* C.W. Daniel Co., Ltd., Essex, England, 1972. This book provides an easy-to-follow outline of the body's force fields and energies and explains how radionics diagnoses and treats this level of anatomy.

RADIX®, also called RADIX Neo-Reichian education, is an educational model by which students learn how to experience, express and manage feelings that are trapped in deep body tissues. RADIX emphasizes personal growth and development toward individual differentiation; students participate fully in the process.

Two central ideas of RADIX are safety and exploration. The principle of safety affords students a trusting, comfortable environment wherein they can investigate deep, personal issues. Exploration grows out of a sense of safety leading into the arena of the somatic experience of emotions.

RADIX was originated by Charles Kelley, Ph.D., and further developed by trainers of the RADIX Institute. RADIX employs techniques from GESTALT THERAPY, BIOENERGETICS, BATES METHOD OF VISION TRAINING, Eidetic Image Therapy and ERICKSONIAN HYPNOTHERAPY.

Students sometimes reexperience earlier traumas and work through them. Work over time facilitates unique experiences of body/spirit that can only be described as ecstatic experiences.

RADIX teachers can be either certified or adjunct. Adjunct teachers are trained to incorporate RADIX into their particular style of work. The RADIX Institute certifies full-time professionals in the RADIX Neo-Reichian educational techniques.

range of motion   a term which describes the movement patterns of synovial joints. These articulations are called synovial due to the presence of a joint cavity and articular cartilage.

The movements of these joints are: **gliding, flexion, extension, abduction, adduction, rotation** and **circumduction.** Gliding, the simplest movement of a joint, is a back-and-forth, side-to-side motion of overlapping surfaces without rotary or angular movements. The carpals (hand bones), tarsals (foot bones), ribs and transverse processes of the vertebrae have gliding articulations.

Angular movements increase or decrease the angle between bones. Among those joint movements are flexion, which decreases the angle, extension and hyperextension, which increase the angle, abduction, which is movement away from the midline of the body and adduction, which is movement toward the midline.

Rotation is the movement of a bone around its long axis, while circumduction, the most complex movement, involves a 360° rotation, flexion, abduction, extension and adduction. During circumduction, the far end of the bone (the distal end) moves in a circular pattern as the close end (the proximal end) remains stable.

Range of motion also includes specialized movements exclusive to particular joints. The feet can **invert,** an inward movement of the ankle, and **evert,** the outward motion. **Protrac-**

tion and **retraction** are forward and backward motions particular to the lower jaw and collarbone (clavicle). The movement of the wrist, palm up is called **supination,** while turning it palm down is **pronation. Elevation** and **depression,** upward and downward, are movements of the lower jaw and shoulders.

Bodyworkers can evaluate the flexibility of a joint by putting it through its range of motion.

rebirthing   a conscious, gentle and connected breathing technique, which helps an individual heighten self-awareness and stimulates the body's natural ability to heal itself. Rebirthing is considered to be a healing process that uses consultation, affirmations and specific breathing techniques to release patterns and beliefs that hold a person back from fully embracing life.

Rebirthers believe that the breath is the bridge that links the conscious and unconscious minds. As the focused breathing enables a person to relax, a greater awareness of the inner breath and inner spiritual source is promoted.

Rebirthing is said to be a long forgotten form of PRANA YOGA, or energy breathing yoga, rediscovered by Leonard Orr in the 1970s. While meditating in his hot tub one day, Orr had, what has become known as, a spontaneous rebirth. He called his experience "rebirthing" because he initially reexperienced his birth and was able to release the trauma associated with it. In addition, many people who underwent this experience reported feeling that their lives were starting over again, with a clearer purpose and greater joy. The name, however, is often misleading. It does not share the religious connotation of being "born again," and Orr has tried to rename it to clarify the distinction. He now calls it "conscious connected breathing" because he realized that more than just birth trauma is released during this process.

A basic concept of rebirthing, or conscious connected breathing, is that any past trauma that is not addressed or released consciously will continue to re-create itself throughout a person's life. The goal of rebirthing is to release these traumas, so they don't continuously resurface, and to create a new life full of joy and passion. Ultimately, rebirthing seeks to achieve and maintain a healthy and harmonious integration of the body/mind/emotion/spirit.

Rebirthing is usually done in a series of 10 to 20 sessions, each lasting one to two hours. A qualified rebirther coaches the individual's breathing. The rhythm of the breathing is a relaxed, uninterrupted, connected flow of inhalation/exhalation through the mouth. The procedure can take place in a hot tub, called **wet rebirthing,** or on the floor, cushioned by a mat, called **dry rebirthing.**

The rhythm of the breath must be intuitive in order to breathe in life energy as well as air. The breath, therefore, should be gentle.

There are two organizations that currently train rebirthers: Rebirth International, founded by Leonard Orr, and Loving Relationships Training International Inc., created by Sondra Ray.

Further Reading

Minett, Gunnel, *Breath and Spirit,* Aquarian/Thorson's, N.Y., 1994. This easy-to-follow book is a guide to rebirthing techniques. Case histories are cited.

Orr, Leonard and Ray, Sondra, *Rebirthing in the New Age,* Celestial Arts, Berkeley, Calif., 1983. The originator and the reknown proponent of rebirthing have written a concise explanation of this system. Breathing exercises are detailed and techniques for deep relaxation are discussed.

Orr, Leonard, *Breath Awareness,* Inspiration University, Stanton, VA, 1988. This is Leonard Orr's latest book about breathing. It is available through Inspirational University's bookstore in Afton, Virginia.

reflexology   the study, science and art of using various touch techniques on specific points of the feet, hands (see HAND REFLEXOLOGY) or ears (see EAR THERAPY) to normalize body function, maintain optimum health and restore energy throughout the body. Reflexologists theorize that points on the feet correspond to particular organs, glands or parts of the body. Their locations on the feet follow a logical anatomical pattern. The goal of the work is to break down

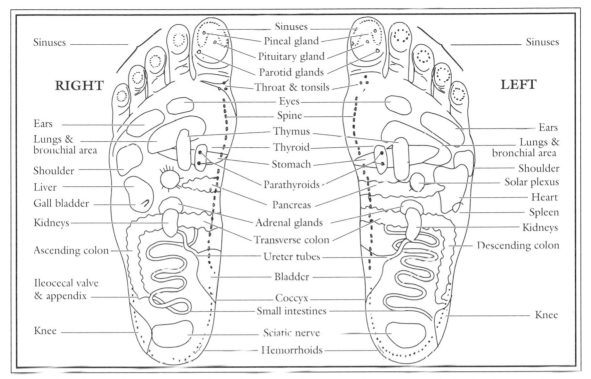

Foot reflexology points are mapped on the feet as they generally appear in the body. Organs that are found on one side of the body show up on the respective foot, such as the heart on the left foot, or the liver on the right.

crystal deposits in the feet and help restore HOMEOSTASIS, or internal balance.[1]

There are several theories how reflexology affects changes. Some practitioners believe that pressure to a foot reflex releases restricted energy flow, improves blood supply and promotes neurological stimulation to the affected area. Others maintain that sensory receptors in the feet are stimulated, sending impulses throughout the nervous system. Since the extremities have a rich supply of nerve endings, stimulation to these points can have far-reaching effects. Another theory postulates that endorphins, the pain-blocking compounds, are released into the bloodstream, providing pain relief and general well-being.

Reflexology is presumably as old as ACUPUNCTURE. Ancient texts indicate that India, China and Japan had their own variations of reflexology based on the concept of enhancing the flow of life energy (QI) through energy pathways (MERIDIANS) in the body.

Western reflexology was developed in 1913 by Dr. William Fitzgerald, an ear, nose and throat specialist. He began research on ZONE THERAPY, which later evolved into the system of reflexology. He discovered that constant pressure on a certain part of the foot relieved pain elsewhere in the body. He divided the body into ten zones, separating it down the middle and creating five zones (one per toe) in each half. The foot was equally divided except for the big toe, which in addition to being a zone in itself, was further subdivided to represent each half of the head area.

Further research was conducted by Eunice Ingham, a massage therapist and an assistant of Dr. Joe Shelby Riley, a pioneer in zone therapy, who felt that zone therapy was to general in its scope and that more detailed foot pressure could treat illnesses more effectively. She developed the "map" of the body, which is currently in practice, thereby refining foot reflexology. She also began experimenting with alternate pressure, replacing constant pressure, which seemed to have more far-reaching therapeutic value other than pain relief. In 1924, Dr. Joe Shelby Riley published his book *Zone Reflex,* which showed an image resembling the human body superimposed on the hands and feet.

Reflexology divides each foot into five longitudinal zones and three lateral zones. The lateral zones represent the shoulder line (across the base of the toes), the diaphragm line (under the ball of the foot) and the waistline (across the arch). In order to locate the point on the foot that corresponds to a particular organ, the reflexologist first locates the longitudinal zone on the foot. Then the organ is defined more specifically by where it lies in relation to the lateral zones. Reflexes can also appear on the sides and tops of the feet.

There are seven basic reflexing, or specific, techniques that reflexologists use to stimulate the points: thumb walking, finger walking, thumb hook and back up, rotating on a point, flexing on a point, pivoting on a point and finger rolling. Thumb walking is performed by bending the first joint of the thumb and moving up the foot. The fingers support the foot on the opposite (top) side. Finger walking is done much the same way. The first joint of any finger is bent, using the thumb as support for the foot on the opposite side. The thumb hook and back up technique is used to stimulate a specific point rather than a broad area. It is a stationary technique where the first joint of the thumb is bent and then straightened. The pressure against the point is constant.

Rotating on a point is done by pressing into a reflex point and rotating the foot. Flexing a point is performed by pressing the point and flexing (bending) the foot repeatedly. Pivoting on a point is performed by thumb walking across the foot with one hand and pivoting (twisting) the foot with the other hand. The tips of the toes (which relate to the head, brain and sinuses) may be stimulated by finger rolling. This is done by rolling the index finger lightly across the top of each toe.

Sessions generally last 30 to 60 minutes. The client is comfortably reclining in a chair or lying on a massage table, propped up with pillows. Each foot may be treated twice. The first coverage of the foot is for general stimulation, followed by more specific point work.

As physical levels of stress are released, the emotional components of these tensions may be released. An intuitive practitioner can provide appropriate feedback to promote the discharge of these emotions and past memories.

There are many reported benefits from reflexology. Clients report feelings of deep relaxation after a treatment, pain may be reduced or eliminated, circulation is improved, there is better oxygen and nutrient supply to the brain and body, detoxification is promoted and there is a normalization of the functions of organs, glands and structures of the body.[2]

A study of obstetrics and gynecology describes the effects of reflexology in treating the symptoms of premenstrual syndrome.[3] Thirty-five women were divided into two experimental groups: an active group and a placebo group. The active group received reflexology on areas of the ears, feet and hands that specifically treat PMS. The placebo group was given manual pressure on unrelated areas of the ears, feet and hands. All women kept daily records of 38 related symptoms for six months. Those women who received the active treatment showed a 46 percent reduction in their distress, while those in the placebo group showed a 19 percent reduction. Unlike hormone treatments and antidepressant medications, reflexology did not produce any unwanted side effects.

Reflexology may be self-administered. Certain tools, such as foot rollers or small balls, may also be adapted for personal use.

Notes

[1] Uric acid, a by-product of cellular catabolism, or lactic acid, a by-product of muscular activity, often solidify into crystalline deposits in the body.

[2] Flocco, Bill, "Foot Hand Ear Reflexology for a Healthy, Vital Life," *American Academy of Reflexology,* Burbank, Calif., no date, p. 40.

[3] Oleson, Terry, Ph.D., and Flocco, William, "Randomized Controlled Study of Premenstrual Symptoms Treated with Ear, Hand and Foot Reflexology," *Obstetrics and Gynecology,* Vol. 82, No. 6, December 1993.

Further Reading

Carter, Mildred, *Helping Yourself with Foot Reflexology,* Parker Publishing Co., West Nyack, N.Y., 1969. Ms. Carter studied with Eunice Ingham and although the writing style may be dated, the substance of her work is detailed. Photographs are used to indicate the position of the reflex points and case histories care cited.

Ingham, Eunice D., *Stories Feet Can Tell,* Eunice D. Ingham, Rochester, N.Y., 1938. This is the first book written about modern reflexology. Photographs and illustrations accompany a detailed text filled with personal anecdotes and case histories. Ingham was Dr. Riley's assistant who mapped the body on the feet.

Issel, Christine, *Reflexology: Art, Science and History,* New Frontier Publishing, Sacramento, Calif., 1993. This updated version, originally published in 1990, provides a fascinating look at the history of reflexology. Chapters explore ancient and modern theories, the art of reflexology as well as a cross-cultural comparison of reflexology charts from all over the world.

Jora, Jurgen, *Foot Reflexology: Visual Guide to Self Treatment,* St. Martin's Press, N.Y., 1991. Full-color illustrations and easy-to-follow instructions offer quick relief for a wide range of health problems.

Kunz, Kevin, and Kunz, Barbara, *The Complete Guide to Foot Reflexology,* Reflexology Research Project, Albuquerque, N.Mex., 1980. This easy-to-use guide details the techniques and applications of foot reflexology. A Table of Disorders provides a quick reference guide for treatment.

Norman, Laura, *Feet First: A Guide to Foot Reflexology,* Simon & Schuster, N.Y., 1988. This popular book is a manual on foot reflexology, which offers information to relieve physical problems and reduce stress. Diagrams help locate the points, and this clear text provides reflexing routines.

Reichian growth work   See MEDICAL ORGONE THERAPY.

reiki   an ancient system of natural healing that works with the HUMAN ENERGY BIO-FIELD. An arduous spiritual discipline was practiced by selective Tibetan monks, 2,500 years ago, which lead to definite spiritual advancement and physical well-being. It was called **raku kei.** Over the centuries, however, the tradition disappeared.

In the late 1800s, Dr. Mikao Usui (d. 1893), a Japanese scholar and Christian monk, began long and exacting research into the miraculous physical healings attributed to Christ and Buddha. During the course of his studies, he discovered a method of healing that shared similar elements to the documented remnants of *raku kei.* He called the healing energy *reiki,* which means "universal life energy." Dr. Usui traveled throughout Japan healing and teaching. The events of World War II wiped out all of the Reiki masters trained by Dr. Usui and his successor, Dr. Chujiro Hyashi (d. 1941) with the exception of Madame Hawayo Takata. She alone held the knowledge of Reiki for over 30 years in her clinic in Hawaii.

In 1974, at the age of 70, Madame Takata taught Reiki to others. Ten years later, she had elevated 22 Reiki masters. These masters in turn, elevated over 2,000 others. It is estimated that there are currently over 200,000 Reiki practitioners worldwide.

Reiki is energy. It is a very high vibrational force, which can influence physical and nonphysical, living and nonliving things. It affects all levels of existence—physical, mental, emotional and spiritual and has an organizational pattern or intelligence of its own, which always works toward a positive end.

Reiki is also the word used to identify the healing modality, which accesses and transfers that energy. (It is also called the Usui System of Natural Healing or the Usui System of Reiki Healing.) To tap into *reiki* energy, the Reiki master **attunes** the person's bio-energy field to accept the *reiki* frequency. Once that process has been accomplished, a person can assess *reiki* for himself or for others at any time, for the rest of the individual's life. *Reiki,* therefore, is channeled energy, and the ability to channel it is what a Reiki master facilitates.

Reiki training is divided into three main levels. In the first level, Reiki I, people are attuned to the energy and instructed in a balanced method of channeling it for themselves and for others. In the second level, Reiki II, people are attuned to a more sensitive level and given the means to intensify the power of the *reiki* energy that flows through them. The third level, Reiki III, is mastership in which a person acquires the ability to initiate people to the use of Reiki.

Reiki is administered with a light touch of the hands upon various parts of the recipient's body in a pattern that promotes optimum energy balancing. Generally, the recipient is in a reclining position during the treatment, which takes between 30 and 90 minutes. There is no need to disrobe and soft music is usually played. The recipient frequently, but not always, has physical sensations of the *reiki* energy, and it is described as heat, cold, tingling or light-headedness.

Reiki accelerates healing of physical injuries, discomforts and diseases. It often significantly lessens physical pain and emotional stress, if not removing them entirely. If the recipient is willing, Reiki will also initiate and promote deeper healing at the emotional and spiritual levels and stimulate personal growth.

Reiki is unlimited in its usages and can be used with animals and plants. Reiki is especially dynamic in the areas of physical well-being and personal growth. It can also be incorporated into a variety of healing arts. Reiki can be administered by a practitioner or by oneself after appropriate training and attunement, provided by a Reiki master.

Further Reading

Baginski, Bodo and Sharamon, Shalila, *Reiki: Universal Life Energy,* Life Rhythm, Mendocino, Calif., 1988. This book explains the history and development of Reiki. Hand positions are shown for a full-body treatment.

David, Jarrell, *Reiki Plus Natural Healing,* Hibernia West, Celina, Tenn., 1991. This book provides instructions in techniques and spiritual philosophy of Reiki and presents the teachings and techniques of Dr. Usui. It also gives insights into the secrets of some of history's greatest healers.

———, *Reiki Plus: Professional Practitioner's Manual,* Reiki Plus Publications, 1995. This book provides healing sequences and treatments for specific ailments.

Horan, Paula, *Empowerment through Reiki,* Lotus Light, Twin Lakes, N.Y., 1992. The author explains how *reiki* energy works, how it can be used, and the effects that can be achieved. Also included is information on how colors, tones, crystals and massage can be incorporated into the Reiki process.

relational dialogue integrates work with voice, breath, body and psychological process to help unearth the meaning contained in people's stories. These stories can hold a lot of significance, which often goes unheeded and whose revelation can harvest deeper meaning.

Relational dialogue was developed by Neal Katz. His interest in somatic therapies began with MEDITATION. He lived in a yoga ashram for a period of time and was looking for a way to bring together awareness practice and his experience of the body. The ALEXANDER TECHNIQUE became that vehicle. Katz taught this technique to theater students and became intrigued in the relationship between voice, emotion and the body.

By slowing down their conversation, students could be taught how tension in their bodies reflected psychological work that needed to be done. He might ask a client, for example, to give him the total weight of their shoulder as they speak. From this, they receive instantaneous feedback, which changes both their physical behavior, such as breathing, voice quality and body tension, as well as their psychological awareness. Their emotional space opens up and their story changes.

Through relational dialogue, the participant may gain new insight into a problem or previously avoided issue.

Release Work®, also known a Deep Emotional Release Bodywork, is a group of techniques designed to promote the release of trauma, anger, phobias and negative beliefs from the physical body. Tremendous amounts of energy and power can be released once these negative emotions are dispersed.

Deep Emotional Release Bodywork addresses the core of emotional blockages, resulting in deep relaxation, clarity of mind and increased self-esteem and confidence. It is believed that many deep emotional traumas are stored within the cellular consciousness, the memory and intelligent awareness of the physical body. In childhood, we are taught to shut down around painful emotions, which in turn result in dysfunctional behavior and repressed feelings.

This system is an integrated system of techniques applied to specific areas of the body. **Amanae therapy,** a system incorporated into Deep Emotional Release Bodywork, is a process that activates very precise zones along the body using hands and pressure. These zones hold explicit emotional memories. When these memories are activated, the body starts to shift into a higher frequency, creating the movement of energy. This in turn permits deep-seated memories to surface and the client to release the charge from the physical body.

Deep Emotional Release Bodywork emphasizes emotional freedom. Once the negative energy is released, a person can start reprogramming his life from a healthier, mature perspective.

Deep Emotional Release Bodywork is not ongoing therapy. Since much can be accomplished in one session, usually no more than five sessions are necessary to experience a sense of completion and reconnection with the body/mind/spirit.

This system was developed by James Hyman, a certified methodologist of Release Work as well as a licensed SHIATSU practitioner. He is a rebirther, instructor of TAI CHI and QIGONG and has been facilitating intensive integrative self-development programs for over 15 years.

resonant kinesiology a bodywork system that acknowledges the idea of vibrational reality. It is a style of bodywork based on the educational rather than the medical model and is considered to be more of a relationship between resonant kinesiologist and student (as clients are called) than a technique. All participants are involved in their experience and do not follow any prescribed modalities.

The foundation of resonant kinesiology is a meditative state called **inclusive attention.** It is a grounded, mindful state in which the resonant kinesiologist is aware of her own somatic, emotional and cognitive experience as well as the surrounding vibrations of the student. This focused, multidimensional state allows the practitioner to attend specifically to the aspect of the experience with which the student opts to work. Resourceful attention to a body permits response and change. Since this change originates from the student himself, it is more likely to be permanent.

Resonant touch, resonant movement and resonant sound are experiential, integral parts of the overall system. They are used to reach a communication as close as possible to direct communication between people. These facilitate meeting someone very close to who and where they are at the present point in their life. In resonant touch, the primary focus is on the student's body and the touch is done with specific attention. As soon as there is a response, or resonance in a body part, there is potential for change.

Resonant movement is considered to be another form of attention, which evokes response and education. The practitioner touches the student, asking "what is willing to move?" She then follows the movement as it presents itself. The movements can be either subtle or big, but are adequate enough to bring habitual movement patterns or restrictions to a person's conscious awareness.

Resonant sound, or singing tones, is a useful way to vibrationally touch small or especially sensitive body parts. It is also a way to expressively acknowledge a person's emotional state. Teaching people to sound, to resonate within their own bodies, helps them continue with their internal learning process.

Resonant kinesiology was developed by Susan Gallagher Borg, who has a background in music and movement. While in school, Borg recognized that she was a kinesthetic learner, someone who understands by sensing through the body, rather than a visual or cognitive learner. Borg realized that she could help others learn through their bodies as well as she could.

The resonant kinesiology training program for practitioners consists of 12 topics presented over a two- or three-year period.

Borg has developed a fundamental philosophy of resonant kinesiology. She believes that each person has all the resources needed to thrive, although they may not yet be available to conscious awareness. People always make the best choice available at the time. Since our minds evolve in response to physical experience, learning initiates change. Finally, she supports the idea that healing is a form of learning.

Great emphasis is placed on the importance of approaching the participant with respect, curiosity and clear intention. The purpose of the work is not to cause change, but rather to bring attention to the place where the change occurs.

Rolfing® is a unique system of bodywork designed to change the way people relate to gravity by systematically lengthening and repositioning the body's entire connective tissue matrix in a highly-detailed, 10-session series causing deep changes in the body which are physical as well as emotional. Before and after photographs of once slouching clients who appear to have grown an inch or two are evidence that, at the very least, the technique improves posture and elongates the body. The view of gravity's impact on human structure is the hallmark of Rolfing and distinguishes it from all other types of bodywork.

Developed by Dr. Ida P. Rolf (1896–1979), the work was originally called Structural Integration but the public preferred the eponymous title and the name remained. The official name of this work, however, is Rolfing Structural Integration and it has influenced the culture to the extent of being one of the only types of bodywork other than massage defined in the dictionary.

Ida Rolf was born in New York and graduated from Barnard College in 1916 with a bachelor of science degree. In 1920 she received her doctorate in biochemistry from Columbia University's College of Physicians and Surgeons. During the 1950s, after 25 years of developing her revolutionary work, Dr. Rolf presented Structural Integration in the United States, Canada and Great Britain, primarily to osteopaths and chiropractors. All deep-tissue therapies developed in this country have been influenced by Dr. Rolf's work. In the 1960s, she was invited by Fritz Perls, founder of GESTALT Therapy, to teach at Esalen Institute in Big Sur, California. During this time, Rolfing® rose to unprecedented popularity and, possibly, because many in the Gestalt movement flocked to Rolfing, it developed a reputation as a desirably cathartic form of emotional processing and release. To this day, most university psychology texts include a description of Rolfing.

Science has known for years that proper physiological function and anatomical structure are related. Dr. Rolf agreed, along with her peers in osteopathy and CHIROPRACTIC, that the body as a whole functioned better when local areas of dysfunction were resolved, when bony segments were in proper alignment and when joints exhibited proper mobility. But she realized that a long-lasting and profound transformation in our bodily being, alignment and overall sense of well being and freedom required a more far reaching understanding of the impact of gravity on our bodies. Dr. Rolf was not only concerned with creating a system of manipulation that could ease the pain and stresses of human life by properly aligning the body, she was also profoundly interested in creating a system that could transform the whole person at every level.

Beginning with the insight that the human body is a unified structural and functional whole that stands in a unique relation to the uncompromising presence of gravity, Dr. Rolf asked this fundamental question: "What conditions must be fulfilled in order for the human body to be organized and integrated in gravity so that it can function in the most economical way?"[1]

The "gospel" of Rolfing is that when the body gets working appropriately, the force of gravity can flow through. Then, spontaneously, the body heals itself.[2]

The medium that is so radically influenced by gravity is fascia. FASCIA is a continuous web of thin, elastic (connective) tissue throughout the entire body. It binds muscle fibers together, attaches muscles to bones and to each other, covers organs and blood vessels and provides the individual shape of the human form. Eighty percent of the body's protein is utilized to create and maintain this intricate system. Fascia can be distorted due to injury, emotional trauma and poor postural habits. It adapts to these insults by contracting and bonding, thereby shortening and thickening. Basic physical movements become complicated and too much energy is then required for simple tasks. Rolfing Structural Integration attempts to reverse this process by systematically and sensitively freeing fascial adhesions and, then, introducing more efficient movement options which reinforce the structural change. The proactive nature of the work is another characteristic that distinguishes the process from other deep-tissue techniques.

The most common misconception about Rolfing is that the technique consists of gratuitous pressure that is applied to the client, but the Rolfer's eyes, more than his hands, are the primary tools used to "see" the structural patterns that have emerged over the course of a person's life. And, rather than merely doing something *to* the body, Rolfers approach their objective to introduce options for change with finesse. Each of the ten sessions has a number of structural goals addressed individually according to each client's pattern. Rolfing Structural Integration is an on-going process of change that continues after the ten sessions. Advanced sessions are available after a period of integration.

An abridged look at the series continues with the second session, which concentrates on getting the legs and feet grounded. The third focuses on getting the internal relationship of shoulders, ribs and pelvis aligned. The fourth session works deep into the body's core, from the inside of the ankles to the pelvic floor, hamstrings, back and neck. The fifth session concentrates on releasing deep abdominal muscles. The sacrum is the focal point of the sixth session, while the seventh concentrates on balancing the neck and head on the spine. The eighth, ninth and tenth then integrate the more differentiated body through a more proactive, movement related "review" of previous sessions goals.

Rolfing Movement Integration is a system of movement education that continues the process of change by promoting more harmonious and efficient movement within gravity, thereby continuing the process of embodiment.

Rolfing practitioners and movement teachers are trained and certified at the International Rolf Institute in Boulder, Colorado.

Photos are taken after the work is completed and are compared to the first set of pictures to see how the body has changed.

Rolfing does not diagnose disease or cure symptoms, per se, but provides a more flexible, resilient, high-energy system, which is better able to ward off illness and overcome stress. Rolfing is an ongoing process that continues after the work has been completed. Advanced sessions are available if additional work is needed.

Rolfing Movement Integration is a system of movement education based on the ideas developed by Dr. Rolf. This work focuses on developing balance and support for action in the gravitational field, learning to move harmoniously with gravity and promoting an open and responsive body. Rolfing movement can be studied by itself or in conjunction with Rolfing sessions.

Rolfing practitioners and movement teachers are trained and certified at the Rolf Institute in Boulder, Colorado.

Notes

[1] Prevention Magazine, *Hands-On Healing,* Rodale Press, Emmaus, Pa., 1989, p. 262.

[2] Feitis, Rosemary, ed., *Ida Rolf Talks about Rolfing and Physical Reality,* Rolf Institute, Boulder, Colo., 1978, p. 31.

[3] Ibid., pp. 209–210.

Further Reading

Anson, Brian, *Rolfing: Stories of Personal Empowerment,* Heartland Personal Growth Press, 1991. This book, written by an advanced Rolfer, is a collection of 85 stories, including 149 photographs, of Rolfing clients. These people range in age from babies to octogenarians.

Fahey, Brian W., Ph.D., *The Power of Balance: A Rolfing View of Health,* Metamorphous Press, Santa Rosa, Calif., 1989. This book, written by a certified Rolfer, expands upon Dr. Rolf's ideas and includes self-help and awareness exercises.

Feitis, Rosemary, ed., *Ida Rolf Talks about Rolfing and Physical Reality,* Rolf Institute, Boulder, Colo., 1978. This book contains excerpts from Dr. Rolf's early class lectures.

Maitland, Jeffrey, Ph.D., *Spacious Body Explorations in Somatic Ontology,* North Atlantic Books, Berkeley, Calif., 1995. One of the world's four advanced Rolfing teachers explores the nature of being and bodily experience within the context of Rolfing, Buddhism, Phenomenology and Alchemy.

Rolf, Ida P., Ph.D., *Rolfing: Re-establishing the Natural Alignment and Structural Integration of the Body for Vitality and Well-Being,* Rolf Institute, Boulder, Colo. This illustrated book, originally titled *Rolfing—The Integration of Human Structure,* is considered to be the definitive work on the theories and principles of Rolfing.

The Rosen Method of Bodywork and Movement^{SM}

a system of bodywork and movement that helps the client experience himself in a more accepting and loving way through nonintrusive, subtle touch, awareness of breath, movement exercises and gentle verbal coaxing.

Marion Rosen, the developer of the system, has said that "the body tells the clearest what we want to hide the most."[1] All childhood traumas are stored in the body and may create short breathing patterns and tense muscles. There is often an emotional component to body holding. Muscular overactivity, when it is not required for support, indicates a deeper reason for the holding, which has more to do with feelings than with physical support.

While the client is lying on a massage table, the practitioner locates muscular tension using a light exploratory touch and by watching the client's breathing. Localized body temperature, color and skin texture are also indicators of internal tension. The practitioner looks for the original holding, which gave rise to the client's present physical condition. She may press slightly deeper into a tense area to facilitate release. When a release is experienced, the muscles relax and breathing is deepened.

There may also be an emotional expression accompanying muscular opening. The use of verbal interaction directs the client's awareness to the physical changes that have taken place. The practitioner may ask the client what he is experiencing, what memories or images come to mind, or simply to acknowledge that a transformation has occurred. The realizations are not necessarily sudden; they may result from an accumulation of small, often unnoticeable changes.

Marion Rosen became a physical therapist in Sweden during the 1940s and was a student of physical therapist Lucy Heyer. She gave massages and breath work exercises to her patients. She taught her first movement class in 1956 in Berkeley, California. Her method of movement is a system of RANGE OF MOTION and stretching exercises designed to lubricate the joints, expand the chest, loosen the diaphragm and restore movements of early childhood, when activity was free and unencumbered. This technique, accompanied by music, provides deeper breathing, muscular lengthening and relaxation, which allows clients to reclaim their health by releasing habitually held muscles.

Reshaping and reeducating the body in a gentle way is the goal of her work. Rosen Bodywork and Movement is for healthy people who want to discover themselves on a deeper level or for physically ill people who want to understand their chronic conditions.

Note

[1] "Rosen Method Bodywork and Movement" workshop brochure, no date.

Further Reading

Rosen, Marion, and Brenner, Sue, *The Rosen Method of Movement,* North Atlantic Books, Berkeley, Calif., 1991. This book, written by the developer of the system, provides an overview of the Rosen Method and offers detailed exercises. The book has illustrations and photographs of the exercises for easy clarification. A special section on disabilities is included.

Rubenfeld Synergy® Method a powerful healing system that synthesizes the body/mind/emotions/spirit integrating elements from the ALEXANDER TECHNIQUE, FELDENKRAIS METHOD®, GESTALT THERAPY and ERICKSONIAN HYPNOTHERAPY and develops them into a new educational paradigm. This system provides a unique approach to dealing with memories and emotions locked in the body, which create energy blocks, tensions and imbalances.

The Rubenfeld Synergy Method was founded and developed over 35 years ago by Ilana Rubenfeld. After many years of research, study and practice, she began the first professional Rubenfeld Synergy Training Program in 1977. As a graduate of the Juilliard School of Music, a trained classical musician and conductor, Rubenfeld developed back problems from her arduous rehearsal schedule and performances. Her studies with Pablo Casals and Leopold Stokowski did not include balanced use of her body during these stressful times. Prescription drugs brought only some temporary relief, but no cure. Musician friends recommended the Alexander Technique.

She found Judith Leibowitz, an Alexander teacher, who taught her much about her body-mind and showed her more efficient ways of using her body posture—thus avoiding injury. The gentle touch used evoked deeply embedded emotions. One day, Rubenfeld began crying and expressing her feelings during a lesson. Leibowitz, untrained to process these emotions, recommended an analyst to help her. Rubenfeld took her advice, but by the time she talked to the analyst, the intense feelings were gone.

For the next few years, she saw Leibowitz who touched, but wouldn't talk. She then proceeded on to her analyst who talked, but would not touch. She knew how powerful it could be to have the same person do both. It was then that she decided to develop what was to become the Rubenfeld Synergy Method. The body held many stories that needed to be released and heard. The concept that the body, mind, emotions and spirit are all connected was just beginning to surface in the late 1960s.

Rubenfeld continued studying and training in the Alexander Technique. She then became a teacher/trainer of this technique. However, Rubenfeld felt that the emotional process was still missing and only addressed half of her clients' needs. This changed in 1965 when she met Dr. Fritz Perls and began to train in Gestalt therapy at the Esalen Institute. In 1970, she met Moshe Feldenkrais, was introduced to his innovative work of touch and exercises and completed his first United States training program in 1979. These bodymind methods and psychotherapy became the foundation and harmonics of the Rubenfeld Synergy Method. The name was suggested to her by Buckminster Fuller, engineer and inventor, who witnessed her work and felt that she had passed beyond integrating therapies into a true, new synergy.

Some techniques Rubenfeld uses include: verbal dialogue, breathing patterns, movement, body posture, imagination, sound and caring touch to assess the reservoirs of blocked feelings. Rubenfeld believes that compassionate touch is an especially powerful form of communication because it precedes talking. The synergist, a certified practitioner of this method, supports clients by creating an atmosphere of safety and trust so that the emerging feelings can be expressed and integrated without fear.

In Rubenfeld Synergy, the goal is to *educate* people to recognize, understand, express and deal with what is going on inside of their bodies. Synergists are not trained to tell their clients what is wrong with them. Rather, they are present to support their clients to contact their own ability to heal themselves and recognize their emotional history that may have caused and contributed to the present, painful problem in their lives. This method is designed so that clients continually learn how to use new tools of their own in order to change.

Rubenfeld believes that practitioners must know how to take care of themselves in order to help clients. After many years of practice, she concluded that the "body tells the truth." Through a specially trained "listening" touch, the synergist can tell whether a client's words are congruent with her body state and verbal message.

A session usually begins when a client—fully clothed—is invited to lie down on a special table. She is reassured that if there is anything said or done that disturbs her, she can stop the session. This is empowering for the client so that she can gently reenter her body in order to release traumas and reclaim herself. Intentionality of the synergist is very important. The synergist continues the session by sensitively touching the client with an "open and listening hand"— enabling her to sense the client's present physical/emotional condition.

By simultaneously adding the verbal dialogue, the synergist establishes the connections and congruency between the body's story and the mind's thoughts. If the client's back is like hard steel, and she talks of soft love, there is a clear contradiction. Only when the client becomes aware of this difference can she begin to express the feelings of her body and eventually change and integrate this insight.

Lightly palpating muscles can also provide information about past traumas and injuries. Rescripting the original scene of the trauma by positive visualizations often changes and releases the past and present pain. Being totally present and intuitive are important elements and attributes of this work. If synergists are busy thinking and figuring out what to do, they lose contact and miss obvious clues to what is happening in the moment with the clients.

Rubenfeld outlines some key elements and philosophies of the Rubenfeld Synergy Method:

1. Becoming aware is the first step in the change process
2. Ultimate responsibility for change rests with the client. Clients are the authors of their self-willed releases.
3. Each time a change is introduced at one level, it affects the equilibrium of every part of the whole person
4. A gentle, caring touch sends messages of nonviolence, trust and respect for the client's boundaries
5. The quality of touch reflects a nonverbal "listening stance"
6. While clients communicate verbally, their bodies may portray another story, which reflects their authentic state
7. Sensing the body's energy field is important
8. Human beings have a natural capacity for self-healing and self-regulation
9. The synergist's self-care is emphasized during the session by paying attention to posture, breathing, physical environment and maintaining professional boundaries
10. Using appropriate humor to lighten painful places and memories
11. Allowing spiritual themes to unfold and letting clients deal with their "soul" issues
12. Touch and movement may create a powerful altered state of consciousness, expanding the dialogue with the unconscious mind
13. Going beyond technique and developing artistry. Sessions become a shared adventure in a universal drama.

Every session has a four-stage metaprocess: **awareness, experimentation, integration** and **reentry.** These stages occur separately and simultaneously on all levels of body, mind, emotion and spirit. This metaprocess does not follow a linear course but rather one that is cyclical and parallel.

The Rubenfeld Synergy Method provides a highly effective, holistic paradigm for bringing the body/mind/emotions/spirit together in a present, trusting whole. This psychophysical journey of synergist and client seeks harmony, empowerment, freedom and integration of life.

Says Rubenfeld, "At its best, the relationship of faith and trust created between client and synergist elevates our spirits and breaks through barriers that otherwise seem impenetrable!"

Russian massage   also referred to as Russian medical or Russian SPORTS MASSAGE, is a form of bodywork that uses the basic stroke forms of classical massage (SWEDISH MASSAGE is based on classic massage). Russian massage has considerably changed each classic stroke performance, so that each stroke provides the patient with the least invasive and most comfortable treatment.

Within Russian massage technique there are over 50 various strokes, which are further divided into **main strokes** and **substrokes.** Russian massage EFFLEURAGE has 11 strokes and substrokes; FRICTION is made up of 10 different forms; PETRISSAGE has 14 variations, and VIBRATION over 18 strokes. While many massage systems work with the body's anatomical structure, Russian massage concerns itself with the body's physiology. Each stroke of Russian massage has a known physiological effect on either a healthy or dysfunctioning body. This approach allows the Russian massage practitioner to provide an appropriate massage for either a particular person, need or dysfunction.

Practitioners of Russian massage maintain that this system is not corrective, but rather it respects the concept that the body is its own healer. The goal of each treatment is to introduce the body to the solution it lacks and needs and to produce effects that will resolve the physical problem. It is painless, yet if pain should occur, it is recognized as a sign to adjust the treatment.

Russian massage began as a part of medical practice during the 1870s. At the beginning of the 1900s, Russian physiologist Dr. I.Z. Zabludovsky (d. 1913) established the connection between dysfunctioning organs and related dermatomes. He immigrated to Germany where he continued his work. The German CONNECTIVE TISSUE massage technique, BINDEGEWEBSMASSAGE, has its roots in Zabludovsky's research.

Although used in clinical settings for over 50 years, Russian massage received greater recognition and prominence after World War II due to economic need and medical energy situations. Wounded Russian veterans were given massage when pharmaceuticals were scarce and of poor quality to treat pain and promote healing. Its efficacy in speeding recovery time promoted massage to a major form of treatment in traditional Russian medicine.

The (former) USSR put physiatrists, medical doctors with physical therapy education, in charge of discovering the effects and benefits of natural healing techniques. The doctors researched the effects of each stroke on the body and specific systems. Their research measured the reaction to massage on healthy individuals and groups of people with different dysfunctions. They found that certain effleurage strokes increased leukocyte (white blood cell) and erythrocyte (red blood cell) count in the blood and was a powerful agent in pain control. Effleurage strokes also proved to be sedating to the central nervous system.

Some friction strokes proved to increase the heat of tissues, improving local circulation up to 140 times. Russian friction can also calm irritated nerves, such as in cases of neuritis (inflammation of a nerve), neuralgias (pain along the course of a nerve) and radiculitis (inflammation of spinal nerve roots, such as sciatica). The Russian massage form of petrissage (which has no gliding as in Swedish massage) reversed muscle atrophy (shrinkage) and increased muscle size.[1]

There are four groups of Russian massage. Effleurage and friction can be relaxing, while petrissage and vibration can be stimulating. Within each stroke category are variations that are either superficial or deep in their pressure. The massage strokes send messages to the nervous system to excite or sedate the body and to restore the body's function in cases of dysfunction.

Russian massage is used medically to treat dysfunctions or expressly to improve athletic performance. The sports massage treatment employs the same basic strokes but uses different patterns for pre- and postevent care, as well as general sports and training massage.

Therapeutically, Russian massage can increase muscle elasticity, flexibility and strength, reduce swelling after injury, minimize pain and increase circulation of blood and lymph.

It has been used to treat high blood pressure, sciatica, joint dysfunctions, headaches and migraines. It can treat diseases of the cardiovascular, neurological, gynecological, dermatological and musculoskeletal systems.

Doctors prescribe massage regularly in Russia and massage therapists are highly trained professionals. It is not uncommon for the largest department in a hospital or clinic to be the massage therapy department.

Its application as a sports treatment is vastly documented. The Russian Olympic teams used massage for their pre- and postgame preparations as early as 1900. Dr. Sarkizov-Serazini, a physician who worked almost exclusively with competing athletes during the 1930s, researched the effects of massage on performance and found very positive results.[2]

A study by Dr. V.E. Vasilieva, professor of sports medicine with the USSR National Academy of Medicine, compared hydrotherapy, electrical stimulation, vitamin therapy, pharmaceuticals, sauna and massage to see which system provided the best results for postathletic event restoration. Massage placed first, followed by hydrotherapy. She found that massage can prevent trauma and serious injury, accelerate healing and help the athlete regain normal body function much faster.[3]

Russian massage is gaining popularity in the United States. Its major proponent is Zhenya Kuroshova Wine. She was trained in the Soviet Union as a physiotherapist and specialist in medical and sports massage and hydrotherapy. She immigrated to the United States in 1980. She now heads the Kuroshova Institute for Studies in Physical Medicine in Rock Island, Rhode Island.

The massage technique also places emphasis on the therapist's comfort level. It is normal for therapists to treat up to 28 people per day, so their hands must be protected and proper body mechanics enforced. To that end, the massage does not use single digit pressure or wrists. Instead, large lever joints, such as the shoulders or elbows, are the primary sources of strength for deep work without causing injury to the therapist.

Notes

[1] Kuroshova Institute, General Information Sheet—*Russian Massage,* Rock Island, Rhode Island, no date, p. 2.
[2] Mower, Melissa, "Russian Clinical Massage—The Kuroshova Method," *Massage,* Issue No. 43, May/June 1993, p. 3.
[3] Wine, Zhenya Kuroshova, "Russian Sports Massage: Post-Event Massage," *Massage,* Issue No. 41, January/February 1993, p. 56.

The text and videos are available from the Kuroshova Institute, Rock Island, R.I.
Clinic Massage
Russian Clinical Massage
Sports Massage, Vol. I, II, III

Further Reading

Wine, Zhenya K., *Russian School of Massage Therapy,* Kuroshova Institute, Chapel Hill, N.C., 1988. Describes the physiological aspects of massage in general and Russian techniques specifically. Explains over 50 strokes of the Russian system and their use. Clearly illustrated.

S

sacro-occipital technique (SOT) an advanced, gentle, corrective CHIROPRACTIC procedure, which recognizes the sacroiliac joint (the articulation between the sacrum and ilium) and pelvic girdle as the structural foundation of the body. With this system, the chiropractor concentrates on stabilizing or balancing the body starting with the pelvis and its dural connection to the occiput (bone in the back of the skull), the atlas (first cervical vertebra) and the axis (the second cervical vertebra). An unsteady pelvis often creates problems in many associated regions and organs of the body.

SOT uses the body's own gravitational pull with noninvasive, precise manipulation to center, or align, the pelvis. Once the pelvis is adjusted, the rest of the spine can be treated.

SOT uses a strategy of structural mapping, called the **category system,** to establish an effective method of diagnosis and treatment. This system also uses wedges, or blocks, placed under the pelvis to restore balance.

The categories of sacral-occipital technique list three divisions of pelvic involvement. Category I is a twisting or torquing of the spinal membranes, at the sacroiliac joint. The technique used in this instance restores the normal flow of neurological information between the brain and the nerves to promote healthy organ function.

Category II is a failure of the sacroiliac joints to bear the weight of the body. The category may be expanded further to include misalignment at the pubis symphysis (the suture joint at the front of the pelvis). Techniques for this condition relieve the swelling and inflammation at the joints and reduce the neural interference.

Category III is an unstable sacroiliac joint that increases the stress on the disk causing it to swell or protrude. Severe low back pain and/or sciatica usually result, causing the body to lean to one side, away from the pain. The treatment for

category III involves blocking and traction to alleviate the back pain and sciatica.

Sacro-occipital technique and the pelvic block technique were developed by Dr. M. Bertrand DeJarrette, D.C., a pioneer in chiropractic, in 1925. He also developed a color film process for Eastman Kodak during the 1930s, which provided him with considerable earnings, enabling him to concentrate on his research and treat patients without charge.

When strategically placed under a client's hips, the innovation of the blocks allows each respiration to adjust the joints of the pelvis. Since the lower spine is recognized to be an important structure for promoting health and strength throughout the body, this noninvasive technique allows the entire spine to return to its regular respiratory motion.

In addition, the use of the blocks releases compromised intervertebral disks (the cushions between each vertebra filled with gelatinous fluid), allows the upper back to realign, neutralizes pelvic rotation and eases stresses in the musculature of the back.

One way to determine the correct placement of the blocks is to measure the length of the legs with the client in a prone (face down) or supine (face up) position on a chiropractic table.

In addition to the sophisticated category system, this technique uses many **indicators,** in the form of neurological signs, weak muscles or active reflexes to evaluate a client's condition.

Sacro-occipital technique includes other evaluation tests to determine where the problem originates. The cervical stair step technique analyzes whether the vertebrae of the neck (the cervicals) are acting in pairs or are subluxated. The chiropractic manipulative reflex technique stimulates internal organs and isolates the source of the problem. Soft tissue regional orthopedics diagnoses and treats musculoskeletal and organ dysfunctions by correcting the disruptive nerve reflexes at specific points. Extremity procedures treat the joints of the limbs, which may also be out of alignment.

For Sacro-occipital technique practitioners, the cranium (skull) is considered one of the two most important areas in terms of structural influence on the body. The other is the sacroiliac. The cranium does indeed have microscopic respiratory motion and is subject to SUBLUXATION, which subsequently affects the entire body. Cranial adjusting techniques, many of them intra-oral, restore the flow of information to the brain and therefore can have prolonged effects.

Sacral-occipital technique uses no force, yet the results in correcting pelvic and, subsequently, spinal misalignments are testimony to its power.

Safe Touch® an approach to touch for health care professionals in all disciplines who treat survivors of childhood incest and other forms of abuse. Bodyworkers, physical and occupational therapists, nurses, physicians, chiropractors, et al., who physically touch their clients/patients, may attend these sensitivity trainings to gain an awareness of the effects of abuse on the body/mind of their survivor clients in the clinical setting. Safe Touch Seminars, Ltd., also presents workshops for the survivors themselves.

The seminars and workshops combine lectures, interactive and experiential learning to educate participants how to work with their survivor clients and, for the survivors, to better connect with their bodies and to understand the impact of their loved ones.

Bodywork professionals are taught a number of skills to help them recognize the signs and symptoms of adult survivors: to recognize if they are ready to work with intent; how to cope with spoken and unspoken limitations or expectations of the survivor client; how to work with a client who has not disclosed his/her history; massage techniques to avoid; how to speak appropriately with the client; how to develop a professional rapport with the client's psycho-

therapist; what a body memory is and how to handle flashbacks; how it feels—or doesn't feel—to be in a survivor's body and how to handle various situations through the use of vignettes and hands-on exercises.

Workshops for survivors are educational in nature and expose participants to new ideas, which encourage further growth. They are intended for people in active psychotherapy but not as a substitute.

In these workshops, survivors seek to gain understanding from their partners through various exchanges. The **ice test** helps partners of survivors safely experience some of the physical sensations and corresponding emotions of how a survivor feels when being touched. **Soft armor** demonstrates the effect of disassociation on the body of the survivor.

No spots turns the tables, so the survivors experience what it is like to avoid certain areas on their partner's body while doing a challenging physical and mental exercise. There is also an interactive. discussion of sexual boundaries, recognizing the current status of the sexual relationship and setting goals to improve sexual intimacy.

Safe Touch provides a safe and caring learning environment where clients are respected and their boundaries recognized.

seifukujitsu See OKAZAKI RESTORATIVE MASSAGE.

sensory awareness a practice in which people learn to pay attention to proprioceptive patterns as a way toward rediscovering natural balance and oneness in themselves and with others. Words such as "method" or "system" are avoided because they carry with them general connotations contrary to the sensory awareness approach, since there is no set rules for achieving preconceived results. It is neither a method nor a system, but rather an exploration. It is an "un"training of constricting, conditioned responses.

Through sensory awareness, people may become aware of their relationship with others, with the earth, air and environment; with this awareness, they can become more direct and appropriate in all their actions and daily activities.

The originator of sensory awareness was Elsa Gindler (1885–1961) of Germany. As a young woman, she developed tuberculosis. Unable to afford a sanitarium for treatment, she took care of herself. She gave full attention to what happened in her organism during every daily activity and recognized that during this kind of attention, negative thoughts and worries subsided. Her constant focus resulted in *Gelassenheit,* a sense of calm, which can be a state of being in balance, grounded, and feeling deep confidence in the world and in oneself.[1] As her lungs healed, she learned that regeneration was "fundamentally an orienting process, which could become perceptible to us at any time."[2]

From 1917 on, she was continually developing a practice she called *Arbeit am Menschen,* working on the human being, which was a way of perceiving the organismic process of movement, mood and thought.

In the 1920s, she met the innovative musician and educator, Heinrich Jacoby, who became her colleague in an ever-deepening exploration of human being. Jacoby was a very important influence in the practice. In Europe, sensory awareness is often referred to as the Gindler-Jacoby work. Only his records of classes remain. His heir, Sophie Ludwig, has been bringing out books from his records during the last few years.

Gindler remained in Berlin during World War II and worked with Jewish and other persecuted people (and anyone else who sought her guidance) to help them survive and live as best they could no matter what their subsequent fates might be.

The word student is used in place of client. In the Gindler-Jacoby work, one studied to rest and move without interference from compulsive thought, to perceive the inner and outer environment with greater clarity and experience a deeper connection with others. This was work toward transformation to the core of a person; deep change was in the experiencing. The heart of the work is being in the present. "Life," Gindler claimed, "is the playground for our work."[3] "If we would have the strength at our disposal that we use in hindering ourselves, we would be as strong as lions."[4]

The work was brought to America and made widely known here by Charlotte Selver, who coined the term sensory awareness in 1955. The basic assumption is that people have not realized their full potentials because they have been habitually hindered by themselves—and society—against being consciously aware of sensation. The goal of the work is to move toward full functioning of the organism, the indivisible body/mind.

Breathing is a vital center of sensory awareness. An interference with total functioning may be discovered by noticing breathing patterns. Being conscious of breathing can help one experience the unity of the organism. Through attention to breathing, the experimenter may discover how respiration is affected by every happening, such as the touch of oneself or one's partner on some area of the body—the chest, or abdomen for example. Touch can also help the student become aware of unneeded tensions, where they are and if they could release.

The "exercises" of the practice are called **experiments.** The movement involved in any activity is consciously followed in order to discover what happens in the body during and in response to that movement. Muscular tensions and somatic attitudes, before and after each experiment, are compared every time the activity is tried out with awareness of the most subtle changes. The student is asked not to think about what is being done, but simply to experience during the experiment. Charlotte Selver calls this "being in the moment," or feeling each movement without trying to control it.[5]

Aspects of this work have been incorporated into many other practices. ESALEN MASSAGE has adapted many of Selver's principles into its treatments, such as permitting organic physical changes to happen naturally, rather than working to make them happen.

Notes

1 Roche, Mary Alice, "Sensory Awareness—The Basic Connection," *Study Project in Phenomenology of the Body Newsletter,* Vol. 2, No. 1, Spring 1989, p. 25.
2 Ibid., p. 25.
3 Selver, Charlotte, "A Taste of Sensory Awareness," Sensory Awareness Foundation, Muir Beach, Calif., Summer 1989, p. 5.
4 Ibid., p. 7.
5 Roche, Mary Alice, "Sensory Awareness—The Basic Connection," *SPPB Newsletter,* Vol. 2, No. 1, Spring 1989, p. 28.

Further Reading

Brooks, Charles, *Sensory Awareness: The Rediscovery of Experiencing through the Workshops of Charlotte Selver,* Felix Morrow, N.Y., 1986. The husband, student and colleague of Charlotte Selver has written the only book about sensory awareness. It was originally published by Viking in 1974 and has been translated into many languages.

Service Through Touch   a unique approach to bodywork for HIV-infected persons. The guidelines for this work were established by Irene Smith, founder and director of Service Through Touch, a nonprofit organization dedicated to the idea that touch and massage are integral components of health care for the seriously ill. Trainings are provided worldwide for people involved personally or professionally with individuals facing a serious illness.

Smith reports that there are many benefits of skilled touch for people with HIV infection. Physically, muscle aches and pain are controlled; increased oxygen to the brain reduces confusion and disorientation and provides a reference of physical reality; the increase in blood circulation stimulates toxin release; the increase in lymph circulation strengthens the body's defense against infection; and the skilled touch encourages greater physical mobility.

The benefits are also realized in the psychological and psychosocial aspects of the illness. Skilled touch validates life and gives hope; it reduces fear and isolation; it encourages emotional expression; it provides emotional safety

and nurturing, particularly to those people who do not have access to their family or other personal support systems. Skilled touch can reinforce a more positive body image that may be lost due to debilitation and disease; it helps the client to develop a more positive relationship with his or her illness; and it gives the family and support team a tool for communication and bonding.

Smith also maintains that the health care staff is helped. By easing the physical and attitudinal symptoms of the patient, skilled touch may ease part of the emotional burden under which health care workers must operate.

The provider: Emotional preparation for the provider is recommended before beginning bodywork. Working with the seriously ill means the provider is working with his or her own feelings concerning physical and emotional pain. This requires a personal commitment to do personal growth work. This may include psychotherapy, meditation, visualization or movement therapies. Everyone works differently. Training in the areas of death, dying and grief is necessary in order to cope with the psychological impact of working with the seriously ill. Support groups based on the sharing of feelings are a necessity, not an option.

The touch session: A careful assessment of the client's physical condition precedes the bodywork. This may include verbal, visual and tactile evaluations. Since the client's body is constantly undergoing dramatic changes, this assessment must begin each session.

With seriously symptomatic persons, the skilled touch provider is working with weakened elimination systems, so many of the bodywork techniques used to enhance toxin release are inappropriate. They may overburden the physical body. Less stimulating forms of bodywork should be used. The rhythm is slow, the pressure is gentle and the treatment time is tailored to the client's tolerance level.

The person with HIV infection may be physically, emotionally and spiritually traumatized. The approach to the client in general, and the actual approach of the hands is slow, gentle and mindful of such trauma.

Smith lists five steps of approaching the skin: enter the field slowly; begin by touching with the fingertips first, without movement or pressure, to give the cells a chance to relax under the touch; place the palms next to give the client a chance to experience the feeling of the hands, without movement or pressure; apply the pressure, if any; and add movement—if any. When departing from the body, depart from the skin in the same five steps.[1]

Smith suggests short touch sessions, such as hand massage or simple stroking of the forehead or hair if the practitioner has no specific training in providing skilled touch to bedridden clients.

Current information reports that in order to transmit the HIV virus, three factors of transmission must simultaneously occur. The virus must have a **proper environment,** such as blood, semen, vaginal fluids and mother's milk. **A sufficiently large quantity** of the virus must enter the system. Blood, semen and vaginal fluids may have a virulent concentration of the virus. The virus must also have a **port of entry,** or a way for the virus to enter the body.

However, infection precautions should always be strictly followed when providing bodywork to all persons. Bodywork tables should be wiped down with a solution of two drops of Clorox (bleach) in a gallon of water, if blood products are in question. Otherwise, a spray-on alcohol solution should be used.

The primary infection precaution is **thorough hand washing,** which is accomplished by scrubbing vigorously with soap. The gentle friction that occurs as the soap lathers is part of the microbicidal action. It is important to include the area between the fingers, the thumbs, the wrists, and even the forearms if necessary. A fingernail brush will assure adequate cleansing of the fingernails. Thorough hand washing should be accomplished before and after each massage session, as well as during the session if this is deemed necessary. Thorough hand washing before giving direct care protects the client who is susceptible to infection, while cleansing after rendering care protects the caregiver and any subsequent client.[2]

The use of gloves is always a secondary infection precaution and never replaces the need for thorough hand washing. Gloves function as an additional layer of protection. Either latex or vinyl gloves may be used, although the permeability of latex is affected with mineral oil-based products. If mineral oil-based products are to be used, it is suggested to wear vinyl hand coverings instead.

Sterile gloves may be used when there is a concern for the susceptibility of the client to infection; when handling blood products and other bodily fluids; if the provider has a cut or open sore on his or her hand; whenever requested by the client; or when working with someone who is suspected of having tuberculosis (the added precaution is also to wear a mask). Double gloving may be used when added protection is thought to be necessary.[3]

The contraindications of touch and special concerns: Skin conditions are common among HIV-infected persons. Rashes may be fungi or allergic reactions to drugs. Some rashes may spread to other parts of your client's body by touching them, and allergic reactions may become irritated by touch. It is best to limit touch to unaffected areas of the body. This is also a good guideline for fungi, psoriasis and eczema.

When working with a client with an unidentified rash, it is advisable to postpone bodywork until there is identification. In some cases, an unidentified rash may simply suggest the use of gloves or touching over a sheet during the session. This does not change the guideline of touching only unaffected areas of the body.

Open sores, cuts, abrasions and puncture wounds, such as recent IVs or blood testings, are very vulnerable areas for an immunodeficient client. The risk of infection is high. Allow these areas to fully heal before incorporating them into the bodywork.

Pain may be a signal of internal injury. Acknowledging the painful area by simply laying the hand on without pressure or stroking is suggested.[4]

Kaposi's sarcoma (KS) is a cancer that, before AIDS, was seen primarily in older Mediterranean males. As an HIV-related opportunistic illness, it continues to predominately affect the male population. KS can be an extremely visual illness, manifesting itself in the appearance of brown, dark red or purple lesions. These lesions may be the size of a mole, or as large as a palm. They can be internal and/or external, open and weeping, or closed and dry. They might itch, hurt, or be sensation free, and the feeling may change from day to day.

Gentle bodywork can be performed over closed lesions, depending upon the degree of sensitivity. Pressure on or near the lesions is contraindicated. In extreme cases, touching unaffected areas of the body is suggested. KS is not contagious, therefore gloves are not necessary. Due to its visual appearance, KS can be quite isolating for the HIV client, so touch can provide an excellent coping system.

A new lesion is traumatic. You may feel fine with your client's new lesion, but he or she may not. This is a very intimate process and requires sensitivity, flexibility and grace of the provider.[5]

Smith stresses that to work with bedridden or seriously symptomatic persons, hands-on training is needed. She states, "This work begins where most schools end."[6]

Workshop and educational material is available from Service Through Touch, San Francisco, California.

Notes

[1] Smith, Irene, *Bodywork for People with HIV Infection,* Service Through Touch, San Francisco, Calif., 1994, pp. 6–7.

[2] Ibid., p. 4.

[3] Ibid., p. 5.

[4] Ibid., p. 10.

[5] Ibid., p. 12.

[6] Smith, Irene, Personal letter, June 1995.

Further Reading

DaJin, Zhong, *Treatment of AIDS with Traditional Chinese Medicine,* Shandong Science & Technical Press, Jinan, China, 1992. This small book describes the treatments from mainland China for AIDS patients, including treatment principle, acupuncture, moxibustion and Chinese herbs.

Kübler-Ross, Elisabeth, *AIDS: The Ultimate Challenge,* Simon & Schuster, N.Y., 1993. Written by the preeminent authority on death and dying, Kübler-Ross explains the special needs of these patients. A chapter by Irene Smith on the massage care of these patients is included.

Ryan, Mary Kay, and Shattuck, Arthur, *Treating AIDS with Chinese Medicine,* Pacific View Press, Berkeley, Calif., 1993. This couple has been treating HIV/AIDS patients for almost 10 years in their Chicago clinic. This book includes a discussion of organizing and funding clinics, AIDS from a Chinese medicine perspective, herbal treatments, acupuncture, massage and dietary recommendations for AIDS patients.

Smith, Irene, *Bodywork for People with HIV Infection,* Service Through Touch, San Francisco, Calif., 1994. This clear, concise booklet describes the HIV virus and the factors of transmission. Smith then outlines the benefits of massage and appropriate precautions for the provider.

Zhang, Qingcai, *AIDS and Chinese Medicine,* Oriental healing Arts Institute, Long Beach, Calif., 1990. For the clinician, this book describes AIDS/ARC treatment with Chinese herbs and provides relevant pharmacological data.

SHEN^{SM} an acronym for Specific Human Energy Nexus, a physioemotional release therapy, is a unique HUMAN ENERGY BIO-FIELD intervention system that releases painful emotions directly from the body in order to regain emotional and physical health.

Holding contracted emotions and painful memories perpetuates their presence in the body and can affect social behavior, thoughts and overall health. During a SHEN session, the practitioner gently rests her hands near or on the participant's clothed body and amplifies the recipient's naturally occurring energy through the emotion centers in a carefully planned pattern. The duration of this noninvasive touch is long enough for the energy from the practitioner's hands to flow through the client. The subtle process gently releases trapped emotions and uncovers the powerful emotions of joy and confidence, often resulting in the expression of pivotal memories.

This touch is repeated on several areas of the body. It usually takes a series of sessions to break through the emotional blocks before they are realized. Sessions usually last one hour with little dialogue between practitioner and participant.

SHEN was developed over a 10-year period by Richard Pavek, who has a background in chemistry, electronics and aeronautics. At a workshop about "subtle energies," which Pavek attended in 1977, he and his partner shared a unique experience on how powerful emotions held in the body could surface by working in the human energy bio-field. He considered that this field would have to follow similar principles of apparent motion that apply to other fields in physics, such as magnetism. Once the system was understood, the phenomenon could be repeated. His research resulted in the development of SHEN. Pavek based SHEN on the disciplines of physics, biology and psychology, coming from years of study, which found logical causes for the effects within the energy fields.

Healing within the human energy bio-field has a rich history. Ancient Egyptian, Chinese and Indian scholars documented evidence that describes energetic healing techniques.

SHEN is a noncognitive process that can affect involuntary and preverbal experiences. It recognizes that correlation of specific somatic dysfunctions with particular emotions. For example, the emotions of love, grief or sadness have somatic effects in the heart. Contracted emotions could lead to congestive heart failure, hypertension or angina. The emotions of anger, fear or anxiety manifest in the solar plexus, often resulting in digestive disorders anorexia or ulcers. Guilt, shame, security, confidence and helplessness are rooted in the navel/pubic region. Somatic disorders might include premenstrual syndrome, irritable bowel syndrome or chronic low back pain. Mortal fear, located in the groin or perineum (the region between the anus and vagina or testicles) could cause psychogenic shock.[1]

Involuntary tensions occur in the body to contain the painful physical symptoms of organic or glandular dysfunction. Specific treatment, like SHEN, is directed at deep relaxation

of local tissue on the site of the suppressed emotion and somatic disorder. As local tension eases, the organic function is restored. SHEN theory maintains that biological and emotional treatments are the same.

A major focus of SHEN is work on these physioemotional problems to remove the traumatic emotions. Another major focus is empowerment of the self by removing the residue of painful, inhibiting emotions trapped in the body. It also promotes relaxation, speeds up healing and may be used in conjunction with other therapies and bodywork systems.

Practitioners of SHEN are trained and certified worldwide through the International SHEN Therapy Association.

Note
[1] Pavek, Richard, *Handbook of SHEN,* The SHEN Therapy Institute, Sausalito, Calif., 1987, p. 33.

Further Reading
Pavek, Richard, *Handbook of SHEN,* The SHEN Therapy Institute, Sausalito, Calif., 1987. Pavek's book on SHEN therapy is easy to follow and full of helpful suggestions to relieve tensions in the body and their accompanying emotional counterparts. Refinements in SHEN practice outdate the book. Trainings are the most effective way to learn SHEN.

shiatsu an ancient Japanese bodywork system that uses hand, knuckle, palm, elbow or foot pressure on specific points, called TSUBOS, located along energy pathways, called MERIDIANS, to promote the free flow of *ki* (CHI) energy. The word *shi* translates to mean "finger" and *atsu* means "pressure."

The origins of bodywork in Oriental medicine were first recorded in the *Huangdi Nei Jing* (The Yellow Emperor's Classic of Internal Medicine), which was written between approximately 300–100 B.C., and is still in existence today. The emperor referred to in this medical text allegedly ruled approximately 2697–2596 B.C., almost 4,500 years ago.

During the Qin dynasty, in the third century B.C., Oriental bodywork therapy was called "moshou," hand rubbing. This healing art advanced to such a high level, that a doctoral degree was created in the fifth century A.D. at the Imperial College of Medicine in Xian.[1] All doctors were required to learn the bodywork techniques to help them develop the keenly sensitive touch they needed for ACUPUNCTURE.[2]

CHINESE MEDICINE was brought to Japan about 1,000 years ago by the Buddhist priest Gan Jin Osho. From these teachings, shiatsu/*amma*, Japanese acupuncture, MOXIBUSTION and palpatory diagnoses were developed.[3]

The Edo period (1603–1867) is regarded as the time when these therapies reached a peak.[4] Most of the *amma* practitioners were blind (*Amma* is an ancient pressing and rubbing massage technique) and provided treatments in their patients' homes.[5]

By the end of the 19th century, European medicine had been introduced to Japan and adopted by the aristocracy. They disallowed the continued teaching of native healing methods and the evolution of massage techniques came to an abrupt halt.[6]

During the Taisho period, in the 1920s, the first law to regulate ancient therapies was introduced in Japan, prompting practitioners to create new names for their work in order to avoid the licensing laws. The publication of *Shiatsu Ho* (Finger pressure therapy) in 1919 by Tamai Tepaku, which described a massage system that combined *amma*, AMPAKU (HARA massage), acu-point therapy, DŌ-IN (self-massage) and Western anatomy and physiology, stimulated great interest in shiatsu. In 1925, the Shiatsu Therapists Association was created in order to distinguish between shiatsu practitioners and the general relaxation work of the *amma* "shampooers."[7]

Since that time, shiatsu practitioners have been considered experts in treating minor ailments in Japan. One of the most renowned and influential practitioners was Tokujiro Namikoshi. His successful treatment of a well-known politician helped launch the recognition of shiatsu as separate from *amma*. Other famous shiatsu practitioners are Katsusuke Serizawa,

who developed TSUBO POINT THERAPY, and Shizuto Masunaga, who created ZEN SHIATSU.[8]

After World War II, shiatsu gained full recognition in Japan. In America, in 1950, Toshiko Phipps became one of the first qualified Japanese shiatsu therapists. She is still very active with the American Oriental Bodywork Therapy Association and is the originator of INTEGRATIVE ECLECTIC SHIATSU.

Oriental medical theories maintain that disease occurs because of a stagnation or blockage in the free flow of *ki* energy. Balance must be established in order for health to be restored. Shiatsu uses pressure techniques to affect the interrupted energy flow throughout the meridians and related organs.

A shiatsu treatment generally takes less than an hour. Before the work begins, however, the practitioner uses many of Japanese and Chinese medicine's diagnostic techniques to evaluate the client's energetic, emotional and physical condition.

Assessment of the spinal areas and the *hara*, the area of the abdomen considered to be the center of the body's strength, provides information on the energetic condition of the visceral organs. PULSE READING and visual assessments may be used to evaluate the constitution as well as health of the 14 major meridians.[9]

Once an assessment has been made, the practitioner can determine which tsubos need concentrated work, whether the energy point is *kyo* (deficient, or empty) or *jitsu* (excessive, or full), the balance between the FIVE ELEMENTS and how to establish harmony and balance within the meridian system.

The treatment begins with the client laying on a padded mat or futon, dressed in loosely fitted clothing. The shiatsu may begin on the *hara* and then move to the legs, arms, neck, head and face. The client will turn over and the back and legs are treated. The hand techniques may include finger pressing, palm pressing, holding and vibration, rubbing, shaking with hand or foot, patting, tapping and kneading, to name some. Joints are often put through their RANGE OF MOTION to increase their flexibility. Specific points are held for approximately 3 to 10 seconds. The pressure can be shallow or deep.

Shiatsu has many beneficial effects. In addition to balancing *ki* energy and the five elements to prevent disease, this ancient system reduces muscle tension, promotes the functioning of the internal organs, prompts peristaltic contractions of the intestines, is deeply relaxing and is useful in treating symptoms with no or slight organic malformation. Shiatsu bodywork can also be adapted for self-help purposes.

Shiatsu is contraindicated in the presence of contagious diseases; for patients with serious organ disorders in the heart, liver, kidneys or lungs; with patients who are susceptible to internal bleeding; in the presence of stomach, intestinal, uterine cancers or sarcoma; and on the site of broken bones or varicose veins. It should also be avoided if the client is under the influence of drugs or alcohol; if a fever is present; immediately after a full meal or if the client is extremely hungry; immediately before or after exercise; and in the acute stages of any disease. Abdominal treatments should be avoided in cases of pregnancy, high blood pressure or heart disease, since they may raise blood pressure.

Notes
1 Dubitsky, Carl, O.B.T., L.M.T., "History of Shiatsu/Amma," *Massage Therapy Journal*, 1992, p. 1.
2 Ibid., p. 1.
3 Ibid., p. 1.
4 Ibid., p. 2.
5 Yamamoto, Shizuko, and McCarthy, Patrick, *The Shiatsu Handbook*, Turning Point Publication, Eureka, Calif., 1986, p. 15.
6 Serizawa, Katsusuke, *Tsubo—Vital Points for Oriental Therapy*, Japan Publications, Inc., Tokyo, 1976.
7 Dubitsky, Carl, O.B.T., L.M.T., "History of Shiatsu/Amma," *Massage Therapy Journal*, 1992, p. 2.
8 Ibid., p. 3.
9 The 14 meridians of shiatsu are lungs, large intestine, stomach, spleen, heart, small intestine, bladder, kidney, heart constrictor (pericardium), triple heater, gall bladder, liver, governing vessel and conception vessel. Seven are YIN and seven are yang.

Further Reading
Goodman, Saul, *Book of Shiatsu*. Avery Publishing Group, Wayne, N.J., 1990. This book, with over 300 photographs, provides easy-to-follow instructions for a full-body shiatsu treatment. It also presents ways to evaluate physical condition and provides dietary and holistic lifestyle suggestions.

Jarmey, Chris, and Mojay, Gabriel, *Shiatsu—The Complete Guide*. Thorsons, San Francisco, 1992. This book explains the concept of *ki* energy, shiatsu techniques, the meridians and provides case studies.

Namikoshi, Tokujiro, *Shiatsu: Health and Vitality at Your Fingertips,* Japan Publications, Tokyo, 1969. Written by one of shiatsu's foremost authorities, this book has 100 black-and-white photographs and 90 illustrations, which clearly depict the locations of the treatment points. The book describes the history of shiatsu and provides information on the maintenance of better health, sex related shiatsu and treatments for specific illnesses.

———, *Shiatsu Way of Health*. The history of shiatsu is explained along with treatment points for specific ailments.

Yamamoto, Shizuko, and McCarty, Patrick, *The Shiatsu Handbook,* Turning Point Publications, Eureka, Calif., 1986. This illustrated guide, written by one of shiatsu's innovators, explains the foundation of shiatsu's history and philosophies, provides information on macrobiotic principles and offers treatments for particular problems.

———, *Whole Health Shiatsu,* Japan Publications, Inc., 1993. This book examines a macrobiotic shiatsu approach to healing and health. Pictures and illustrations clearly explain the techniques.

Shintaido™
a modern system of body movement whose roots lie deep in the traditional arts of Japan. Shintaido translates as "new body way," but it is more than a simple health exercise. It is an art form, akin to brush calligraphy performed with the entire body. Relaxed and flowing, or bright and expansive, Shintaido practice liberates and replenishes energy.

Shintaido is meditation in movement, an emptying of one's being, a life exchange with others and an opening of the self to nature and the universe. While Shintaido is a highly sophisticated form of physical culture, its simple, uncluttered forms of movement can be practiced by people of all ages and physical conditions.

Shintaido has been called "the light in the shade and the sun in the shadow."[1] As a mood or sensation, Shintaido is more religious and artistic than scientific, and involves cooperation more than competition in its movements. Yet it is the cooperation with others that emphasizes individual expression.

As a martial art, contrary to a fighting art, the emphasis is on getting the most effective results by using the least amount of energy and transforming negative and destructive energy into positive and constructive energy.

Shintaido was researched and developed by almost 40 professional martial artists in 1965. This group, brought together by Hiroyuki Aoki, was called the Rakutenkai Group. It also included musicians of various ages and physically challenged participants. This diverse group set out to create something new, although their actual goals were unclear.

Three years later, their development work was complete. The result, this new art of movement and life expression, was intended for an international audience. Shintaido was introduced in the United States by Haruyoshi Ito and Michael Thompson, who, in 1976, cofounded Shintaido of America. The Shintaido curriculum is extremely rich and varied.

A typical Shintaido class begins with stretching, warm-up movement, and preparatory exercises followed by vigorous jumping or other locomotive movements specially designed to activate the lower part of the body, free the entire body of unnecessary tension and to develop a soft, strong, unified, movement for the body as a whole. This is followed by unique Shintaido techniques that are often accompanied by sustained vocalizations.

There are partner exercises based on the unique philosophy of life exchange, which cultivate a goal of true communication rather than to defeat an opponent. Life exchange is a concept that transcends the usual notion of self-preservation or self-protection. In Shintaido, we recognize that an opponent does his best to attack with pure intention; this helps us fight back with the same intensity, making his victory more difficult.

Note
1 Aoki, Hiroyuki, *Shintaido,* Shintaido of America, San Francisco, 1982, p. 21.

Further Reading
Aoki, Hiroyuki, *Shintaido,* Shintaido of America, San Francisco, 1982. This book explains the history of Shintaido and provides step-by-step photographs of the movements of this martial art.

shortwave diathermy a deep heat therapy used in physical therapy or other rehabilitative modalities, elevates the temperature of the body's tissues by passing a high-frequency, shortwave current through a particular body part. Heat is produced when these tissues resist the electrical current. These waves penetrate deeper than INFRARED RADIATION but do not produce the same physiological head sensations.

Electrodes are placed on each side of the body area, separated from the skin by an insulating material. This method is called the **condenser field method.** As the current is applied, an electromagnetic field is created between the electrodes. The tissues of the body absorb the heat that is produced.

Shortwave diathermy can cause healing effects on the muscles, visceral organs and fat. It can also penetrate the body to its deepest tissue level and therefore has some effect on bone.

The dosage of the current depends upon the client's comfort level and tolerance, and treatments should never exceed 30 minutes. Before a session begins, all metallic objects should be removed from the client and the general treatment area.

Shortwave diathermy has been effectively used in the treatment of chronic arthritis, musculoskeletal conditions that are accompanied by pain, spasm or infection, sciatica, colic, lumbago (lower back pain), mastitis (inflammation of the breast), SUBLUXATIONS and headaches.

It is contraindicated in cases of pregnancy when the lower half of the body requires treatment, during menstruation, in the presence of acute inflammation, over wet skin, near any metal objects and with clients wearing pace-makers.

small intestine meridian a bilateral YANG MERIDIAN that governs the entire body through the assimilation and absorption of food. This meridian is also responsible for separating the pure from the unpure in the body. Mental anxiety, emotional excitement, nervous shock and anger can affect blood circulation in the small intestine, causing blood stagnation. Dis-harmonies in this pathway may cause abdominal pain, diarrhea or constipation. This meridian governs the spine and shoulder girdle.

Beginning on the outside tip of the small fin-ger, this meridian runs up the outside of the arm and ends outside the ear. There are 19 ACUPUNC-TURE points in the small intestine meridian.

soft tissue a term used to describe the types of structures treated in many hands-on bodywork systems, particularly muscle tissue and certain CONNECTIVE TISSUE, such as tendons, ligaments and fascia.

Soma bodywork See SOMA NEUROMUSCULAR INTEGRATION.

Soma Neuromuscular Integration™ also called Soma bodywork, is a 10-session system of body/mind therapy that changes people physi-cally and psychologically. These changes are achieved by structurally balancing the body in gravity and integrating the nervous system to allow more freedom of movement, spontaneity and creativity in our responses to the environ-ment.

Mental and emotional states are reflected in the physical structure of the body, and appro-priate bodywork facilitates significant psycholog-ical growth. Changes in the structure are accom-plished primarily through manipulation of the FASCIA (connective tissue) and muscles, whereas the neurological work occurs on both physiolog-ical and psychological levels. This work affirms

the unity of the body/mind, so work in each area will have a profound effect on the other.

By working on the fascia, Soma practitioners can free the musculature. (The fascia is a thin network of connective tissue that wraps around each individual muscle and muscle group. Myo-fascia refers to the combined muscle and fascial systems.) Chronic pain in the joints or muscles is generally reduced once the myofascia is structur-ally integrated.

The work on the muscles balances the tone among muscle pairs. Muscle tone is vital to the healthy process of the **proprioceptive feedback loop,** which tells us where the body is and what it is doing. The nervous system receives the proprioceptive input through small structures in muscle tissue called **spindles.** Soma Neuromu-scular Integration uses these spindles as switches to reprogram the nervous system and balance and maintain healthy muscle tone, thus en-hancing structural integrity. As the body struc-ture discovers new, more comfortable and appropriate positions in space, new options for experience become available. Clients report feeling greater self-reliance and more flexible physical and psychological responses.

Soma Neuromuscular Integration was devel-oped in 1978 by Dr. Bill M. Williams, Ph.D., one of the first students of Ida Rolf. Soma owes its roots to ROLFING theories. Williams's work indicated a departure from some of Rolfing's invasive work. Williams believed that the most intrusive work of Rolfing created the least amount of positive change. This discovery led to refinement of the original Rolfing approach. The differences between the two systems today focus on the results of the work, the way the work is presented to the clients and the practitioners' training.

The Soma clients are encouraged to be ac-tively involved in their own process. Their level of awareness can greatly influence the experience of the work. To promote this involvement, a number of learning tools are provided, such as AUTOGENIC TRAINING (a deep relaxation technique), personal journal writing, individual movement education and written material corresponding to each session.

Soma practitioners, effect changes in the nervous system through tissue manipulation and techniques, which are unique to Soma. These techniques are based on the **three-brain model,** a way of understanding human consciousness and the activity of the nervous system. It is based on neuropsychiatric research which explains the functions of the left and right hemispheres of the brain. The third "brain" is the **corebrain,** which consists of nerve plexi located in the abdomen. This core is responsible for graceful, coordinated movement. It is the source of bodily energy and the means by which the left and right hemispheres translate cognition into activity.[1]

The three-brain model permits the Soma practitioner to synthesize specific bodywork with movement education and learning materials to create an experience with the client of greater conscious access to the body/brain.

The Soma approach applies pressure to the body in a way that evokes as little pain as possible. The body is treated gently and respectfully. Practitioners work with, rather than on the body.

The results of Soma bodywork are progressive rather than permanent. The body continues to improve long after the processing is over. The change initiated by the work gives people the opportunity to transform their lives into paths of greater fulfillment and creativity.

Through its multidimensional approach, Soma Neuromuscular Integration offers the opportunity to live a freer, more effective life, by giving one the capacity to move and respond more appropriately. The result is that one is not only more energetic, creative and coordinated, but one's behavior itself, rather than a fixed reaction, becomes a fulfilling, spontaneous expression of one's authentic self.

Note
[1] In Chinese medicine, the HARA, located at the site of the corebrain, is the center of the body's vital energy—*chi*.

somatic psychotherapy an evolving term that represents psychotherapists and bodyworkers who recognize the inherent unity of the human body/mind and have worked to develop clinical approaches that reflect this belief. Among these practitioners are body-centered psychotherapists, body-oriented psychotherapists, somatic psychotherapists and counseling bodyworkers, to name a few.

Placing the body/mind at the center of the healing process, represents both a return to ancient traditions and a natural evolution of Freudian work. In his early days, Dr. Sigmund Freud was interested in the body and even did massage. Along with one of his teachers, Dr. Breuer, Freud was interested in the relationship of emotions and the somatic process. They did a great deal of work with hysterics and physical symptoms that stemmed from emotional roots.[1]

Dr. Wilhelm Reich, one of Freud's students, was an innovator in psychoanalytic thought (see REICHIAN GROWTH WORK). He pursued the physical manifestations of the sexual response and the physiological and emotional functions of the orgasm. Nonverbal dimensions of the personality, emotional distress and body armoring were among his many theories.

In Norway, Dr. Ola Raknes, a contemporary and teacher of Reich's, was involved in the body and energy theory.

In more contemporary times, many methods and techniques comprise the field of somatic psychotherapy. In addition to those who concentrate on one particular approach to body/mind integration, there are also eclectic practitioners who combine different modalities.

Some of these approaches include, but are not limited to, REICHIAN THERAPY, BIOENERGETICS, CORE ENERGETICS, PESSO BOYDEN SYSTEM PSYCHOMOTOR, HAKOMI, EMOTIONAL-KINESTHETIC PSYCHOTHERAPY, FOCUSING, RUBENFELD SYNERGY, INTEGRATIVE PSYCHOTHERAPY and RELATIONAL DIALOGUE.

Note
[1] Marks, Linda, "Psychotherapy That Includes the Body: A Consumer's Guide to Somatic Psychotherapy," *Spirit of Change Magazine,* Grafton, Mass., 1995.

somatics an integrated discipline that combines psychology, various bodyworks, movement therapy and spirituality. The works of Sigmund Freud, Elsa Gindler (see SENSORY AWARENESS), F. Mathias Alexander, Wilhelm Reich and Moshe Feldenkrais are incorporated with bodywork systems such as ASTON PATTERNING, HAKOMI, LOMILOMI and ROLFING. The somatic approach to healing emphasizes the role body processes play in character and personality development.

The spiritual aspects of somatics is derived from non-Western traditions including yoga, breathing exercises and meditation.

SomatoEmotional Release[SM] a therapeutic process that helps rid the body/mind of the residual effects of past trauma associated with negative experiences. From 1977 to 1980, the joint research of osteopathic physician John Upledger and biophysicist Dr. Zvi Karni at Michigan State University Department of Biomechanics in East Lansing, led to the discovery that the body often holds on to physical forces rather than release them. Accidents, injuries or emotional traumas may contribute to the retention of the trauma by creating a dysfunctional, isolated area, which they have called an **energy cyst.**

This cyst may inhibit normal somatic functioning, and it may compromise tissue vitality. This problem often worsens over time, eventually making it difficult to overlook.

Drs. Upledger and Karni found that clearing negative memories and emotions that are related to past experiences was helpful, but this clearing process did not always resolve the physical problems. Sometimes it seemed that a naturally programmed biological process had been triggered and interrupted. In these instances, the process could often be completed in the patient's imagination with positive therapeutic effect. They have called this technique, which makes use of therapeutic imagery and dialogue, **the completion of biological processes.**

The SomatoEmotional Release process requires extreme sensitivity on the part of the therapist and a positive attitude and trust from the client. The therapist acts as a facilitator, encouraging the positive aspects of the individual to surface and discovering harmful, negative patterns. By helping the individual to relive the trauma, one of many energy cysts may be released.

The therapist touches the individual in a gentle manner and intuits what the healthy body wants to do. He or she then helps the individual achieve effective positions or movements. Generally, the body gets into the position it was in at the time of injury. As this happens the energy cyst is exposed and resolved. A sensation of heat usually generates at the (former) site of the energy cyst as the underlying tissues relax. An emotional component often accompanies this physical release.

The name energy cyst was suggested by Dr. Elmer Green of the Menninger Foundation after witnessing the process. SomatoEmotional Release was coined by Dr. Upledger.

Sôtai a unique method of aligning the body by addressing each joint and vertebra. It is made up of a series of exercises designed to bring about muscular relaxation by harmonizing the breath and movements. Sôtai stretches concentrate on moving in the direction opposite to the physical discomfort.

Integral to the Sôtai practitioner is a deep understanding of the human body/mind. The alignment is achieved by using the client's own strength, while the practitioner is guided by the feeling of the client. According to Sôtai, distortions and misalignments in the body are reflective of any mental, physical and emotional problems that may be present.

Sôtai was developed in Japan by Keizo Hashimoto and is recognized there as an effective method of treatment. Sôtai can be done with the aid of a practitioner or on one's own.

Further Reading
Hashimoto, Keizo, Herman, Aihara, trans., *Sôtai: Natural Exercises,* George Ohsawa Macrobiotic Foundation, Oroville, Calif., 1990. This book describes the exercises and

stretches of this Japanese system for the relief of common discomforts and to maintain optimum health.

sound healing or sounding, a powerful technique that uses different pitches of sounds over the CHAKRAS (energy centers), organs and bones for healing purposes. Each chakra vibrates at a particular frequency. When disease is present, or the chakra is not functioning as it should, sounding specific pitches into the HUMAN ENERGY BIO-FIELD can be a powerful method of correcting the vibration.

When the right sound is generated, the chakra responds to it by tensing up, brightening in its color emanations and beginning to spin rapidly and evenly.[1] There is a vibrational resonance in the energetic body of the recipient, which can cause a profound inner experience.

The facilitator's mouth or other tuning devices, are placed about 1 inch from the chakra's location. Sometimes, the recipient uses her own voice to generate sound, thereby sending a vibration through the tensions and blockages in various parts of her own body from an internal source.

The theory of sound healing is reflected in the use of chanting found in many spiritual practices. Many cultures regularly use song and sound as part of their healing and religious rituals.

Note
[1] Brennan, Barbara Ann, *Hand of Light,* Bantam Books, N.Y., 1988, p. 241. People with high sense perception, or the ability to see auras, can see the changes in the chakras.

Spinal Touch Treatment™ is a nonforce, preventive and restorative treatment that balances the pelvis and spine, improves posture, eliminates pain and promotes optimum health through muscle relaxation. The therapist lightly touches key areas of the spine to redirect the healing energies of the body. This process causes the affected muscles to relax and repositions the pelvis and spine.

This system, which used to be called Aquarian-Age Healing, is the study of distortion, its causes, effects and corrections.

Facilitators maintain that the pelvis is the area of the body most responsible for disturbed mechanics. Ideally, when the pelvis is stabilized and integrated, the spine above would be straight and the lower limbs would be even. Internal organs would be in their normal positions, and the body would be functioning perfectly. There would be no strain or tension anywhere in the body.

However, this is not the case for the vast majority of people. The **elastic limit,** or the level of allowance for the body to absorb stress, is generally exceeded, producing a distortion of the pelvis and its far-reaching deleterious effects on the body.

Correction to the pelvis is performed without force or the use of tools. The pelvis is positioned and health is restored to the degree of pelvic alignment.

The treatment lasts from 5 to 25 minutes and is a nonmanipulative technique that brings the spine into mechanical balance through muscular release. It corrects distortions of the body in a minimal number of sessions. Very little force is employed, contrary to deep tissue work.

Spinal Touch Treatment can be used in conjunction with other massage therapies.

spirit releasement therapy provides a process for releasement of an unwanted spirit, which has become attached to an individual.

The possibility of spirit possession, the full or partial takeover of a living human by a discarnate being, has been recognized in most cultures throughout history.

Spirit attachment may be random, although there are certain times when people are more vulnerable to this possibility. Occultists believe that a majority of the population are affected or influenced by spirit entities. They may be either helpful guides or destructive entities.

Spirits remain in the earth plane because they don't recognize their own death. Earthbound spirits, the surviving consciousness of deceased humans, are the most possessing spirits to be found. Attachments may not produce any symptoms, but they do consume the host's energy, and unhealthy behavior patterns and habits may develop.

Spirit releasement therapy helps the client achieve greater personal integration by releasing the unwanted spirit. This system was developed by William J. Baldwin, Ph.D., of the Center for Human Relations in Enterprise, Florida.

spiritual healing, also called divine, energy, faith or psychic healing as well as LAYING ON OF HANDS, is the summoning or channeling of universal healing energy from a higher, spiritual source to a person in need. It is believed that the healer is able to transmit God's or universal positive energies, which have the capacity to heal the body/mind/spirit of an individual.

The most recognized method of energy transference is through the hands, although prayer is another popular form. Spiritual healing with the hands can be composed of many bodywork systems, such as AURA BALANCING, CHAKRA BALANCING, Laying on of Hands, POLARITY, THE RADIANCE TECHNIQUE, REIKI or THERAPEUTIC TOUCH, to name some of the more common methods.

A mother's loving touch is probably the first experience we have with spiritual healing. When a child is hurting, the mother touches or kisses her child on the injured body part and tells him that the pain will go away, making it "all better." The child's belief in his mother's healing words and touch reassures him and, indeed, the pain goes away.

Throughout history, "miracles" occurred at healing rites and rituals because people believed in them. Beyond mere belief, however, stand the metaphysical reasons for the changes in a person's health, such as energy transference. The earliest healers were witch doctors, shamans, medicine men and priests whose chants and rituals attempted to influence the spirits causing disharmony or illness.[1] In the sixth century B.C., spiritual healing was an integral part of therapeutic pursuits. The Essenes of today's Middle East were considered to be a powerful group of healers.

Royalty was often called upon to heal the sick, since it was believed that the "king's touch" could cure the ailing. King Louis IX of France was canonized after his death in 1270 for his healing abilities.

In spite of Jesus' healing talents and prophesies of even greater healers to come, the practice of healing was restricted to ordained ministers once the Christian Church started to gain in power. Church policy associated healers with old pagan religions and persecuted them or put them to death. Psychics and healers were linked with the devil, and by the time the King James Bible became used in England, over 300,000 healers had been executed in a time span of 200 years. In 1735, Parliament's Statute of Persecution was repealed, putting an end to the systematic annihilation of physics and healers.[2]

By the 18th century, spiritual healing began to revive. In the United States, the Christian Science Church, founded by Mary Baker Eddy (1821–1910), became one of the largest proponents of faith healing. Mainstream religious services now include prayers for the ailing.

Spiritual healing, according to the Jewish Association of Spiritual Healers, a nondenominational healing organization, can encompass present or absent (distant) healing. God's energy is used to stimulate and assist the innate healing powers of the body/mind/spirit. Spiritual healing brings into harmony the spirit, mind and body, effecting a total physical, mental and emotional improvement. Jewish spirituality maintains that a healing and healthy body must be an integrated whole. It may be effective in one session or require several sessions to secure health.

Healers often place their hands gently near the site that needs healing, where intuition guides them, or over the individual's head for general healing.[3] Regardless of where the hands are placed, the body is perceived as an integrated form and healers believe that the energy will go directly where it is needed.

Many of the aforementioned bodywork systems deal with balancing the energy that surrounds and permeates the physical body. The alteration and reparation in the HUMAN ENERGY BIO-FIELD explains the healing effects of spiritual healing.

Prayer is another component of spiritual healing, although religious faith is not a prerequisite. Many modern hospitals are hiring chaplains with special training in counseling and interfaith understanding, recognizing that the spirit as well as the body is an integral part of a person's total health. The power of belief can have positive physiological effects, promoting recovery, assisting in overcoming fears and anxieties and maintaining health.

Notes
[1] Angelo, Jack, *Spiritual Healing: Energy Medicine for Today,* Element Books, Rockport, Mass., 1991, p. 7. The word "witch" came from the Anglo-Saxon root word "wit," or wise person. Seven African dialects translate "witch doctor" to "wisdom doctor." (The modern word "quack" comes from "quacksalver" and has its etymology in two Dutch and low German words: *kwakkelen,* a verb meaning to be sick or ailing, and *zalver,* a noun meaning a man who saved or healed. Thus, its true meaning is "a healer of the sick.")
[2] Ibid., p. 8.
[3] Healers, unless licensed to do so, do not touch.

spleen meridian   a bilateral YIN MERIDIAN that governs the blood, general nutrition and the process of transformation. This meridian is responsible for digestion and blood production. Certain bodily fluids, such as saliva, gastric bile and secretions from the small intestines, are influenced by this energy pathway. It is also responsible for maintaining organ and muscle shape and tone.

Mental fatigue adversely affects the spleen meridian, and a lack of exercise can cause malfunctioning digestive and hormonal secretions.

The spleen meridian starts at the medial side of the big toe, runs up the leg and ends on the side of the body, 6 inches below the armpit. There are 21 ACUPUNCTURE points in the spleen meridian.

sports massage   a specialized, and often eclectic, form of (SWEDISH) MASSAGE THERAPY, which focuses on enhancing athletic performance and

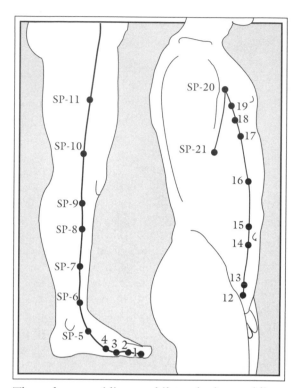

The spleen meridian, a bilateral yin meridian, starts at the big toe and runs up the leg, ending on the side of the body, six inches below the armpit. It governs blood, general nutrition and the process of transformation, or fermentation.

facilitating post-event recovery from the professional or amateur athlete, dancer and exercise enthusiast. Practitioners of this system concentrate on working the whole body but pay particular attention to those muscle groups that are involved in a specific activity.

Sports massage, whether pre-event or post-event, has numerous benefits. In addition to the benefits derived from a general massage therapy treatment, sports massage keeps the whole body in optimum physical condition. It can prevent injuries by increasing flexibility and elasticity to the joints. It can elevate athletic performance and boost endurance. Sports massage promotes faster recovery to injured tissues and can be a major factor in extending an athletic career.

Many professional athletes push themselves to an extreme and are often required to perform with an injury. Sports massage can reduce pain, minimize muscle fatigue and be restorative after injury.

Sports massage therapists use strokes that may not be incorporated into a general massage treatment, but are of particular value to the athlete. The four basic strokes of sports massage are **direct,** or TRIGGER POINT **pressure,** CROSS-FIBER FRICTION, **compression** and **percussion.** Two supplementary strokes, EFFLEURAGE and PETRISSAGE are applied as the need arises.

Direct, or trigger point pressure, is fingertip or thumb pressure directly into a tight or sensitive area. The point should be pressed for a count of five and then released. This stroke can be repeated several times. The trigger point, a hypersensitive area in the myofascia (muscle and connective tissue), which often causes radiating pain, is often recognized as a nodule within the muscle. Releasing the trigger point encourages increased circulation to the area, permitting the underlying tissue to soften.

Cross-fiber friction, also known as deep transverse friction, (see CYRIAX MASSAGE) stems from direct pressure. It is a back and forth motion, which is applied perpendicularly, or across, the direction of the muscle fibers. For example, if a muscle is vertical, such as the hamstring in the back of the thigh, pressure is applied horizontally. This stroke loosens the muscle fibers, breaking down spasms and adhesions (muscle fibers that stick together), promoting flexibility, realigning the muscle fibers in a parallel fibrillary network and creating soft and pliable scar tissue (scar tissue torques as a muscle contracts). The stroke may also be applied in small circles around a joint. In this case, it is referred to as circular friction.

Deep compression strokes are produced by a rhythmic, pumping action. The muscle is compressed against the underlying bone with the therapist's palm, loose or angled fist, or fingertips, to spread the muscle fibers and increase circulation. This stroke releases histamine and acetylcholine (a substance found in tissue that relaxes peripheral blood vessels), creating a durable hyperemia, which prepares the athlete for all-out competition. The stroke is performed on the "belly" (widest, central aspect) of a muscle, up and down or in and out, depending upon the angle. Deep compression is used before an event or workout. The purpose of the post-event treatment is to relieve DOMS—delayed onset of muscle soreness.

Percussion, also called TAPOTEMENT, is made up of a rhythmical, alternative striking movement and is used in sports massage as either **beating** or **hacking.** Beating is an alternate movement with loose fists, while hacking is performed with the (ulnar) sides of the hands. When applied for less than 10 seconds, percussion is stimulating. A longer application will sedate the muscle. Percussion is not a heavy-handed stroke, but rather a light one. The full weight of the hands should not be felt, and the rapid pace reverses the stroke almost upon impact. This technique may be used for the pre-event treatment, restoration rehabilitation, training and conditioning phases.

Effleurage, a long, gliding stroke, which spreads the lubrication and prepares the muscles for deeper work, and petrissage, a squeezing, lifting motion used to relax the muscles, are both used as preparatory strokes in the post-event and rehabilitation phase. Oil is used primarily in the post-event, restoration and rehabilitation phases. Its use earlier on in treatment could clog the athlete's pores, creating a barrier to perspiration, which could lead to hyperthermia (overheating). Effleurage also has the ability to facilitate reabsorption of waste products after a strenuous workout. It is therefore applied as the follow-up stroke to the friction stroke, which loosens waste products.

Many of the current sports massage techniques were developed in the former Eastern Bloc countries, especially the former Soviet Union (see RUSSIAN MASSAGE). Massage was a daily ritual for many top athletes. It helped them recuperate faster and prevented many injuries from occurring or worsening. The Olympic teams of these countries always traveled with a sports massage therapist. The benefits of sports massage quickly became apparent to the West. Consequently, many professional teams employ sports massage therapists before and/or after each game.

The pre-event massage helps the athlete avoid serious injury by warming and stretching tendons and ligaments and making joints more flexible. CONNECTIVE TISSUE, which does not have its own blood supply, warms up more slowly and is therefore more susceptible to overstretching and injury. The massage gently stretches these tissues, minimizing the risk of harm. Post-event massage is restorative, reduces soreness, loosens muscle spasms, maintains flexibility, enhance reabsorption of waste products and reduces cramping.

HYDROTHERAPY and ICE THERAPY are adjunctive systems used in sports massage. Hydrotherapy includes the use of water, in all its forms, for therapeutic purposes. Jacuzzis, hydroculators, whirlpool baths and steam rooms are common applications of hydrotherapy. Ice, in the form of gel packs, cubes or crushed, is applied directly on a particular area to reduce swelling and minimize pain.

A session of sports massage, whether pre- or post-event, can take less than one hour. If only a particular muscle group is being worked on, the treatment, which is rather vigorous, might only take 15 minutes.

Sports massage may also be used by people who overexert themselves to relieve the microtraumas in the muscles. Although this system is more advantageous when performed by a licensed therapist, some of the techniques can be self-administered.

Further Reading

Hungerford, Myk, Dr., *Beyond Sports Massage: Injury Prevention and Care through Sports Massage,* Sports Training Institute, Costa Mesa, Calif., 1991. This book is considered to be the most comprehensive text on the subject.

Meagher, Jack, and Boughton, Pat, *Sports Massage,* Dolphin Books, Garden City, N.Y., 1980. The first book on the subject provides an overview of sports massage and details the massage techniques. Clear illustrations show the locations of important trigger points. Fifteen sports injury and treatment sites are described.

spray and stretch technique a technique that treats TRIGGER POINTS by providing a gentle, passive stretch to a muscle after the sensitive region has been sprayed with a coolant. The coolant often used is Fluori-Methane. (The trigger point is usually a localized, congested area of a muscle that has a specific pattern of referred pain.)

Some medical doctors may actually inject the trigger point with saline or procaine.

This technique was pioneered by Dr. Janet Travell, who had mapped previously unrecorded patterns of **referred pain** from trigger point areas. (She is also known for being John F. Kennedy's doctor when he was a senator and president.)

Once the area has been sprayed (or injected), massage techniques are used to restore blood and lymph circulation to prevent further development of trigger points.

St. John Neuromuscular Therapy, also called St. John Neuromuscular Pain Relief or the St. John Method of Neuromuscular Therapy, is the science by which HOMEOSTASIS (balance) is brought about between the nervous and musculoskeletal systems.[1] This system recognizes five physiological principles that govern the activity of the nervous and musculoskeletal systems as the predominant forces that create balance. However, other supporting considerations include proper nutrition, elimination of waste products, hormone balance and the role that the mind plays in the health of a person.

These five principles are **dysfunctional biomechanics, postural distortion, ischemia** (lack of blood), TRIGGER POINTS and **nerve compression and entrapment.**

The goal of the neuromuscular therapist is to help clients achieve pain-free and biomechanically correct movement patterns. This includes appropriate movement of the extremities to ensure proper locomotion by the legs and dissipation of momentum in the upper torso. The body is a whole proprioceptive mechanism that is always attempting to self-correct dysfunctional patterns in order to meet the demands. Malfunctions in muscle tone often lead to dysfunctional joint movement, which creates a cycle of greater muscle tension. Joint surfaces often wear away because of the increased intrajoint pressure as a result of muscle tightening. The soft tissues have to be released, articulation pressure decreased and the client has to be reeducated in proper movement patterns.

Postural distortion, or the imbalance in muscle tone, results in body postures that are out of alignment. The St. John Method of Neuromuscular Therapy looks at how communication between the body's center of gravity in the sacrum and the vestibular system, or the balance system, in the center of the ear occurs in order to maintain structural homeostasis. When the body is posturally distorted, the muscles assume the function of the bones. In other words, they attempt to compensate for body weakness by acting as a support for the body. This creates muscle tension and fibrosis (abnormal formation of fibrous-connective tissue) and decreased intramuscular circulation. The body is analyzed for abnormal amounts of tilt, torque, rotation and projection that distorts the spine, pelvis and sacroiliac joints. Postural distortion always translates into dysfunctional biomechanics. Conversely, when the body is aligned, health can be maintained.

Ischemia, or lack of blood, usually accompanies muscle constriction. The resulting poor circulation increases friction within the muscle, which can increase irritation and inflammation.

Upon palpating the area, the ischemic muscle will feel tight. There is a decrease in natural irrigation of the tissue and a build-up of metabolic waste products. Some of these wastes can irritate muscle tissue, resulting in either swelling or further vasoconstriction. Dysfunctional biomechanics and postural distortion lead to ischemia and vice versa.

Trigger points, tight, hypersensitive areas in soft tissue, which cause referred or reflected pain in other parts of the body, are the fourth principle of St. John Neuromuscular Therapy. Trigger points are areas that have changed from high neurological activity to low neurological activity.[2] When trigger points from one muscle fire their high intensity impulses into another muscle, the result is a somatic-somatic reflex arch. In other words, the pain travels elsewhere in the body. If the muscle refers to an internal organ, then a somatic-visceral reflex is created. There might also be a visceral-visceral reflex, when one organ or gland affects another. A fourth possible response is the visceral-somatic reflex. High intensity impulses in the organ are referred to muscles, as in the case of menstrual cramps, where signals from the uterus affect the muscles of the lower back.[3]

Nerve compression, pressure on a nerve by a bony or cartilagenous structure, usually occurs along the spine as intervertebral disks compress the spine. Pain, numbness or paralysis and eventually atrophy (shrinkage) may result. Nerve entrapment is the pressure and intrusion on a nerve by the increased tightness of soft tissues. As the muscle continues its pattern of increased tension, the nerve strangulation becomes greater. To relieve the entrapment, appropriate and specific soft tissue manipulations must be performed.

St. John Neuromuscular Therapy was created during the 1970s by Paul St. John as a result of his own constant physical pain. He had sustained a serious back injury in high school, survived a helicopter crash in Vietnam and was severely injured in an automobile accident in 1974.

After spending thousands of dollars on medical doctors and medications, St. John was still in pain. In 1976, he received a treatment from a friend of his who was studying CHIROPRACTICS that offered relief. The system, "receptor tonus technique," was developed by Dr. Raymond

Nimmo and later called the Nimmo Technique. St. John studied with Dr. Nimmo and continued his research of the pain mechanism. He began teaching his own technique in 1978.

The St. John Method of Neuromuscular Therapy is a form of soft tissue manipulation designed to correct the neuromuscular components to the five principles described earlier. Lubrication is only used when treatment indicates, since palpation may be difficult if lubrication is present.

A moderate stroke rate ensures the proper palpation of the underlying tissues. The pressure varies on an individual basis, depending upon the extent of the trauma, the individual's age, general health, toxicity level and abnormal posture patterns. It is suggested that the therapist use just enough pressure to elicit moderate discomfort.

Eight to twelve seconds of pressure is long enough to produce a therapeutic response in the tissues. The highest degree of success is achieved by going back to the trigger point three or four times. The use of the thumb is preferred over other fingers or body parts.

St. John Neuromuscular Therapy addresses the cause of most pain, rather than concentrating on its effects.

Notes
[1] St. John, Paul, L.M.T., "Physiological Principles That Explain Pain Mechanisms," St. John Neuromuscular Pain Relief Institute, Palm Beach Gardens, Fla., p. 1.
[2] Ibid., p. 2.
[3] Ibid., pp. 2–3.

stomach meridian   a bilateral YANG MERIDIAN that relates to the functioning of the stomach, esophagus, duodenum, reproduction, lactation, appetite and the menstrual cycle. It transports food nutrients and participates in the transformation of QI energy.

The stomach meridian emerges under the eye and descends down the body and leg, ending at the lateral side of the second toe. There are 45 ACUPUNCTURE points in this energy pathway.

strain-counterstrain therapy   a treatment designed to relieve muscle dysfunction and pain. It was developed by Dr. Lawrence Jones, D.O. He named it strain-counterstrain to describe the origin of painful somatic conditions and the treatment.

Dr. Jones described strain as ". . . overstretching of muscles, tendons, ligaments and fascia with the attendant neuromuscular strain reflexes."[1] He emphasized treatment at the neuromuscular reflexes rather than the tissue stresses.[2] His method applies counterstrain to the neuromuscular reflexes that caused the condition. Counterstrain is described as ". . . a mild strain or overstretching applied in a direction opposite that false and continuing message of strain from which the body is suffering."[3]

Dr. Jones developed this technique with a patient who was not improving. This patient was unable to sleep because of pain, so Jones tried to find a comfortable position for him to help him sleep. After several attempts, Jones found a position that relieved the pain. After holding that position for only a brief amount of time, Jones's patient was able to stand pain-free with long-lasting relief.

A position of relief, close to or at the point of the original strain, is found and held for 90 seconds. The structures are then slowly and passively returned to neutral.

Jones developed this technique to relieve painful conditions. APPLIED KINESIOLOGISTS use strain-counterstrain as a way to restore neuromuscular function in the absence of pain by directing treatment to the involved muscle.

Notes
[1] Walther, David S., Walther, D.C., *Applied Kinesiology: Synopsis,* SDS Systems DC, Pueblo, Colo., 1988, p. 191.
[2] Ibid.
[3] Ibid.

Further Reading
Jones, Lawrence, Dr., D.O., *Strain and Counterstrain,* American Academy of Osteopathy, Indianapolis, Ind., 1981. Written by the developer of the technique, this book explains the theory of strain-counterstrain and illustrates

the trigger points of the muscles and the positions for the body to relieve neuromuscular pain and dysfunction.

structural integration another term for ROLFING.

subluxation a CHIROPRACTIC term that describes the misalignment of the vertebrae of the spine. These bones fit together so that nerve impulses from the brain may filter down the spinal cord and out through the nerves.

These neural messages communicate information all over the body in order that growth, repair and healing may occur. When vertebrae are out of their natural position, or alignment, the potential for nerve interference, or spinal nerve stress as it is also called, is great.

When nerves are unduly stretched or twisted (pinched), the critical communication between the brain and the spinal column with the body is impeded.

Subluxations are treated and the spin is repositioned through chiropractic adjustments.

Swedish massage also known as the Western or classic style of massage, is a scientific system of manipulations on the muscles and CONNECTIVE TISSUE, or the SOFT TISSUES, of the body for the purpose of relaxation, rehabilitation or health maintenance.

Swedish massage therapy is probably the most popular and familiar massage system being practiced today and has served as a foundation for many of the massage techniques, which have developed over recent years. Swedish massage is comprised of five basic strokes and their variations: EFFLEURAGE, PETRISSAGE, FRICTION, TAPOTEMENT (or **percussion**) and VIBRATION.

Effleurage, the long gliding stroke, begins and ends each massage and the work on individual body parts. The pressure of this stoke can be either light or deep, depending on the desired results, and stroking is always performed toward the heart to increase circulation. As an introductory stroke, effleurage is used to apply the lubricant to the skin and as an evaluation tool of the underlying tissues.

Effleurage manipulation directly increases blood and LYMPH circulation. This increase speeds up the removal of metabolic waste and the by-products of tissue damage and inflammation. In addition, the delivery of oxygen and nutrients to the cells of the body is enhanced as circulation is promoted.

The increase in blood circulation works predominately upon the veins, which return deoxygenated blood back to the heart. Blood flow in the arteries is indirectly affected by the same movements that assist venous blood flow.[1]

Local blood flow changes occur due to three different effects of massage, particularly effleurage: the direct physical effects on the blood vessels, the release of vasodilators, which relax the blood vessels, and the reflex response of massage on the autonomic nervous system due to tissue stimulation.[2]

Petrissage, or kneading, is the second manipulation of Swedish massage. The pressure also can be light or deep, depending upon the desired result. In most cases, petrissage lifts the skin from the underlying structures.

There are many variations of this stroke. **Circular kneading** can be performed using fingertips, palms or thumbs in a centrifugal direction, away from the center.

Fulling compresses the skin between the thumb and index finger in a pinching manner. It acts upon the skin and the underlying tissue. In **rolling,** the tissues are compressed against underlying structures in a forward and backward motion. Fingers are held straight and close together. **Wringing** is performed by grasping the limb with both hands and squeezing in opposite directions.

Chucking is a form of petrissage wherein the limb is supported by one hand while the other hand firmly grasps the fleshy portion of the muscle and drags it up and down. Movements are made about six times at each aspect of the limb, helping to elongate contracted muscles and act upon blood vessels and nerves.

Pick up is an alternate hand lift and twist performed on the fleshy aspect of a muscle. Pick up is beneficial for improving muscle tone and containing atrophy (muscle shrinkage). Petrissage, along with effleurage and friction, enhance circulation. Petrissage is also involved with tissue nutrition and cellular respiration. It increases the absorption of inflammatory exudate. When petrissage is done on the colon, it can improve the tone of the intestinal wall and promote peristaltic activity.[3] The strokes of petrissage produce localized heat.

Friction, the third stroke, is an important manipulation in Swedish massage as well as MEDICAL and SPORTS MASSAGE techniques. It is either applied across the fibers of the muscles and soft tissues (transverse friction—see CYRIAX CROSS-FIBER FRICTION), or circularly into a joint with centripetal pressure. Generally, this deep stroke is followed by effleurage to help reabsorb the waste products broken down by the application of the stroke.

Friction is performed with open palms for broader work, or fingertips and thumbs for deeper, more specific work. When applied to the joints, circular friction increases flexibility, elasticity and RANGE OF MOTION. It may break down adhesions and granulations, rendering muscles and joints more supple.

Friction is involved in circulation and promotes the absorption of inflammatory waste and the products of stasis, as in the case of fractures, by spreading them over a wide area and enhancing drainage into the lymph channels.

Light friction over a deep organ diminishes its blood supply by increasing activity to the overlying vessels. This causes blood to go around, rather than through, the organ. Light friction acts on superficial veins by accelerating the flow of blood and lymph to those parts being treated and to subcutaneous circulation.

Neurologically, friction can excite languid nerves or reduce swelling after nerve inflamma-

tion, as in the case of sciatica. The reflex action upon the vasomotor centers results in dilation of small vessels of the skin and an increase in the activity of peripheral circulation.[4]

There are at least five variations of tapotement, or percussion: **beating, hacking, slapping (clapping), cupping** and **tapping.** Beating is a rapid, alternate manipulation using the ulnar (little finger) surface of the fists. Hacking is performed with open hands on the ulnar surface in rapid, chopping strokes. Slapping uses the flat surface of the open palms, while cupping is a dome-shaped hand position using the fingertips and heels of the palms as the contact surfaces. Tapping is a fingertip percussion, usually applied to smaller surfaces.

Light percussion, for a period of less than 10 seconds, causes contraction of the blood vessels, permitting a quicker access of blood and the interchange of nutritional and waste material. Prolonged percussion, over 10 seconds, causes the blood vessels to dilate.

Muscle contraction can also be affected by the length of application. Contractibility can increase when tapotement is used over a short period of time. In this instance, tapotement may counteract muscle atrophy (shrinkage) and restore normal power to weakened muscles. Conversely, abnormally contracted muscles relax when tapotement is applied for a longer duration. Tapotement increases the irritability of nerves and can arouse sluggish sensory or motor nerves.

The final stroke of Swedish massage is vibration. It is a strong, rhythmic shaking or trembling of the hands or fingers in a stationary or "running" position. Generally, vibration is used to increase the contractibility of muscles. Over a prolonged period of time (more than 10 seconds), vibration may assist in the breakdown of muscle spasms.

Vibration stimulates glandular activity, nerve plexi and the peristalsis of the intestines. In cases of nonacute inflammation, vibration promotes the absorption of waste material.

Swedish massage, the cornerstone of many soft tissue manipulation systems, has a long and distinguished history. The Chinese wrote about massage as early as 2,500 years ago in the extant medical text *Huangdi Nei Jing* (The Yellow Emperor's Classic of Internal Medicine). Ancient texts of the Egyptians, Persians, Indians and Japanese refer to the benefits of massage and other natural healing techniques.

A great advance was made by the ancient Greeks and Romans who first brought massage to Europe. Hippocrates, the father of modern medicine, wrote that every physician should learn massage in order to restore flexibility and elasticity to his patients' joints.

In Athens and Sparta, specialists were employed to provide massage at the gymnasium, which was a state institution granted to any free citizen. It was used to treat asthma, epilepsy (Julius Caesar used massage for this purpose) and neuralgia.[5]

When he was in India, Alexander the Great received massage for the treatment of rheumatism. Legend has it that without these specialized manipulations, he would have been incapacitated and would have failed in his conquests.

During the Middle Ages, massage practice had mostly been forgotten, only to resurface around the 17th century. About 200 years ago, the French began to translate the Chinese books on massage, which accounts for the commonly used French terminology of Swedish massage. The Swedish technique used today was credited to the Swedish fencing master and gymnastics instructor, Per Henrik Ling (1776–1839), who, in 1813, based his massage technique on the scientific views of anatomy and physiology and systematized the five basic strokes. Medical gymnastics, or joint exercises, was initially included as a part of his system. Using what he developed, Ling cured himself of rheumatism.

During the last century, many advances were made in the application of massage. Lucas-Championnière prescribed the use of massage and exercise to treat fractures.[6] In England, James Mennell (see MENNELL MASSAGE TECHNIQUE) and Mary McMillan (see MCMILLAN MASSAGE TECHNIQUE) systemized specific massage manipulations and techniques and applied them to various medical conditions. James Cyriax (see CYRIAX MASSAGE) applied his cross-fiber friction technique for therapeutic purposes.

During the 1960s and 1970s, massage practitioners began incorporating Eastern concepts into their techniques, creating a new genre of bodywork. Medical and sports massage facilities started to spring up as the fitness craze of the 1980s erupted. Massage schools in the United States and Canada are now training large numbers of professionals to fit the growing demands.

Developments and innovations continue to be made (as evidenced by the number of bodywork systems based on Swedish massage in this text) in the field of massage. Massage therapy is currently the third most prevalent alternative health care, behind relaxation techniques and CHIROPRACTIC, in the United States.[7]

A session of Swedish massage usually takes one hour. The lubricant, which may also be a mixture of scented essential oils (see AROMATHERAPY), is warmed between the therapist's hands before being applied to the client. The client lies unclothed on a massage table and is draped with a sheet and towel for warmth and to maintain professional standards. A body part is uncovered only when it is being massaged.

The traditional Swedish massage treatment begins with the client in a supine (on his back) position. Pillows, cushions or bolsters may be used under the client's head, under his knees or to prop limbs. Therapy begins on the right arm, followed by the left, arm, right leg, left leg, face, head, neck, chest and abdomen. A head rest or face cradle may be added to the table for use in the prone position. This optional piece allows the client to keep his neck in a neutral position. In this face-down posture, the massage commences on the left leg, followed by the right leg and finally the back.

Numerous therapeutic effects of massage are produced in three ways: by mechanical pressure, through reflex action or metabolically. During mechanical stimulation, the tissues of the body are passive and are acted upon by the use of pressure. Reflex action stimulates the peripheral and central portions of the nervous system. Impressions are made up on the nerve endings, connected to nerve centers. Messages are transmitted back to the body part being massaged, as well as related areas. Metabolic changes occur as modifications appear in the tissues, either through direct action or reflexively.

Increases in the blood and lymph circulation are perhaps one of the most widely accepted physiological effects of massage. The ability to reduce edema (swelling of limbs from excess fluid) has been demonstrated in many clinical studies.[8] Massage increases red blood cell count, which can be beneficial to people with anemia, and decreases blood pressure.[9,10]

Heart contractions become more powerful due to the increased circulation, developing this muscle, yet blood pressure is decreased.

The physiological response to direct manual pressure influences the distribution in the vascular and lymphatic structures, displacing their contents into areas subjected to less pressure.[11] This mechanical displacement expedites the removal of waste and toxic products from the tissues.[12]

Upon the muscular system, massage can be relaxing, separate fibers thereby breaking down adhesions and spasms and stimulate contractions.[13] Myofascial pain (see FASCIA) is reduced and when massage is used for a pre- or post-athletic event, it can expedite recovery, delay muscle soreness and improve performance (see SPORTS MASSAGE and RUSSIAN MASSAGE). As a rehabilitative treatment, massage can help improve circulation and increase strength to immobilized, injured or denervated muscles.[14]

The contractile response of the muscles to massage is affected by motor nerve activity, not the action of the muscles themselves.[15] Muscle tone is a function of the nervous system, or more specifically, alpha motor nerves.[16] This means that in order for a muscle to relax or contract, higher brain centers must be involved.

Due to its influence on circulation, the muscles receive improved nutrition, expedited waste removal and atrophy is limited.

Myofascial TRIGGER POINTS can be treated and released by direct pressure on these sensitive areas. Fibrosis, an abnormal formation of fibrous tissue from injury, immobilization, inflammation or denervated muscles, can be relieved with petrissage and friction. Fibromyalgia, muscle pain, is also alleviated with massage.

The nervous system receives primary effects of stimulation to the deep nerve trunks and cutaneous sensory nerves. Secondary effects include relaxation and pain relief.[17]

Massage has been used to treat respiratory diseases for many years. The depth of respiration increases and the muscles of this vital system are developed.[18] Tissue respiration is also increased. This cellular response affects the entire body, including brain and liver function.

Massage to the skin (the integumentary system), the largest organ of the body, stimulates both superficial and deep nerve plexi in such a manner as to influence a curative effect at their ends in the brain and spinal cord. The activity of the skin is increased by direct and reflex action to the sweat glands, sebaceous (oil) glands and hair follicles.

The skeletal system is indirectly affected by manual manipulation. Bone growth may be stimulated and the development of a callus, the osseous formation at either end of a fractured bone, is enhanced by increased nutrition to the area. In addition, massage increases the retention of nitrogen, sulfur and phosphorus, essential minerals in healing.[19]

The blood-making process of bone marrow is enhanced by applying tapotement to the ends (epiphyses) of the long bones.[20]

Massage has a profound effect on the entire nervous system, which in turn, influences all the tissues and systems of the body. Massage can be either sedative or stimulating, depending on the length, pressure and choice of stroke. The calmative effects of massage can reduce pain and nervous irritability.[21]

Massage helps digestion and elimination in several ways. The stimulation to the nerves of the abdominal viscera improves circulation and glandular activity. Digestive secretions of the stomach, pancreas, intestines and liver are increased. Massage on the large intestine, particularly petrissage or vibration, promotes peristaltic activity. Massage promotes the absorption of digested nutrients by the blood and lymph and the intestinal walls are strengthened.[22] The organs of elimination, such as the skin, lungs, kidneys and intestines, are activated.[23]

The long list of the effects of massage therapy could not be complete without including the emotional and psychological impact derived from this treatment. Skin stimulation increases endorphin (feel-good compounds) output, which reduces pain, lowers anxiety levels and minimizes tension.[24,25]

The nurturing aspect of massage cannot be overlooked or diminished. The skin is our most sensitive organ, our first means of communication and the earliest sensory system to function.[26] The power of touch, therefore, is basic and can have substantial emotional impact, promoting relaxation, calmness and peace of mind. Heart rate and systolic (the contractile portion of the heart cycle) blood pressure significantly reduce after only 10 minutes of massage, prompting a sedative effect.[27]

It is evident that the effects of massage are prodigious. Its applications are also vast. Massage is indicated for general purposes of relaxation, stress reduction and health maintenance as well as for hundreds of more specific pathological conditions and medical applications.

Although massage abounds in its benefits, there are several instances where either full-body or localized treatment should be avoided. Full-body massage is contraindicated when a fever is present; when there is pain in the body of unknown origin; when the client is nauseous, vomiting or has diarrhea; in cases of heavy bleeding (a heavy menstruation indicates avoidance of abdominal massage); acute phlebitis (vein inflammation), thrombosis (presence of a blood clot) or aneurism (arterial dilation due to pressure or weakened tissue, which forms a blood clot); with jaundice; if there is an abdominal mass; hemophilia; gall or kidney stones; and immediately after the client has had a full meal, is intoxicated or under the influence of drugs.

Localized massage should be avoided at the site of any break in the skin, burns or lesions; directly on varicose veins or the site of a fracture until healing is complete; directly on bruises or keloid scars (thick, ropy scars); and deeply to the abdomen if the client has high blood pressure, ovarian cysts, an ulcer, if an intrauterine device is being worn or if the client is pregnant.

Notes

1 Zerinsky, Sidney S., Ph.D., *Handbook of Swedish Massage*, Swedish Institute, N.Y., 1982, pp. 6–7.

2 Yates, John, Ph.D., *A Physician's Guide to Therapeutic Massage*, Massage Therapists' Association of British Columbia, Vancouver, B.C., 1990, p. 5.

3 Op. Cit., p. 7. Zerinsky, Sidney S., Ph.D., *Handbook of Swedish Massage*, Swedish Institute, N.Y., 1982, p. 7.

4 Despard, Louisa L., *Text Book of Massage and Remedial Gymnastics*, Hodder & Stoughton, London, 1916, p. 226.

5 Swedish Institute, *Basic Massage Manual*, N.Y., 1994, p. 3.

6 Knapp, Miland F., M.D., "Massage," Physical Medicine and Rehabilitation, Vol. 44, July 1968, p. 193.

7 Eisenberg, David M., M.D., et al., "Unconventional Medicine in the United States," *The New England Journal of Medicine*, Vol. 328, No. 4, January 28, 1993, p. 248.

8 Yates, John, Ph.D., *A Physician's Guide to Therapeutic Massage*, Massage Therapists' Association of British Columbia, Vancouver, B.C., 1990, pp. 2–3. A study in 1955 by Martin Waim, Archives Physical Medical Rehabilitation, 48:37–42, showed that simple rhythmic compressions of an edemous limb was effective in cases of posttraumatic edema. Another study, in 1979 by Fujimori Z. Yamazaki, proved, using a plethysmograph (a device that measures variations in the size of a body part due to vascular changes), that edema was reduced and blood flow increased by proximally directed massage.

9 Kresge, Carol A., C.I., R.M.T., "Massage and Sports," *Massage Journal*, April 1985, p. 45.

10 Pemberton, R., and Scull, C.W., *Massage—In Handbook of Medical Physics*, Year Book Publications, Inc., Chicago, Table 1.

[11] Scull, C. Wesler, Ph.D., "Massage—Physiologic Basis," Archives of Physical Medicine, March 1945, p. 159.

[12] Ibid., p. 160.

[13] Kresge, Carol A., C.I., R.M.T., "Massage and Sports," *Massage Journal,* April 1985, p. 45.

[14] Yates, John, Ph.D., *A Physician's Guide to Therapeutic Massage,* Massage Therapists' Association of British Columbia, Vancouver, B.C., 1990, p. 10.

[15] Ibid., p. 10.

[16] Ibid., p. 11.

[17] Scull, C. Wesler, Ph.D., "Massage—Physiologic Basis," Archives of Physical Medicine, March 1945, p. 159.

[18] Despard, Louisa L., *Text Book of Massage and Remedial Gymnastics,* Hodder & Stoughton, London, 1916, p. 222.

[19] Kresge, Carol A., C.I., R.M.T., "Massage and Sports," *Massage Journal,* April 1985, p. 45.

[20] Despard, op. cit., p. 222.

[21] Ibid., p. 221.

[22] Ibid., p. 222.

[23] Zerinsky, Sidney, Ph.D., *Handbook of Massage Therapy,* Swedish Institute, N.Y., 1982, p. 9.

[24] Stillerman, Elaine, L.M.T., *MotherMassage: A Handbook for Relieving the Discomforts of Pregnancy,* Dell Publications, 1992, p. 113.

[25] Yates, John, Ph.D., *A Physician's Guide to Therapeutic Massage,* Massage Therapists' Association of British Columbia, Vancouver, B.C., 1990, p. 29.

[26] Montagu, Ashley, *Touching—The Human Significance of the Skin,* Harper Colophon Books, N.Y., 1971, p. 1.

[27] Yates, op. cit., p. 30.

Further Reading

Bahr, Robert, *Good Hands: Massage Techniques for Total Health,* New American Library, N.Y., 1984. Classical (Swedish) and finger pressure techniques are explained, based in theory, anatomy and practice.

Downing, George, *Massage Book,* Random House, N.Y., 1972. This book of photographs explains how to give a complete massage and how to design a personal massage style.

Hollis, Margaret, *Massage for Therapists,* Blackwell Sci., Cambridge, Mass., 1987. This easy-to-read textbook explains massage procedures and techniques.

Juhan, Deane, *Job's Body,* Station Hill Press, Barrytown, N.Y., 1987. This is a technical book, often used as a textbook at many massage schools, which is still easy to understand. It explains how bodywork effects change in the body/mind/spirit.

Maxwell-Hudson, Clare, *The Complete Book of Massage,* Random House, N.Y., 1988. An illustrated, comprehensive guide to massage techniques, including therapeutic and sensual massage, aromatherapy, massage for birth, infants and children.

Yates, John, Ph.D., *A Physician's Guide to Therapeutic Massage: Its Physiological Effects and Their Application to Treatment.* Massage Therapists' Association of British Columbia, Vancouver, B.C., 1990. This small book is filled with data from numerous scientific studies on the physiological effects of massage.

T

Tai Chi Chuan means "the supreme ultimate fist" (*chuan* directly translates as the potential for the hand to be a fist), or "boxing style," is a system of slow, centered movement based on more than 4,000 years of Taoism and Confusian thought and philosophy. It is a system of exercise and health, which integrates the body/mind, a martial art form and meditation. In Tai Chi Chuan, the heart/mind is kept at the *tan den* (see *hara*), or the center of the body. The CHI, life's vital energy, follows the mind and the body follows the *chi*. By keeping the heart/mind in tan den, a practitioner can move "centered" or clearly move the *chi*. This system is comprised of many facets, styles (usually derived from the family that developed it) has far-reaching benefits.

Tai Chi Chuan, also spelled Taijiquan, is composed of a series of postures, each called **a form,** performed in a slow, continuous sequence. Each form varies in its complexity, with some consisting of a dozen or so postures and others more than one hundred. This flowing movement is dancelike in nature and takes a long time to master. The focus of this fluent movement is on *tan den* and the weight is down.

The postures develop flexibility, stamina, energy and grace and promote imagination, concentration, confidence, self-control, serenity, awareness and power. Tai Chi is an ancient method of self-care, which is designed to cultivate *chi* energy, life's vital force, circulate it all over the body and remove energy blocks. As a result of increased *chi* energy, stresses, tensions and organic weaknesses are relieved.

As a self-defense system, Tai Chi is considered to be the greatest of all the arts of the fist, yet it is an internal system of kung fu, which emphasizes the development of vital energy rather than fighting techniques. It is not competitive and there are no degrees or belts awarded students of this discipline. Instead, practicing with a partner or in a group sensitizes students to each other's energy and teaches them how to respond effectively in a variety of situations.

As an exercise, Tai Chi creates and stores energy rather than depleting the body, reserving it for other activities. It also fosters an aerobic effect by promoting deep, slow breathing and centered one-pointed balance. Tai Chi can be used as an adjunct to other sports and forms of exercise to enhance physical efficiency and reduce injury.

Tai Chi is active MEDITATION, a way of moving to become closer to the inner self. It also promotes a more harmonious relationship with natural processes, enabling the student to maintain calmness and serenity despite life's tribulations.

Many older people enjoy the benefits of this slow-moving system. Among its many benefits, Tai Chi can help restore and maintain physical equilibrium, improve circulation and increase *chi* flow, lower the center of gravity in the body, deepen breathing and increase flexibility to joints and muscles. In China, Tai Chi is often begun by people of advanced age because of its reputation for increasing health and promoting longevity.

A study conducted by James Judge and colleagues at the University of Connecticut School of Medicine divided 20 elderly women into two groups. One practiced Tai Chi three times a week along with using leg press machines. The other group stretched and practiced Tai Chi once a week. The first group showed a 17 percent improvement on single-leg balancing, while the latter group demonstrated no improvement at all.[1]

It is a common sight to witness groups of people of all ages practicing Tai Chi in parks at dawn. According to Chinese philosophy, nature's *chi* flows strongest as the sun rises.

The roots of Tai Chi Chuan are obscure. Over 4,000 years ago, ancient Chinese drawings depicted monks in postures representative of Tai Chi. Some historians credit Chang San-feng, a

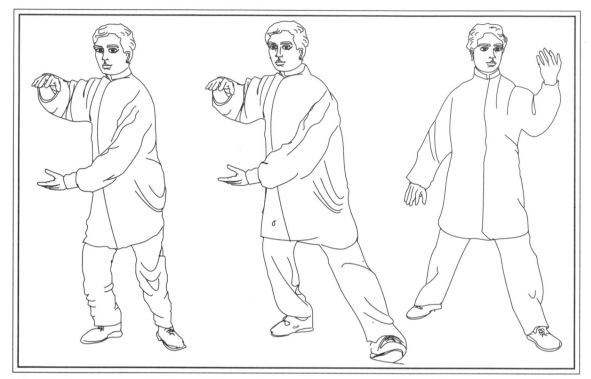

This movement system of ancient China translates as "the supreme ultimate." It is composed of a series of forms performed in a slow, continuous, dancelike sequence. Although it is a martial art, people of all ages practice Tai Chi Chuan to promote energy and longevity.

monk and famous kung fu boxer, with originating Tai Chi at the end of the Sun dynasty (A.D. 960–1270). The story goes that after witnessing a fight between a bird and a snake, Chang San-feng noticed that the snake avoided its predator's attacks by using fast but subtle movements. Other, more recent theories, ascribe a Chinese general in the 17th century with developing Tai Chi by combining martial arts with the theories of CHINESE MEDICINE.

Tai Chi was deeply influenced by Taoism, "the way," described by Lao-tze, which emphasizes the attainment of harmony with nature and the universe. When balance or harmony is achieved, all things function easily and spontaneously, according to Nature's laws. **Softness** and **suppleness,** two essential elements of Tai Chi, can be attained by cultivating *chi* energy.

The theory of YIN and YANG, the law of complementary polarities is inherent in Tai Chi. (The name of the symbol associated with the yin/yang theory is Taiji Du, or Diagram of the Supreme Ultimate. Tai Chi Chuan is the boxing style based upon the Tai Chi symbol.) For example, an "active relaxation" is essential in movement. Another example are the movements of Tai Chi that turn on a center line from the top of the head down through the foot. When turning on this line, half of the body moves to the left while the other half moves to the right as the center line remains perfectly still.

All movements in Tai Chi describe circles, spirals, arcs and curves, which create energy and calmness. A paradox of form, a term called "curved seeking straightness," refers to the necessary curvature and shape of the limbs. This system's name is also a contradiction. The "supreme ultimate fist" actually purports a principle of softness. Practitioners believe that outer suppleness and inner stability can overcome violent movements, like a blade of grass yielding to the wind.

Tai Chi Chuan is taught in classes, but the movements can be practiced individually at home. Some classes begin with a few minutes of standing meditation to promote tranquility and stimulate the flow of energy. Specific forms are then practiced as a type of moving meditation. Concentration, placed on the *hara,* or the point $1\frac{1}{2}$ to 2 inches below the navel, *tan den* (or CONCEPTION VESSEL 6), is known as centering oneself. This ACUPUNCTURE point is the source and storehouse of *chi* energy. *Chi* is stored in the *tan den* but there are a variety of sources. We are born with *chi,* and take it from the air we breath, food we eat and from the earth.

Movements have names taken from nature, such as "white crane spreads its wings," recognizing the Taoist philosophy of harmony with nature. Movements require the integration of breath and form.

Note
[1] Grimm, Ellen (compiled by), "Beat: Tai Chi Helps Elderly Find Balance," *Natural Health,* November/December 1994, p. 21.

Further Reading

Crompton, Paul, *The Elements of Tai Chi,* Element Books, Rockport, Mass., 1990. This book, for beginner and intermediate students, examines the history, techniques, weaponry, breathing, qigong, *I Ching* and herbology of Tai Chi.

Gallagher, Paul, *Drawing Silk: A Training Manual for T'ai Chi,* Deer Mountain Taoist Academy, Guilford, Vt., 1987. This book contains essays, guidelines and Taoist fiction about Tai Chi Chuan. Included is a list of various postures.

Hine, John, *Yang Tai Chi Chuan,* A&C Black, London, 1992. This book has 250 instructional, photographed sequences of the yang style of Tai Chi.

Man-Ch'ing, Cheng, *T'ai Chi Chuan: A Simplified Method of Calisthenics for Health and Self-Defense,* North Atlantic Books, Berkeley, Calif., 1981. The beginner is introduced to the history, forms and benefits of Tai Chi Chuang. Photos are included of Cheng practicing his form.

———, *Thirteen Chapters,* North Atlantic Books, Berkeley, Calif., 1985. Key principles of Tai Chi are described as well as principles of the state of mind, *chi,* softness and self-defense.

Yen-ling, Shing, *T'ai Chi Chuan Basic Exercises,* Japan Publications, N.Y., 1990. A basic introduction is followed by a 24-movement form and a 48-movement form.

Tantsu™

Tantsu™ or Tantric SHIATSU, follows the same principles as WATSU, except that this system is performed on the land. (Watsu is a combination of water and ZEN SHIATSU stretches.) In addition to providing all the benefits of shiatsu, Tantsu provides both the participant and practitioner a sense of meditative calmness, energy and awareness.

Tantsu, like Watsu, developed by Harold Dull at the Harbin Hot Springs in Middletown, California, is deeply rooted in the impulse to free the body. In Tantsu, the flow of one move into another is called **free form.** Tantsu massage focuses on the CHAKRAS of the body and centers both the participant and practitioner in a system called **co-centering.**

While working on land, the practitioner uses his entire body to hold and cradle an individual. The person remains clothed throughout the session and contact is limited to the supported body part. Focus is placed on stretching and releasing the MERIDIANS and major ACUPUNCTURE points. Tantsu is designed so that released energy is centralized in the spine.

The session begins, while the individual is face down, with a gentle rocking and proceeds with pressure point massage down the spine and legs. The individual remains passive as she is turned over. On her back, the legs are cradled and stretched, while keeping one of the practitioner's hands placed on her HARA (the point in the abdominal region $1\frac{1}{2}$ to 2 inches below the navel. This point is said to be the source and storehouse of vital QI energy.) She is then rolled into a side-lying, fetal position and her chest, chin, arms and legs are cradled and stretched.

Head, neck, chest and upper back Tantsu follows. The joints of the body are stretched and manipulated. The individual is then rolled on to her back again and stretched some more. The *hara* is massaged from this vantage point. The Tantsu treatment ends with a LAYING ON OF HANDS on the person's heart chakra and third eye.

Tantsu stretches joints and improves their flexibility while proving a deeply relaxing treatment.

Further Reading
Dull, Harold, *Bodywork Tantra on Land and in Water,* Harbin Hot Springs Publications, Middletown, Calif., 1993. This book describes the sequence and benefits of Tantsu.

tapotement also referred to as percussion, is one of the basic strokes of SWEDISH MASSAGE. Tapotement is often the last of the strokes before the final EFFLEURAGE signals the end of the massage.

Tapotement is a rapid, alternate percussive movement performed in five different ways: **beating, hacking, slapping** or **clapping, cupping** and **tapping.**

Beating is performed with loose fists, using the ulnar aspect of the hand as the striking surface. Hacking employs the ulnar surface of an open hand, while slapping or clapping is done with a flat hand. Cupping is a form of tapotement that uses the hands in a tentlike position, and tapping is fingertip percussion used on smaller surfaces, such as the face. The pressure of tapotement can be light or deep, depending on the surface being treated and the tolerance of the client.

Tapotement offers mechanical excitation by causing initial contraction of superficial vessels, which then become dilated as the application of the stroke continues. As in the case of VIBRATION, tapotement produces a stimulating reaction to the underlying tissue when it is used for a period of one to ten seconds, while longer treatment creates a sedating response.

Light percussion increases nervous irritability, while deep tapotement can exhaust the nerves, sometimes causing numbness. Tapping, slapping and hacking excite nerve centers. Strong tapotement relieves pain by tiring the nerves and decreasing their sensitivity. This is beneficial when treating neuralgia (sharp pain running along the course of a nerve).

Tetanic contraction (hypertonicity) may be induced by a succession of rapid strokes. Local contraction, independent of nerve stimulation, activates the muscle. The contraction permits a quicker access of blood and the interchange of cellular material, promoting nutrition to weak and wasted muscles. Tapotement often increases local temperature and nutritional activity. It can also counteract muscle atrophy (shrinkage) and restore normal power to weak muscles through its contractile responses.

With each of the tapotement variations, local circulation is improved, and it is particularly beneficial when skin activity is impaired. Liver activity is stimulated when the stroke is applied to the organ. It will promote peristalsis (intestinal movement) when applied over the gluteal and sacral regions. Tapotement to the chest can break up congestion and facilitate expectoration (expulsion of phlegm or mucous).

Beating to the sacrum is a valuable treatment in controlling atony (lack of physiological tone) of the bladder and in cases of sexual problems, such as impotence.

temporomandibular joint therapy a treatment to the joint of the jaw by using any number of bodywork techniques.

The temporomandibular joint is a hingelike joint made up of the temporal bone of the skull and the upper jaw, called the mandible. It connects the jaw to the head, with ligaments, cartilage, FASCIA, an articular disk, muscles, nerves, blood vessels and many tissues running in, around and through the region.[1]

When the mouth opens and closes, the joint behaves like a hinge. During mastication, or chewing, however, the complex movement slides the jaw from side to side, providing the grinding action of the teeth.

When the temporomandibular joint is misaligned or functioning abnormally, a condition

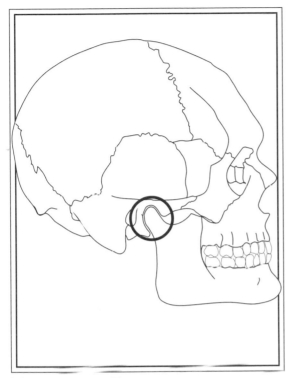

The temporomandibular joint is a hingelike joint made up of the temporal bone of the skull and the mandible, or jawbone. Joint dysfunction may cause headaches, back pain or more serious functional problems throughout the body.

known as **TMJ syndrome** or **TMJ dysfunction** may result. This condition, first identified in 1934 by Dr. J.B. Costen, an otolaryngologist (ear and throat doctor), can cause symptoms ranging from slight to severely debilitating. There may be a popping or clicking sound when the mouth is opened, accompanied by tightness or pain. In some cases, the jaw may actually lock into one position and temporarily be unable to move.

This syndrome can manifest itself in many other painful ways: headaches; migraines; hearing loss; tinnitus (ringing in the ears); facial swelling; shoulder, neck or cheek pain; toothaches; nausea; and blurred vision. Some researchers have linked this condition with throat, sinus and ear infections; asthma; and heart, stomach, intestinal, respiratory and emotional disorders.[2]

Almost 60,000,000 people in the United States have temporomandibular syndrome to some degree, with more women being affected than men.[3]

There are a number of possible causes of this joint dysfunction, including any kind of head, jaw or lower back trauma, birth trauma, improperly fitted orthodontia (braces), bruxism (grinding of the teeth) and stress. Other conditions related to temporomandibular syndrome are **dental distress syndrome** (DDS), brought on by a bad dental bite and **"jawlash,"** a result of an accident or facial trauma. Both can cause pain, muscle spasms, dizziness, chronic fatigue and insomnia, similar to TMJ Syndrome.

Temporomandibular joint therapy treats the cause of this malfunction and seeks to remedy the accompanying symptoms. CHIROPRACTIC techniques, such as SACRO-OCCIPITAL TECHNIQUE, CRANIOSACRAL THERAPY and APPLIED KINESIOLOGY, realign the body and treat the skull/jaw/spinal/ structural relationships. SOFT TISSUE manipulations, such as SWEDISH (or MEDICAL) MASSAGE, TRIGGER POINT THERAPY, MYOFASCIAL RELEASE, FELDENKRAIS METHOD, ROLFING and many other bodywork systems have also been successful in reducing pain and relieving this condition.

Notes
[1] Koren, Tedd, M.D., D.C., "TMJ Syndrome/ Dysfunction," Koren Publications, Philadelphia, Pa., brochure, 1991, p. 1.
[2] Ibid., p. 1.
[3] Ibid., p. 1.

Thai massage or *nuad bo-rarn,* is an ancient Siamese (Thai) bodywork system designed to unblock trapped energy and improve vitality by applying pressure along the MERIDIANS (energy pathways) called *sens.* These pathways carry vital life energy, QI in Chinese, PRANA in Hindi. Although Thai massage recognizes 72,000 *sen,* this system focuses on only ten major pathways.[1]

In Thai, the words translate to mean *nuad*—massage and *bo-rarn*, ancient or antique. It is also sometimes called Thai medical massage.

Thai massage, which is theoretically based on CHINESE MEDICINE and AYURVEDIC MEDICINE, is over 2,500 years old. It is believed that in the second century B.C., the Indian King Ashoka sent Buddhist missionaries to Siam (Thailand). The personal physician of Guatama Buddha, also the doctor to many of the missionaries, brought the massage technique with him to Siam (Thailand). It was enthusiastically adopted by the King of Siam as a great healing method and became a part of the royal court. Great temples were built, which often had stone carvings depicting many of the 104 postures and movements of Thai massage, adapted from Hindu YOGA techniques.[2]

The system became a part of the Thai culture and was passed down from one generation to the next, within families, orally and through demonstrations of the technique.

Thai massage uses slow, often meditative, rhythmic pressing by fingers, thumbs, hands, forearms, elbows and feet (which are used extensively) and yogalike stretches coupled with gentle rocking motions. Joints are put through their RANGE OF MOTION with these stretches.

The massage is performed with the recipient in four different positions: on the floor on his back, front, side-lying and sitting. The recipient is clothed in loosely fitted garments of natural fibers.

It is an accepted belief that the peripheral stimulation of the treatment produces specific internal effects. Thai massage increases overall fitness, stretches joints and balances major muscle groups, increases energy and removes blockages along the *sens* (lines), which may be causing organic dysfunction.

Thai massage makes up one of the four components of Thai medicine, which also includes diet, medicine and herbal remedies, and spiritual or magical practices.

There are two schools of nuad bo-rarn that still exist today. The most famous is at the Wat Poh Temple in Bangkok. This school has many of the remaining ancient medical texts carved in stone on the temple walls. Part of the temple is a medical school and clinic. The Chiang Mai School is located in northern regions.

Notes
1 International Professional School of Bodywork, "Thailand Massage" brochure, IPSB, San Diego, Calif., 1993.
2 IPSB, "Nuad Bo-Rarn" brochure, IPSB, San Diego, Calif., 1993.

thalassotherapy a type of HYDROTHERAPY that uses seawater or salted water along with massage for therapeutic purposes. The word comes from the Greek *thalassa,* which means sea.

Bathing or submerging in seawater is said to have certain medicinal properties. A session of thalassotherapy includes soaking in seawater while receiving a massage or seaweed pack. The massage may be manual or done with strong jets of seawater.

Therapy in a heated pool is contraindicated when a fever is present, with very high or low blood pressure, acute joint inflammations, infectious skin conditions or pregnancy.

therapeutic touch a contemporary approach to healing that is derivative of the ancient practice of LAYING ON OF HANDS. It is based on the idea that human beings are energy in the form of a field (see HUMAN ENERGY BIO-FIELD). In health, the field flows freely, while it becomes imbalanced when disease is present. Therapeutic touch is a gentle yet powerful tool for actualizing the natural capacity within each person to heal and achieve wholeness.

Therapeutic touch was developed by nurses Dolores Krieger and Dora Kunz in the early 1970s. Kunz had been involved with the study of laying on of hands when she invited Krieger to join her at a seminar of the renowned healer, Colonel Oscar Esteban. They both were astonished at the results Esteban achieved and proceeded on their own to develop therapeutic touch.

In her experiments, Krieger proved that therapeutic touch has the ability to significantly raise hemoglobin value (the part of red blood cells that carry oxygen). She believes that most people can train their hands to become sensitive to radiant energy and, therefore, learn to administer therapeutic touch to anyone.

This system is performed as a five-step process. **Centering** is a moment of quiet meditation, establishing the intent and compassion needed to heal. It is important for the provider to be a focused conduit in order to direct the energy.

Assessment is the evaluation of the recipient's energy field. The therapeutic touch provider attunes herself to the energy bio-field by using her hands as sensors. She passes them 2 to 4 inches above the recipient's body from head to toe and front to back. A healthy field will feel whole and evenly distributed. An unhealthy field might be perceived as thickness, pressure, coldness, emptiness, drawing in or sluggish.

Clearing congestion, the third part of the process, is performed by repeated downward, rhythmical sweeping movements. The provider shakes the energy off her hands after each stroke. **Filling the holes** transfers energy back to the recipient, while **Balancing the field**, or "unruffling" the field, smooths roughened spots and reorganizes the energy.

Therapeutic touch has been used by many health care providers to ease pain, promote relaxation, relieve arthritis, reduce headaches and in the treatment of dying and cancer patients. It is currently being taught at universities and nursing and medical schools across the United States.

Further Reading

Kreiger, Dolores, R.N., *The Therapeutic Touch: How to Use Your Hands to Help to Heal,* Prentice Hall, N.Y., 1979. Written by one of the founders of the technique, this book explains the use of therapeutic touch in healing.

_____ , *Living the Therapeutic Touch: Healing As a Lifestyle,* Dodd Mead, N.Y., 1987. This book is an easy-to-follow guide on the healing effects of therapeutic touch and its applications.

_____ , *Accepting Your Power to Heal: Personal Practice of Therapeutic Touch,* Bear & Co. Publications, Santa Fe, N.Mex., 1993. Therapeutic touch is a safe and helpful treatment for many ailments. The developer of the system encourages readers to accept their own healing abilities in this book.

Macrae, Janet, R.N., *Therapeutic Touch: A Practical Guide,* Knopf, N.Y., 1993. This book explains the theories of therapeutic touch and offers easy-to-follow instructions on its use.

Tibetan massage an integral part of Tibetan medicine used for improving general well-being or treating specific medical problems. For the former, oils are used with a full-body massage to rejuvenate, prevent illness and improve vital body functions. For the latter use, ACUPRESSURE is used in place of the full-body treatment, for the relief of physical problems.

There are five stages of massage within this system. The first, **application,** refers to the application of the appropriate oil for that client. It is always heated and then spread to the entire body. The choice of oil or lotion is a significant part of the treatment, often considered more important than the massage technique.[1] The proper use of pure, herbal or medicated oil can make the difference in the outcome of the treatment. For instance, side effects such as sluggishness or nausea may result from an incorrect oleation (oil) treatment.

Rubbing is the technique of using a light upward and downward stroke, similar to the EFFLEURAGE of SWEDISH MASSAGE, while **kneading** is performed on large muscle groups much the same way as kneading dough. SHIATSU, the fourth stage of Tibetan massage, is the acupressure component. Acupressure is used to stimulate certain external points, which are known to be energetically related, through the MERIDIANS, to systems and organs of the body. The acupressure in this form of massage comes from the Chinese system and is called *mDzub gNan* ("zoop noon"), meaning thumb pressure.[2]

The two schools of massage in Tibet use different numbers of points. One employs 78, while the other uses 108. Finger pressure is also diverse, although thumb pressure directly on a point is the most common technique.

Since the Tibetans have combined spiritual practice with acupressure (their contribution to acupressure), the technique also includes releasing the thumb pressure followed by rotating the thumb on the point while reciting a specific mantra.

Cleansing is the fifth stage of massage. It is done after the treatment, first by using a special flour suited to the constitution of the client, to remove the oil. These flours (i.e., chick pea, barley or lentil) help remove the residue of toxins from the skin's surface and rejuvenate and restore the skin. This procedure is usually followed by a shower, sweat bath or herbal steaming to promote continued toxin removal.

Tibetan medicine was first recorded during the 4th or 5th century B.C., when AYURVEDIC MEDICINE, the ancient medicine of India, was brought to Tibet. By the 11th century A.D., Chinese and Greek medicine also began to have an important influence on Tibet. The synthesis of these three classical medical theories was formulated into Tibetan medicine's major text, the *rGyud bZhi* ("gyu sbee").

As in the Indian and Chinese system, Tibetan medicine uses principles of the FIVE ELEMENTS that find their manifestations in the form of the **three humors** (energetic principles): wind, bile and phlegm. Wind is described as dry, cold, light and mobile. Bile is hot, moist, light and mobile, while phlegm is cold, moist, heavy and slow. The three humors are closely related to the body's major systems and organs. The interaction or harmony of these humors is the basis of determining health or illness.

Tibetan medicine also uses PULSE READING (similar to the Chinese method), urinanalysis (Greek in origin), visible examination and the patient's medical history to evaluate the physical condition.

Treatment is determined on the basis of the first, second and third lines. The first line is a naturopathic approach, which consists of diet and behavior recommendations. The second line is generally used in more acute cases or when the first line of treatment fails. This line includes the use of herbal preparations. For chronic or emergency conditions, or when the second line fails, the third line is employed. This line is made up of three parts, used progressively as the condition worsens.

Panch **karma,** or detoxifying, is the first part of the third line. It may include massage, oleation treatment, herbal steaming, enemas, purgatives, blood washes and nasal cleansing. The second part incorporates fomentations or herbal packs. The third part, used if these two fail, includes MOXIBUSTION, ACUPUNCTURE or bloodletting.[3]

Tibetan medicine is strongly influenced by Buddhist philosophy and has a psychological/emotional component to each of the humors. Imbalances in wind may result in desire, bile may create anger and phlegm may cause ignorance.

In Tibetan medicine, massage is used in the first line of treatment for general health as well as the third to treat specific conditions. The massage will also differ according to the body type of each individual (an Ayurvedic influence). For example, a wind individual requires heated oil, particularly on stress areas. Rubbing, kneading, acupressure and cleansing are primarily used for this body type. A bile person would benefit most from acupressure limited to a few specific points, and oil use should be sparse. For the phlegm body type, no oil or a light oil should be used with deep tissue massage, although the primary technique should be cleansing. The Tibetans have many systems of self-massage, which may include the use of herbal packs and remedies.

The time of day, season and even a medical horoscope based on the zodiac sign can tell when the treatment would be most salubrious, according to body constitution.

Notes
[1] Connelly, Marc, "Tibetan Massage with Dr. Lobsang Rapgay," *Massage,* Issue No. 25, May/June 1990, p. 62.

[2] Ibid., p. 61.
[3] Ibid., pp. 60–61.

Further Reading

Rapgay, Lobsang, Dr., *Tibetan Therapeutic Massage,* Passage Press, Sandy, Utah, 1985. Written by the leading expert on Tibetan medicine, Dr. Rapgay is a fully ordained Tibetan Buddhist monk and a doctor of Tibetan medicine with a Ph.D. in Buddhistic psychology. This book describes the history, stages of Tibetan massage and the treatments best suited to the three different body constitutions.

tongue diagnosis   one of the methods of diagnosis, according to CHINESE MEDICINE. This ancient medical system maintains that internal health is mirrored in external appearance. Accordingly, doctors have five ways of evaluating a patient's health: looking, listening and smelling, asking and touching.

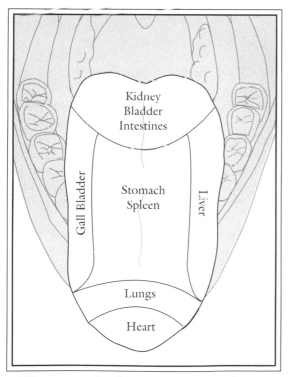

Different areas in the tongue correspond to specific organs. Practitioners use this ancient Chinese diagnostic tool to evaluate a person's physical condition.

The first, observation, is an evaluation of the patient's general appearance followed by a diagnosis of the tongue. There is a close relationship between the tongue and the **three heaters** (the upper heater, which relates to respiration, the middle heater, which relates to digestion and the lower heater, which relates to elimination), organs, QI, blood and fluids of the body.

Tongue diagnosis was used as early as the Shang dynasty (c. 16th century–11th century B.C.) and discussed in the *Huangdi Nei Jing* (The Yellow Emperor's Classic of Internal Medicine).[1]

The tongue and its coating are assessed according to the **Eight Principles of Differentiation.**[2] The tongue can reflect physical changes and be a guide to the effectiveness of treatment. (Tongue color can be affected by colored or spicy foods and smoking, which turns the coating yellow, therefore the practitioner should take these factors into consideration when making a diagnosis).

A healthy tongue has "spirit" or vitality, is a pale red, supple without cracks or ulcers and slightly moist. The coating should be thin and white.

The vitality of color, or tongue spirit, is examined first. A "tongue of death," or a dark and withered tongue, indicates a severe illness or impending death. The body of the tongue is examined next. This is the most important part of the inspection, reflecting the condition of the organs, blood and *qi*.[3]

The body shape is checked for its thickness, swelling, size, cracks and movement. The coating reflects the strength of pathogenic influences—the stronger the influence, the thicker the coating. Tongue moisture indicates the status of the body fluids and the balance of yin and yang.

In order to analyze the corresponding meridians, the tongue is divided into four sections. The tip is considered the **upper burner,** representing the HEART and LUNGS. The middle is the **middle burner,** representing the SPLEEN and STOMACH, while the middle sides represent the

LIVER and GALL BLADDER. The **lower burner** is located at the back of the tongue. Here, one can evaluate the health of the BLADDER, KIDNEYS, SMALL INTESTINE and LARGE INTESTINE.

A pale tongue indicates deficiency, coldness or insufficient *qi* and blood. An abnormally red tongue demonstrates the opposite—too much heat, or YANG, and a deficiency of YIN fluid.

A deep red tongue indicates severe fever or a prolonged illness where yin fluid is depleted. A tongue that appears to be purple or has purple spots, indicates stagnated *qi* and blood. A flabby tongue, larger than normal size, or one which is ridged on the edge from teeth marks, demonstrates a deficiency of *qi* energy. Cracked or ulcerated tongues are evidence of internal fluid loss through excessive heat (yang), loss of kidney or yin deficiency. A thorny tongue, where the papillary buds swell up, indicates excessive heat. A rigid tongue indicates excessive heat and damage to the liver.

The tongue's coating is usually white, but a thick white film may indicate cold digestive disorders. A thin yellow coating means that there is internal heat and dampness, while a dry yellow coating involves the stomach and intestines injured by heat. Grayish black coloration indicates extreme internal cold or heat due to long-term pathology. Sometimes the tongue may appear to have its coating peeled off, leaving a smooth, glossy tongue. This indicates a crisis of a long-term illness and injury to yin.

Tongue diagnosis is a valuable tool in determining a person's overall health and locating the source of any physical problems.

Notes
1 Maciocia, Giovanni, *Tongue Diagnosis in Chinese Medicine,* Eastland Press, Seattle, 1987, p. 1.
2 Ibid., p. 23. The Eight Principles of Differentiation provides a system that differentiates the origin and development of a disease. They are: exterior/interior, hot/cold, excess/deficiency and yin/yang.
3 The yin organs are the kidneys, spleen, liver, heart constrictor (pericardium), lung and heart.

Further Reading
Maciocio, Giovanni, *Tongue Diagnosis in Chinese Medicine,* Eastland Press, Seattle, 1987. This detailed description of tongue diagnosis is clearly illustrated and explained and is considered to be the most comprehensive text on the subject.

toning   See SOUND HEALING.

Touch For Health®   a self-help system of muscle testing, based on Dr. George Goodheart's, D.C. system of APPLIED KINESIOLOGY, which balances and strengthens weak muscles and promotes energy flow to related organs and glands.

Dr. John Thie, D.C. met Dr. Goodheart in 1964 and became extremely impressed with his discovery of how testing muscles and stimulating specific reflex points on them could strengthen and correct weaknesses. Although originally intended as a diagnostic tool for chiropractors, Thie felt that the basic idea of muscle testing was simple enough to be used by lay people. He wrote a manual for his patients, *Touch For Health* (1973), which became very popular. This system can be self-administered or used with other modalities, the latter being more effective.

There are several ways a Touch For Health practitioner examines the body in order to analyze the problems or dysfunctions. The symptoms a person exhibits can be very revealing. Posture can indicate deviations from normal body position, often the first sign of a problem or the result of years of compensation. In addition, PULSE READING, the Chinese diagnostic technique, is often used by Touch For Health practitioners. Imbalances in the MERIDIAN SYSTEM can be exposed from this examination.

Muscle testing is the cornerstone of Touch For Health. The examination determines the strength of the muscle being tested and the results help to indicate where on the body the work needs to be done. A weak muscle often mirrors weaknesses in related organs or glands, even before symptoms manifest. Relief to the weak muscle provides relief to the affected organ.

Muscle-testing procedures take into account the personal aspects of the individual being tested, such as age and relative strength. Testing positions are designed to isolate the muscle from its group with which it normally functions. Since muscles don't work alone, singling one out is a true test of its strength. It is important to test only the first few inches of its range of action, applying and releasing the pressure gradually. In this way, the muscle will either be strong, and be able to resist the opposing pressure of the tester, or fail completely. It is, therefore, important for the practitioner to learn to feel the difference within the first few inches of testing (the range of muscle action). Sometimes a repeated test is necessary to validate the results.

Testing muscles indicates the area of needed work. It is also a part of the treatment itself by directing the body's energies where to go. Retesting a muscle checks the effectiveness of the treatment and realigns the body to a more normal position.

Once the testing has revealed where the weaknesses are, there are many methods of treatment in Touch For Health. One strengthening technique is working on the **origins** and **insertions** of the muscles, or where they attach to other structures at both ends. For example, the insertion (the attachment to the bone it moves) and several places along the origin (the fixed attachment) are gently held. The ends of the muscle are pulled together, with a slight contraction, all over the muscle. Upon retesting, the muscle should be stronger.

Neurovascular holding points, found mainly on the head, require light contact with the pads of the fingers gently stretching the skin. A pulse should be felt a few seconds after contact is made. Once the pulse is felt with both hands, and has become synchronized, the neurovascular points can be held from a few seconds to 10 minutes, depending upon the need. Blood circulation to the muscle and its organ relation seems to improve after stimulation to these points.

Neurolymphatic massage points regulate the energy to the LYMPHATIC SYSTEM. These reflex points, found mostly on the back and chest, act like switches, which turn off when the system is overloaded. They are usually tender to the touch and those which are the sorest require the most amount of work. The deep massage on these points should last 20 to 30 seconds. Once the reflexes have been turned back on, lymph flow will return to the muscle and organ.

ACUPRESSURE is another technique used in Touch For Health to strengthen and balance weakened muscles. Acupressure holding points are used on the same side as the weakness. Arm and leg points are held first, for about 30 seconds or until a pulse is felt. Tracing a meridian, or an energy pathway, is also used to strengthen muscles.

Finally, an **adjustment,** or realignment, of the cranial bones, a technique reserved for doctors, affects the flow of cerebrospinal fluid. In Touch For Health, lay people can release the skull by placing fingertips along the middle skull seam and pulling the (parietal) bones apart. (This technique is also helpful for strengthening the abdominal muscles.)

Choosing which method, or combinations, of treatment to use depends upon each individual's circumstances.

The muscle/organ relationship of Touch For Health is the same as those of applied kinesiology.

Muscle	Organ
Abdominals	Small Intestine
Adductors	Sex
Anterior Deltoid	Gallbladder
Coracobrachialis	Lungs
Deltoids	Lungs
Gastrocnemius	Adrenals
Gluteus Maximus	Sex
Gluteus Medius	Sex
Gracilis	Adrenal
Hamstrings	Large Intestine
Latissimus Dorsi	Pancreas
Levator Scapulae	Stomach
Neck Muscles	Sinuses
Pectoralis Major/ Clavicular Head	Stomach
Pectoralis Major/ Sternum	Liver

Muscle	Organ
Peroneus	Bladder
Piriformis	Sex
Popliteus	Gallbladder
Psoas	Kidney
Quadriceps	Small Intestine
Rhomboids	Liver
Sacrospinalis	Bladder
Sartorius	Adrenal
Serratus Anterior	Lungs
Soleus	Adrenal
Subscapularis	Heart
Supraspinatus	Brain
Tensor Fascia Lata	Large Intestine
Teres Major	Spine
Teres Minor	Thyroid
Tibialis Anterior	Bladder
Trapezius	Spleen
Triceps	Pancreas
Upper Trapezius	Eyes and Ears

Touch For Health may also be applied to test for nutritional deficiencies, allergies and emotional strain.

Further Reading

Thie, John F., D.C., with Marks, Mary, *Touch For Health*, DeVorss & Co., Publishers, Marina Del Ray, Calif., 1973. Written by the originator of the system, this easy-to-follow book has detailed explanations of the technique accompanied by clear photographs illustrating treatment methods.

Trager® or **Tragerwork**, also known as Trager Psychophysical Integration, is an innovative approach to learning and teaching movement reeducation and neuromuscular release. It combines gentle bodywork with a sequence of dancelike movements called **Mentastics®**. The bodywork serves to communicate a quality of lightness to the nervous system, eliciting a similar tissue response. When a body feels lighter, the posture and movements are lighter.[1] The bodywork is a way to reach the unconscious mind, where unhealthy patterns are stored.

Trager was developed over 60 years ago by Dr. Milton Trager, M.D. (b. 1908). He devel-

oped his system almost by accident. As a young man, Trager was a professional boxer. One day, when he was 18 years old, he offered to work on his trainer, who had given him daily rub downs. The trainer was duly impressed with Trager's touch and told him so. Trager went home that day and treated his father, who was suffering from sciatica. After only two sessions, his father's pain was gone. This prompted the young man to pursue, expand and refine his skill.

When he left boxing, he practiced his work while he earned a living as a dancer and acrobat. At the age of 19, he successfully treated his first polio victim, a 16-year-old boy who had been paralyzed for over four years. For the next eight years, Trager worked almost exclusively with people suffering from debilitating illnesses.

In 1941, Trager received his doctorate of physical medicine from the Los Angeles College of Drugless Physicians. After serving in the physical therapy department of the navy during World War II, Trager sought to become a doctor. All the American schools he applied to refused him admission, claiming that, at age 42, he was too old. He was eventually admitted to the University Autonoma de Guadalajara in Mexico, where he worked extensively with victims of polio.

He graduated in 1955 and moved to Hawaii, where he remained for the next 18 years. In 1975, Dr. Trager received an invitation to demonstrate his work at the Esalen Institute, Big Sur, California. This appearance brought wide recognition to Tragerwork.

In 1980, he cofounded The Trager Institute with Betty Fuller, M.A., in Mill Valley, California.

Trager believes that clients should approach the work as if they were learning a lesson, rather than receiving a treatment. The work concentrates on using motion within the muscles and joints to produce pleasurable sensory feelings, so that the feedback loop between the body and mind triggers tissue changes. Each time the feeling is recalled, the change becomes deeper and more permanent.[2]

Trager Psychophysical Integration sessions last from one hour to one and a half hours. Clients lie on a well-padded table, in a comfortable environment, wearing bathing suits or underwear. Lubrication is not used for the bodywork.

A unique component of Trager work is how it is performed. The practitioner works in a peaceful state of consciousness, called **hook-up.** Within this meditative state, practitioners maintain a deep connection with the client, work more efficiently without fatigue and are constantly aware of their client's responses.[3] Trager calls hook-up "like basking in a vast ocean of pleasantness . . . as in meditation, one connects with the energy force that surrounds all living things."[4]

Trager purports that it is the hook-up that creates the results. Mental blocks, which cause physical tensions, are removed within this tranquil state.

The practitioner contacts the client's body with a light touch. Intrusive deep work is never performed, since Trager believes that invasive work makes people tighten up. The bodywork consists of three levels: **mobilization, relaxation** and **movement reeducation.**

A series of rhythmic, gentle movements, similar to general mobilization, or range of motion, provides manual cervical (neck) and lumbar (lower back) traction. The bodywork is profoundly relaxing. The client's body is rocked, which allows for the release of physical and mental tensions. The movements also provide reeducation to the body.[5]

The three levels of bodywork, combined within the session, provide the means for neurophysiological changes. Clients report feeling less pain, a reintegration of their body and a stronger connection of the mind within the body.[6]

After the table work is completed, the client is given instructions in Mentastics. This is a series of effortless movements developed by Dr. Trager to maintain the sensations of flexibility and lightness that were felt during the table work. Trager calls them "mental gymnastics" or "a mindfulness in motion."[7]

Practitioners are certified by The Trager Institute in Mill Valley. The course takes a minimum of six months to complete and is made up of a six-day beginning training, a five-day intermediate training and a six-day anatomy and physiology training. Students must document at least 60 Trager sessions without charge and receive at least 20 sessions. In addition, evaluation tutorials with trained practitioners are required before certification is awarded.

Notes
1 Juhan Deane, "The Trager Approach: A Comprehensive Introduction," Trager Institute, Mill Valley, Calif., 1993, p. 1.
2 Ibid., p. 1.
3 Ibid., p. 1.
4 Leviton, Richard, "Moving with Milton Trager," *East West Journal,* January 1988, p. 3.
5 Witt, Phil, "Trager Psychophysical Integration," *Whirlpool,* Summer 1986, p. 5.
6 Ibid., p. 6.
7 Juhan, Deane, "The Trager Approach: A Comprehensive Approach," Trager Institute, Mill Valley, Calif., 1993, p. 1.

Further Reading
Trager, Milton, M.D., and Hammand, Cathy, Ph.D., *Trager Movement as a Way to Agelessness: A Guide to Trager Mentastics,* Station Hill Press, Barrytown, N.Y., 1989. The movements in this book provide a way to move with grace, freely and energetically. This movement series may also offer pain relief and preventive care.

transpersonal bodywork and psychology are syntheses of energy-based bodywork techniques and psychospiritual counseling which recognize non-ordinary states of consciousness.[1]

Transpersonal bodywork combines energy work, LAYING ON OF HANDS, somatic psychology, AURA and CHAKRA BALANCING and clairsentience to harmonize the body/mind connection and release blocked emotions. This system recognizes and works with body memories, psychic scanning and various types of touch to free the client's energy flow.

Transpersonal psychology is the validation and acceptance of non-ordinary states of consciousness and how they can be applied in the healing journey. It is a combination of HOLOTROPIC and INTEGRATIVE BREATHWORK, a discipline that integrates modern science with great spiritual traditions, BIOENERGETICS, to facilitate recognition and release of blocked emotions and GESTALT THERAPY, a holistic organismic therapy that utilizes body awareness, breath, imagery and the power of the "here and now" to bring awareness, expression of feeling and release of locked memories.

Joanne Rossi, director of the Center For Transpersonal Body/Mind Studies, has traveled to many Third World countries in Central America and the Caribbean to study and live among indigenous healers/shamans and share a cross-cultural perspective on healing. Rossi maintains that much of our awareness and connection of our own energetic life force has been lost due to the disembodiment of a highly technological society.

The healers and shamans with whom she worked believed strongly in the existence and power of an invisible world, a world that can be accessed through non-ordinary states of consciousness. The work of Dr. Stanislav Grof (Holotropic Breathwork) and Jacquelyn Small (Eupsychia), both leaders in the field of transpersonal psychology, shares congruent beliefs with the shamans: that most people have lost their rootedness and connection to themselves.

Transpersonal bodywork and psychology seeks to reconnect individuals with their "beingness" through body/mind energy work.

Note
[1] Non-ordinary states of consciousness are often accessed during shamanistic rites/rituals of indigenous healers. According to transpersonal bodywork and psychology, this level of awareness can be attained and experienced through focused breathing, select rhythmic music and energy based bodywork.

Trauma Touch Therapy™ a bodywork system specifically designed to meet the needs of clients with trauma or abuse histories. This innovative work allows clients to discover "the gift" within the wound, encouraging empowerment and choice, which promotes safe access to their physical issues. The work is very individualized and almost always done in conjunction with the psychotherapeutic process.

Clients of Trauma Touch Therapy deal with many different trauma issues, such as physical/emotional/mental/sexual abuse; holocaust and postwar traumas; environmental traumas; surgical, injury and accident traumas; childhood traumas; and posttraumatic stress disorder, a serious result of any number of possible stress factors. Conservative estimates reveal that one out of three women and one out of six men have been victims of child molestation, rape or incest before their 18th birthday.[1]

Therapists of this system support their clients in discovering the power of conscious touch and transforming negative experiences into positive growth experiences. A strong partnership of trust and appreciation develops between client and therapist, which honors the innate wisdom of the body.

Many survivors of trauma/abuse find it equally difficult to relax during a MASSAGE and to communicate their fears about being touched. Since the late 1980s, massage therapists have been making a strong, affirmative impact on those men and women seeking a positive experience of touch in a safe environment. Massage therapy has had considerable success because it is nonthreatening, nonabusive, respectful and supportive.

The benefits of this work are numerous. Clients feel more alive with heightened physical sensations and are willing to accept appropriate touch. Symptoms are alleviated and improved sleeping patterns develop. Emotionally, clients learn to trust and can enjoy better quality relationships accompanied by an enhanced ability to experience joy and pleasure. A greater sense of self-awareness and acceptance develops from this work.

Trauma Touch Therapy recognizes the importance of appropriate table side manner. The therapist must be able to set clear boundaries around safety and trust. Clients are asked to define the level of disrobing for themselves as well as the depth and areas of touch. Attention must be paid to the environment, including room lighting, temperature, odors and sounds. Therapists of Trauma Touch Therapy have an awareness that the power differential is inherent in the massage setting—the vulnerability of an unclothed, reclining client as compared to the clothed, standing therapist—which could set the stage for revictimization.

It is important for the therapist to be aware of his own feelings regarding sexuality and sexual abuse. He must explore if his feelings are being telegraphed and whether they are helpful or potentially harmful.

Telltale signs in a client's reaction to touch may indicate abuse. A therapist should always be on the lookout for clients who disassociate on the massage table. They may "space out," or go numb. If the latter should occur, it is important to discontinue the treatment and discuss their feelings with the therapist. A client may hold on to or stop breathing, potentially indicating fear. Breathing keeps us in our bodies, while holding it cuts us off from physical and emotional associations.

Trauma Touch Therapy is owned and operated by the Colorado School of Healing Arts and was codeveloped by Chris Smith and Roberta Gibson Thompson. Both instructors have trained extensively in the field of bodywork and trauma. Chris Smith is the director of education at the Colorado School of Healing Arts, and has been a Certified Massage Therapist since 1988. She has trained in HAKOMI INTEGRATIVE SOMATICS, and teaches massage, focusing on DEEP TISSUE and EMOTIONAL RELEASE WORK. Her background includes dance and movement, and she is currently studying the interface between psychotherapy, spirituality and bodywork.

Roberta Gibson Thompson is the former Director of CSHA, a CMT for 14 years and teaches massage, REFLEXOLOGY and energy work. Roberta is an author and poet, has written numerous published articles on the role of bodywork in recovery from trauma and is currently writing a book on the subject. Her background also includes the use of dolphin therapy for cancer patients.

The 100-hour certification program is offered at the school and is designed to familiarize and educate therapists in the particular needs and issues of the trauma/abuse survivor client.

Note
[1] Thompson, Roberta Gibson, with Smith, Chris, "Trauma Touch Therapy," Colorado School of Healing Arts, Lakewood, Colo., no date, p. 1.

Further Reading
Blume, Sue E., *Secret Survivors,* Wiley, N.Y., 1990. This book talks about the silence and reticence inherent in coming forward as a survivor of childhood abuse or incest.
Braddock, Carolyn, *Body Voices, the Power of Breath, Sound and Movement to Heal and Create New Boundaries,* Atrium Publications, Santa Rosa, Calif., 1995. With an understanding of how an individual can suppress the experience of childhood abuse or incest, this author offers healing methods to explore the pain and move beyond it.
Davis, Laura, and Bass, Ellen, *The Courage to Heal,* Harper-Collins, N.Y., 1990. This book talks about people who are willing to face the demons of their childhood, relive the traumatic experiences and move ahead with their lives in a rich manner.

trigger point therapy the use of various methods to relieve or eliminate **trigger points.** A trigger point is a hypersensitive area in the muscle, its tendon or in FASCIA, which can be palpated as a fibrous area. Usually, the trigger point is not in the area of pain, yet digital pressure over the trigger point will elicit pain in the referred area.[1]

Trauma is a common cause of trigger points, either by direct injury, excessive stretching or contraction. Once these sensitive regions form, repeated muscular stress or even a lesser degree will activate the pain in a reference zone.

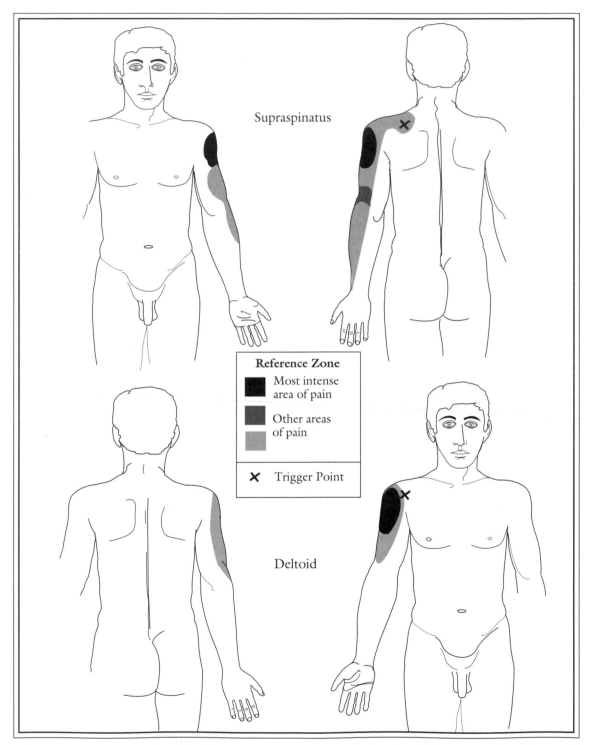

Trigger point charts, developed by Dr. Janet Travell, indicate the location of the trigger point, the muscle involved and the pattern of referred pain. The *X*s show the location of the trigger point and the shaded area indicates the pain pattern in these shoulder and arm muscles.

The person most often associated with trigger point therapy is Dr. Janet Travell (1901–?). She described trigger points as ". . . a small, hypersensitive region from which impulses bombard the central nervous system and give rise to **referred** pain."[2] Although the pain is not necessarily located in the **dermatome** of the muscle, there is a consistent pattern, which led Dr. Travell to develop trigger point charts that indicate the location of the trigger point, the muscle involved and the referred pain pattern. These charts have become the primary method used to diagnose trigger points and their referred pain.

The pattern of pain is called the **reference zone** and the trigger point may be located within that area, although it is usually either on the edge of or removed from the pain site.[3]

It is possible to have more than one trigger point associated with a particular condition. One point is generally the major one, while **satellite** involvements are more difficult to ascertain. A search-and-find approach is used to locate these other trigger points.[4]

Dr. Janet Travell graduated from Wellesley College in 1922 and entered Cornell University Medical College, graduating in 1926 with the Polk Memorial Prize for the highest scholastic class standing.

She is credited with the innovative work on trigger points, but is perhaps best known for being John F. Kennedy's physician when he was a senator and president.

Her work with trigger points began in 1939 when she injured her right shoulder and applied self-massage techniques to relieve the pain. She reproduced the pain previously felt in her arm, and she realized that this referred pain was directly related to the point she was massaging— the trigger point.

Dr. Travell is credited with developing the SPRAY AND STRETCH technique, wherein trigger points are injected with procaine or a coolant spray, while the related muscle is passively stretched.

Finger pressure, such as ACUPRESSURE, can also be effective in relieving trigger points. Five to seven seconds of direct pressure usually sedates the point and reduces pain in the referred area. Once the point is eliminated, massage can be applied to remove the waste products and restore circulation to the area.

Trigger point therapy is used by medical doctors, massage therapists, physical therapists and chiropractors to treat musculoskeletal problems and certain internal organ pain, such as trigger point therapy to the abdominal wall. BONNIE PRUDDEN MYOTHERAPY™ is a technique of trigger point therapy, which employs direct finger, knuckle or elbow pressure to the trigger point.

Trigger point therapy should be carefully applied when treating internal organs, since the possibility of a visceral pathology may be present.[5]

Notes
[1] Walther, David S., D.C., *Applied Kinesiology Volume I— Basic Procedures and Muscle Testing*, SDC Systems, Pueblo, Colo., 1981, p. 173.
[2] Ibid., p. 171.
[3] Ibid., p. 171.
[4] Ibid., p. 172.
[5] Ibid., p. 180.

triple heater (triple warmer) a bilateral, supplemental YANG MERIDIAN. It serves as a complementary function of the SMALL INTESTINE. It also controls the spirit and environment of the visceral organs by circulating energy to the entire body. This pathway protects the function of the LYMPHATIC SYSTEM and is linked to the immune system. The triple heater is a thermal regulator based on water metabolism and is often thought of as the organ of the CONNECTIVE TISSUE.

It begins at the outside tip of the ring finger and runs up the arm to the outer edge of the eyebrow, on the temple. There are 23 ACUPUNCTURE points along this energy pathway.

tsubo is the term given to the treatment and diagnosis points of Japanese SHIATSU. *Tsubos* are found along the energy pathways, called MERIDIANS, and are treated with finger, hand, elbow or foot pressure in a similar fashion to the needling techniques of Chinese ACUPUNCTURE.

Tsubos are normally sensitive to the touch, but hypersensitivity may indicate CHI energy stagnation in that region or related organ. The *tsubos* on one meridian are connected to related areas of the body, but energy has a greater tendency to stagnate in some points more than others.

They are named according to their location on a particular meridian or body part, such as triple heater 14, *ken ryo* ("top of the shoulder") or according to their function or organ relationship, such as heart constrictor 8, **ro kyo,** which means "palace of anxiety" and is used to treat nervous tension and insomnia.

tsubo point therapy   the use of the invisible, vital points called *tsubos,* found on the surface of the body along the MERIDIANS (energy pathways), for therapeutic purposes. Many physical problems can be relieved by pressing, rubbing, massaging, using ACUPUNCTURE or MOXIBUSTION on these points. Each *tsubo* has a specific relationship with a particular body part, so stimulation to the point releases energy blockages, promoting the free flow of healing energy to that region.

There are approximately 365 *tsubos* in the body.[1] The meridians are created as a result of the organization of *tsubos* along these pathways. According to Oriental medical theory, all diseases and their symptoms are created by problems in the circulation of KI-(*qi*) **ketsu,** vital energy. The *tsubos* are the places where the energy gets stuck. If they are manipulated, the energy is released and the symptoms may be alleviated.

In locating a *tsubo* for the treatment of a specific symptom, the cause of the condition is a primary consideration. For example, a headache point may not be very effective if the cause stems from LARGE INTESTINE dysfunction and the *tsubo* treatment point is on the LIVER meridian.

The easiest way to treat a *tsubo* is with the use of one's fingers, although acupuncture and moxibustion are quite effective. There are four techniques used in *tsubo* point therapy: **rubbing**
and stroking, general massage, localized massage,** and **pressure.**

Rubbing and stroking uses the **amma** method, considered to be one of the therapeutic techniques of CHINESE MEDICINE. *An* means "press," which effectively sedates over stimulated muscles and nerves. *Ma,* or "rubbing," normalizes functional integrity of body systems. In order to perform the rubbing, one palm is placed against a point with a moderate amount of pressure.

In the general massage, the whole palm or fingers draw small circles and knead the muscles along the meridians.

Localized massage removes tension around the *tsubo* and the hand pressure stays steady.

Pressure, either SHIATSU or ACUPRESSURE, is the *an* portion of *amma*. These manipulative techniques use the fingers or whole palm with gradually increasing point pressure. Each point is pressed for three to five seconds.[2]

Finding the exact *tsubo* takes practice to develop sensitivity. There are three ways to locate these treatment points: lightly rubbing the skin, pinching the skin while moving it back and forth or gently pressing the skin with the thumb or fingers.[3]

Notes
[1] Serizawa, Katsusuke, *Effective Tsubo Therapy: Simple and Natural Relief without Drugs,* Japan Publications, Inc., Tokyo, 1984, p. 19.
[2] Ibid., pp. 23–24.
[3] Serizawa, Katsusuke, *Tsubo: Vital Points for Oriental Therapy,* Japan Publications, Inc., Tokyo, 1976, p. 41.

Further Reading
Serizawa, Katsusuke, *Tsubo: Vital Points for Oriental Therapy,* Japan Publications, Inc., Tokyo, 1976. This clearly illustrated book demonstrates where the *tsubos* are found and what physical problems they treat. The chapters are divided into overview, general treatments and specific treatments.
———— , *Effective Tsubo Therapy: Simple and Natural Relief without Drugs,* Japan Publications, Inc., 1984. This book concentrates on locating treatment points by each of the 14 regular meridians. Part two is divided according to symptoms.

tui-na   an ancient Chinese system of massage/ bodywork. Legend has it that China's first physician, Pien Jue, used tui-na in the spring and autumn of 500 B.C. References were made to it as early as 300 B.C., in the *Huangdi Nei Jing* (The Yellow Emperor's Classic of Internal Medicine). By A.D. 591, a department of massage had been established at the Imperial College of Medicine.

Tui, which means "to push," and *na,* which means "to grasp," is an integral part of Chinese medicine, along with ACUPUNCTURE, MOXIBUSTION, herbal medicine and QIGONG. Traditionally, *tui-na* was passed down from one generation to the next as a beneficial form of self-healing. Today, it is taught in all traditional medical schools in the People's Republic of China. In the hospitals, massage is often used in conjunction with herbal compresses and osseous manipulations and is as popular as acupuncture or herbal medicine.

There are a variety of styles and specific manipulations within *tui-na,* which came down from different medical lineages or traditions. Throughout history, five major remedial schools of Chinese therapeutic massage are recognized.

The **one-finger school** uses one finger to stimulate acupuncture points along the MERIDIANS. Force is concentrated through the tip of the thumb. This system, which is still practiced in medical *tui-na,* is effective in the treatment of internal and gynecological problems.

The **rolling school** came out of the one-finger school. This method covers larger body surfaces and is used to treat soft tissue symptoms.

Flat-pushing method is a combination of *nei kung* exercises and a massage treatment where QI energy is channeled to the client.

POINTING MASSAGE is a form of acupressure that is used as a first aid, in emergencies and in the treatment of pain.

Bonesetting is made up of eight forms of manipulations: joining, holding, lifting, pushing, pinching, pressing, rubbing and feeling and is mainly used in orthopedic wards.[1]

Tui-na is used to treat injuries to the soft tissues, internal disorder, joint and CONNECTIVE TISSUE diseases and to balance the flow of *qi* (life's vital force) energy.

According to Chinese medicine, disease is the result of impeded *qi* energy flow. This vital energy courses through the body within the meridians. Along these energy pathways are specific acupuncture points that relate to specific organs or glands. The aim of *tui-na* is to harmonize the flow of YIN/YANG energy and improve the functioning of related organ systems.

Tui-na uses a variety of hand techniques, such as grasping, rolling, pressing, rubbing, vibrating, pushing, squeezing, twisting, and tapping and dragging. It is a gentle but vigorous treatment, usually lasting for 20 to 30 minutes. The practitioner can use his fingers, thumb surfaces, knuckles, palms and elbows in order to stimulate the acupoints, affect the meridians and treat the soft tissue.

One major technique is the rolling method, which rolls the back side of the hand side to side in hundreds of fast repetitions over a problem area. This stroke can also be employed along a limb or the entire torso.

Tui-na is used to treat many ailments, among them: injuries, back and neck pain, headaches, high blood pressure, menstrual irregularities, asthma, hay fever, arthritis and sore throats.

Tui-na is the only massage system that has a separate and totally different pediatric massage system. It was developed during the Tang dynasty (A.D. 600–900). Pediatric *tui-na* is gentler than the adult version and treats acupoints that are located in places other than where adult points are found. Pediatric *tui-na* is primarily used to treat childhood illnesses.

Note
[1] Wolfe, Honora Lee, "China," *Massage and Bodywork Magazine,* Vol. 1, Issue 4, 1986, pp. 25–26.

Further Reading
Changye, Luan, *Concise Tuina Therapy,* Foreign Language Press, Beijing, 1994. This book is divided into five parts. Part one contains a brief discussion of the benefits of *tui-na.* Part two discusses fundamental maneuvers. Part three is about the principles of *tui-na.* Part four describes

routine manipulations on parts of the body. The final part offers specific treatments for 43 conditions.

Chengnan, Sun, ed., *Chinese Bodywork: Complete Manual of Therapeutic Massage,* Pacific View Press, Berkeley, Calif., 1993. Based on the teachings of the Shangdong school, this book incorporates the use of *tui-na* to treat disease.

Flaws, Bob, *Turtle Tail and Other Tender Mercies,* Blue Poppy, Boulder, Colo., 1984. An English primer on pediatric *tui-na.*

Lew, Share K., and Helm, Bill, *Tui Na: Chinese Healing and Acupressure Massage.* This illustrated book clearly describes the *tui-na* massage technique.

U

ultrasound therapy is a deep heat therapy that is generally used in conjunction with CHIRO-PRACTIC, OSTEOPATHY or PHYSICAL THERAPY treatments. These sound waves, which are inaudible to human hearing, generate heat and can relieve edema (swelling of the extremities), increase metabolism, provide immediate relief from pain through localized anesthesia and offer a deeply penetrating micromassage.

The apparatus is made up of a generator, which provides a high frequency current, and an applicator, also called the sound head. The electrical oscillations produced by the generator cause the transducer in the applicator to vibrate and create sound waves.

Ultrasound radiations cannot pass through the air, so close contact must be established between the applicator and the body. In order to create a tight bond, the skin is covered with oil or water over the area of treatment. When using water as a medium of contact, the body part and applicator are usually submerged.

As the sound waves pass through the body, some of the motion is transformed into a uniform heating pattern, called **volume heating.** When these waves are impeded by certain physical structures, the localized heating is called **structural heating.** The effective beaming characteristics of ultrasound radiation produce better localized heating than most other forms of heat energy.

Treatments usually start for 5 minutes and progress to 10 minutes on localized areas. A series of ultrasound treatments is considered to be up to 12 sessions. It has been used to treat bursitis (inflammation of the bursas—the sac or pouch in connective tissue usually found around joints), fibrositis (inflammation of the white fibrous CON-NECTIVE TISSUE anywhere in the body), herpes zoster (an acute, inflammatory and infectious disease of the skin), myalgia (muscle pain), joint pain, Raynaud's disease (a vascular disorder causing constriction in circulation to the extrem-

ities), TRIGGER POINTS, sprains, strains and varicose ulcers.

Ultrasound therapy is contraindicated in cases of acute infection, on malignant lesions, near pacemakers, over bony prominences, over reproductive organs, over the eye, on the brain, on the heart or nerve plexi or near hearing aids. Extreme caution must be exercised when treating any inflammatory conditions.

ultraviolet radiation is the part of the electromagnetic spectrum which falls between visible light and X rays used for therapeutic purposes. Ultraviolet rays, which are absorbed by the skin, produce chemical reactions. (Conversely, INFRARED RADIATION produces a reaction of heat.)

There are three types of ultraviolet lamps: **hot quartz, cold quartz** and **sun lamps.** The hot quartz lamps are further subdivided into a **mercury,** or **high vapor lamp,** which is the most common type used in treatment. It produces a bluish glow and is placed 15 to 30 inches from the body, and the treatments can last for a few seconds to several minutes.

The **kromage** lamp, the other hot quartz ultraviolet source, is a water-cooled lamp used solely for local radiation. It can be put in contact with the body or can be used to radiate into the interior of the body, such as the nose, throat or mouth. The duration of treatment is extremely short, 2 to 10 seconds, depending upon the proximity of the source.

The cold quartz lamp stays relatively cool throughout the treatment. It is placed near the body and is used primarily as a bactericide.

Sun maps are either **fluorescent** or **reflector** lamps. Both can produce localized skin reddening, or **hyperemia,** within a few minutes. Tanning salons use modified sun lamps.

Since ultraviolet rays produce chemical reactions and are absorbed by the skin, the reactions occur at skin level. There is an increased blood supply (hyperemia) to the area, an irrigation and destruction of cells, capillaries and arterioles dilate and cellular fluid passes into the tissues. **Erythema,** or reddening of the skin, usually occurs as a delayed reaction to exposure, but that can be altered by a strong dose of rays.

Ultraviolet rays create a reaction in the skin where vitamin D is formed. The body's resistance to infection is increased because ultraviolet rays stimulate production of antibodies. Ultraviolet rays also produce a general tonic effect, which improves appetite, promotes sleep and minimizes irritability. (Airports are using ultraviolet radiation as a way to reduce the effects of jet lag.)

There are certain sensitizers that increase the effectiveness of ultraviolet radiation: coal tar ointment and a prior exposure to infrared radiation. Certain drugs and food can unintentionally enhance the effects of ultraviolet radiation. Clients should be cautioned against the excessive erythematic reactions of the following: gold, when used as a rheumatoid arthritis treatment, insulin, quinine, tetracycline and thyroid medicines. Strawberries, eggs and lobsters also increase ultraviolet reaction.

Ultraviolet radiation is contraindicated in cases of hypersensitive skin, when a client is taking the aforementioned drugs, wherever an X ray or X ray therapy has been recently performed, lung tuberculosis, severe sunburns, hyperthyroidism, diabetes, acute eczema or other dermatitis, lupus erythematosus or severe cardiac, pulmonary, hepatic or renal pathologies.

Ultraviolet treatments should be given with a medical prescription. The lamp is heated for at least five minutes prior to use, and the direction of the rays is 90°. The skin is cleaned and only the area to be treated is exposed. Both client and operator should wear protective eye goggles.

UNTIE® developed in the United States in the early 1980s as an alternative to exerting force into soft tissue, which may already be painful to the touch. UNTIE emphasizes that pain and limitation of movement are frequently caused by imbalances in the musculoskeletal system. It combines comprehensive soft tissue evaluation with a specialized method of light manual pressure to normalize the soft tissues (muscles, tendons, ligaments and FASCIA) and restore balance to the musculoskeletal system, in accordance with the individual needs of the patient.

It is basic to UNTIE, that soft tissue dysfunction, no matter how deep within the body, can be felt in the skin. These **patterns** of dysfunction are palpable once the proper awareness and sensitivity have been developed.

Patterns are like snowflakes, no two are identical. A pattern is an infinitely variable expression of a specific soft tissue dysfunction and it is synergistically related to the dysfunction. The physiological mechanism by which patterns appear in connection with dysfunction is yet unclear. Although we know that the skin and the central nervous system develop from the same embryological layer and are thus intimately connected, the multidimensional aspect of this dynamic connection has still not received scientific attention. Yet the skilled practitioner can readily access dysfunction in even the deepest layers of soft tissue, by working with the patterns that are associated with the dysfunction.

Initially, a three-stage evaluation is used to objectively determine soft tissue imbalances. Special attention is paid to the interplay between overt signs and underlying causes. Once the imbalances have been determined and the patterns are identified through palpation, they are released by precisely applied, sensitive movements of the practitioner's fingertips along the surface of the skin. The movements of the fingers are coordinated with the changes in the patterns, without any application of force, will or preconceived routine. The fingers move in perfect concert with the patterns, gently, slowly, flowing.

Pressure is regulated so that the force of the practitioner's fingertips into the skin is slightly less than the resistance of the skin against the fingertips. With the use of a small amount of lotion, this pressure allows the fingers to move along the surface of the skin in a friction-free manner, increasing sensitivity to the changes that take place in the patterns. Changes in the patterns are stimulated by the presence of the practitioner's fingers and determined by the body's natural desire to reach HOMEOSTASIS. Once the patterns release, the soft tissues are reevaluated to confirm that they have normalized in response to the manipulations.

Although other approaches may not specifically address soft tissue patterns, the patterns are affected, since there is contact with the skin when the soft tissues are manipulated. The more thorough the method used, the more likely it is that the pattern will be released. Because the foundation of UNTIE is sensitivity, it readily deals with the unique patterns of the individual. It is a procedure for working "with" the body—not "on" the body.

V

vibration one of the basic strokes of SWEDISH MASSAGE. It can be performed with the flat of the palms or with the fingertips. It can be a stationary stroke to treat a specific muscle, or executed in a "running" manner, such as down the spine, for general stimulation.

Vibration acts directly upon the nerve trunks stimulating peripheral nerves and all nerve centers with which the trunk is connected. When applied to the nerve trunk, vibration is a valuable stroke in the treatment of neuralgia (sharp pain running the course of a nerve), neurasthenia (a sense of weakness or exhaustion) and most disorders of diminished nerve impulse. Deep vibration acts on deep organs and nerves. When applied along the spinal column, vibration is used to treat sclerosis (hardening) and other degenerative conditions of the spinal cord.

Vibration to the extremities relieves coldness from spasms of small vessels due to vasomotor disturbances, numbness, tingling, etc., and it can help relieve pain. It produces reflex effects, which include muscular action, vascular and glandular activity and general tissue change.

Strong and rapid vibration will cause tetanic contractions (hypertonic) of a muscle. Normal tetanus requires impulses to be received at the rate of 10 to 20 per second. In order for vibration to be effective in creating muscle contraction, the rate of impulse must be faster. Mechanical vibrators are often substituted to produce such results.

Vibration is instrumental in breaking down spasms and hard, resistant areas. It can help treat insomnia when it is applied to the spine for more than 10 seconds. In nonacute inflammatory conditions, vibration promotes the absorption of the by-products and waste materials. When applied to the colon, vibration increases its peristaltic action (wavelike movement during excretion).

Vibration for 1 to 10 seconds produces a stimulating effect, while longer application becomes sedating and relaxing.

vibrational healing encompasses the use of energy systems for therapeutic purposes. These systems may include CHAKRA BALANCING, POLARITY THERAPY, AROMATHERAPY, MERIDIAN THERAPY, AURA BALANCING, MAGNETIC THERAPY, CRYSTAL HEALING, THERAPEUTIC TOUCH, PSYCHIC HEALING and VIBRATIONAL HEALING MASSAGE THERAPY.

It is generally believed that the body is surrounded by an energy field (the HUMAN ENERGY BIO-FIELD) made up of several layers or bodies. These bodies interpenetrate and surround each other in successive layers. Each succeeding layer vibrates at a higher frequency than the body it surrounds.

Illness and disease is caused by an imbalance or deficiency in the rate of vibration in any of the layers. Vibrational healing, employing any of the energy bodywork systems, seeks to realign the human energy field, promote the free flow of energy and restore health.

Further Reading

Davidson, John, *Subtle Energy,* Beekman Publications, Woodstock, N.Y., 1987. Higher levels of energy and their roles in nature, healing and illness are discussed. Vibrational science, polarity balancing therapies, earth energies, auras and biomagnetic healing are also described.

Gerber, Richard, *Vibrational Medicine,* Bear & Co., Santa Fe, N.Mex., 1988. This textbook provides an extensive exploration into energy-healing systems, including homeopathy, flower essences, crystals, therapeutic touch, acupuncture, electrotherapy, psychic healing, herbs and therapeutic radiology.

McNamara, Rita J., *Toward Balance: Psychophysical Integration and Vibrational Therapy,* Weiser, York Beach, Me., 1989. Using radiesthesia to detect electrochemical imbalances in the chakras, the appropriate polarity treatment, aromatherapy, homeopathic remedies and meridian therapy for each chakra is provided. Meridian therapy is stressed as a powerful way to align postural imbalances and emotional blocks.

Vibrational Healing Massage Therapy™ a form of bodywork that moves the emotions and works the body deeply, yet gently. It allows for the release of patterns, behaviors and recurring pains and illnesses that have kept people stuck in unhealthy conditions and situations.

This work includes educating individuals in the **Fluid Model®**, a new way to think about the body as a living process rather than a solid thing. Incorporating the Fluid Model in one's life promotes health, flow and ease in the body as well as in all daily activities.

Unlike traditional SWEDISH MASSAGE, clients may be clothed during a session. There is no need for oils or lotions unless the practitioner and client choose to combine Vibrational Healing Massage Therapy with another type of massage. Sessions can last anywhere from 10 minutes, as a first-aid treatment or for stress relief, to a full-body massage lasting 60 to 90 minutes. The work can be received in many ways: with the client in a chair, on the floor, on a massage table and even outdoors.

Specific skills and techniques are designed to restore communication and orchestrate the release of shock waves and tensions in the body. **Stretches** are made up of decompression (traction)/compression, rhythm, repetition and holds, and are used to open up and lengthen the joint areas. **Shakes** are comprised of very small and large movements to unlock stored vibrational waves throughout the whole volume of the body. **Push-pulls** are performed using opposing hand positions from joint to joint, or one area to another, to create relationship and connectedness. **Rebounding** is joint work that allows the joints to reconnect themselves and become more relaxed, flexible and spacious. To really encourage the vibrational flow, shakes are often used inside stretches, push-pulls and rebounds.

Rocking and rolling can be subtle or large to relax and soften the whole body. **Lifts** employ leverage to the client's arms or legs to free deep pelvic or shoulder tensions. **Kneading** is especially good for ribs, joints and vertebrae. **Squeezing, pinching, twisting** and **milking** are used on the limbs, while **rotating** is applied to the joints. All techniques are performed with the intention of encouraging flow and freeing energy

that has been stopped. The reverberations and emanations from these releases are profound and transformational. It is like playing the human body as the fine-tuned instrument it is.

Vibrational Healing Massage Therapy has been in development since 1981 by Patricia Cramer, the founder of the World School of Massage and Advanced Healing Arts in San Francisco, California. She created this system after four years of private study with Pierre Pannetier in POLARITY THERAPY. This work goes beyond the notion of balance within the polarity principles into arenas of profound sensing of vibrational awareness and expansion.

This system recognizes that almost all of the 206 bones of the body are flexible with movement at the joints. The body is, therefore, a moving, fluid process, alive and flowing from moment to moment. The goal of this work is to teach people to experience and live within the Fluid Model. When a body is fluid, vibration occurs naturally throughout the organism and the energy can flow freely. This system offers clients access to others' authentic feelings. The work allows for clearing and freeing the body/mind/spirit, so the individual can receive and feel in a new manner.

Vibrational Healing Massage Therapy also brings forth the **Language of Healing®**, teaching that the body feels and responds to every word that a person says or thinks. In order to enhance healing, a new language of harmony must be learned. Phrasing words According to the desired behavior or result allows an individual's mind to imagine a new way of behaving. For example, instead of saying I have a "bad knee," one could say "my knee has room to release here." This new awareness and use of body communication creates access for true holistic healing.

This system combines well with other forms of massage and bodywork, and brings quick and simple restoration to the natural flows of the body, releasing innate healing capacities.

Aspects of Vibrational Healing Massage Therapy can also be performed by nonprofessionals. Families and children as young as seven years old can master the techniques.

A new form of the work that is becoming popular is what is called **"New Dance."** New Dance is really teamwork, dance and touch, all combined to create a fun and healthy experience for the participants. Two or more people "work" on a person who is on a massage table, while they are actually dancing with each other. Principles of rhythm, repetition, synchronicity and play are part of the techniques. People receiving get the benefits of several people working on them at one time and really let go into relaxation. The "workers" have the pleasure of touching, healing, playing, teamwork, dancing and enjoying a fun, new recreation.

Visceral Manipulation   a hands-on therapy that works that the interconnected synchronicity between the motions of the visceral (abdominal cavity) organs and other structures of the body.

When the body undergoes stress, the skeletal (voluntary) muscles, as well as the involuntary muscles associated with the viscera, respond by developing abnormal tone and becoming fixed. In addition, the membranes that support the various organs are also affected. These CONNECTIVE TISSUE may dry up and adhere (stick together).

When the organs cannot move in harmony with the neighboring viscera, their functions are impeded, often resulting in distress.

The Visceral Manipulation technique consists of manual adjustments that promote normal mobility and inherent tissue motion of the viscera and their connective tissues. Since these tissues is extremely delicate, small, precise and direct force is used for maximum results. Practitioners work with a balanced pulse in each organ (similar to the pulsation of CRANIOSACRAL TECHNIQUE) or sometimes with more direct techniques.

Visceral Manipulation courses at the Upledger Institute, Palm Springs Gardens, Florida, were developed by Jean Pierre Barral, R.P.T., D.O. Barral bases his treatment method on the theory that each internal organ rotates on a physiological axis. The program has been expanded by Frank Lowen, a protege of Dr. Barral.

Further Reading

Barral, Jean Pierre, R.P.T., D.O., *Visceral Manipulation I, II.* Eastland Press, Seattle, 1989. These texts detail the theories and techniques of Visceral Manipulation.

———— , *Urinogenital Manipulations,* Eastland Press, Seattle, 1992. Manipulations of the internal organs in the urinogenital area are explained.

———— , *The Thorax,* Eastland Press, Seattle, 1993. The author and developer of Visceral Manipulation discusses the organs and structure of the thoracic region and how to free constricted organ movement.

———— , *Manual Thermal Diagnosis,* Eastland Press, Seattle, 1995. Using sensitive hand techniques, the author explains how to palpate the body for heat differences and what they might mean.

visualization   See GUIDED IMAGERY.

Dr. Vodder's manual lymph drainage

See LYMPHATIC DRAINAGE MASSAGE.

W

Wassertanzen a HYDROTHERAPY technique performed underwater in a heated pool. It is done in conjunction with WATSU and was developed in Switzerland by Arjana C. Brunschwiler and Aman P. Schroter in 1987. This advanced system combines Watsu, akido, baby rocking, massage, dolphin movements and dance.

The client is stretched, twisted and bent while in motion underwater. The sequences are done rhythmically above and below the surface of the water. Deep meditation, relaxation and trances may occur during a Wassertanzen session. Old traumas may be released in this nurturing environment.

Watsu® or water SHIATSU, is a system that employs the stretches of ZEN SHIATSU in a pool of warm water.[1] The pool provides a deeply relaxing environment where weight and pressures are removed from the body. The client is floated and rocked as the spine is gently pulled and stretched, following the precepts of Zen shiatsu.

Aquatic bodywork was developed by Harold Dull, the Director of the Harbin Hot Springs in Middletown, California. He discovered that the effects of the stretches, which include stronger muscles and increased flexibility and joint RANGE OF MOTION, were amplified when performed in a pool. Physical therapists corroborated these findings since they too often work with physically challenged and rehabilitating patients in water.

Freeing the spine is the focus at the onset of each Watsu session. The weightlessness of the body in water provides expanded stretching and flexibility while it opens the energy pathways. Zen shiatsu's principle of continuous support takes on a new dimension while the client is being floated and rocked in the water.[2]

The sessions can affect people on all levels. The **water breath dance** helps clients connect with their breath and very often with their emotions. In this basic move, the client is floated in the practitioner's arms and sinks a bit as they both exhale. On the inhalation, they both rise. The water breath dance is repeated at the beginning and throughout each session to create a connection which can be carried into the stretches that follow.

The **flows** of Watsu are the way one movement extends into another and creates a sense of continuity.

TANTSU (Tantric Shiatsu) coordinates stretching and rocking while the CHAKRAS and ACUPUNCTURE points are held. This system was also developed by Dull to re-create Watsu's nurturing flow on land. Clients are cradled and supported while put through a series of movements.

WASSERTANZEN is a form of hydrotherapy done by guiding a client underwater. It was developed in Switzerland by Arjana C. Brunschwiler and Aman P. Schroter in 1987. It is an advanced technique that combines Watsu, akido, baby rocking, massage, dolphin movements and dance.

The client is stretched, twisted and bent while in motion. The sequences, which are done above and below the surface of the water, are performed rhythmically, depending on breathing capacity. Deep relaxation, meditation and trances may occur. It is a powerful tool in releasing old traumas.

The Watsu pool has many varying depths in which to work. In a pool with only one depth, the best condition is a depth of about four feet. The larger the pool, the more space there is to move and turn. The Watsu pool is 10 feet in diameter and holds four feet of water, almost 4,000 gallons. The ideal temperature for the water is the same as the body's skin temperature, 94°F. In an outdoor setting, if the air is cold, the water temperature can be slightly warmer, but no more than the body's internal temperature,

98.6°F. Replenishing body fluids is very important when working in water, so it is advisable to drink copious amounts of water.

Although Watsu is ideal for people of all ages and physical abilities, there are some contraindications. Watsu should be avoided with fevers over 100°F, uncontrolled epilepsy, cardiac failure, significant open wounds, respiratory disease of vital capacity of less than 1500 cm, severe urinary tract infection, respiratory tract infection or blood infection, tracheotomy, bowel incontinence, menstruation without internal protection and infectious diseases. Necessary precautions must be taken in case of skin infections, small open wounds, uncontrolled blood pressure, unstable cardiac rhythms, multiple sclerosis (depends upon the client), chlorine sensitivity, vertigo or vestibular disorders and inappropriate behavior.

Range of motion precautions include hip replacements, recent spinal surgery, acute ligamentous instability, recent bone fracture, arthritic cervical (neck) spine, herniated vertebral disks, fibromylagia and frequent ear infections.[3]

Individual differences must be considered in order to provide an appropriate treatment. The client's size, flexibility, buoyancy and holding are all taken into account when designing the best course of treatment.

Watsu begins with the client standing with her back against the wall of the pool. Her right arm is placed behind the practitioner's back and her neck is gently placed in the crook of the practitioner's left elbow. The right hand is placed on the client's heart chakra where it stays for a few breaths. The practitioner's left knee is lifted under her hips, floating her away from the wall, his right hand lifting her up at the base of her spine.

Watsu continues with basic moves interspersed with the **transition flow,** a graceful shift from position to position. Joints are stretched and put through their range of motion. At the conclusion of the session, the client is returned to the wall where the neck is slowly released.

One hand is placed on her heart chakra and the other on the third eye and crown chakra. The practitioner's hands are quietly lifted, as he backs away, his hands now in a prayer position, honoring the client, the space between them and the work.

Notes
[1] These stretches, dating back at least to the development of acupuncture, release blockages along the meridians, or energy pathways.
[2] The "mother" hand always stays in place while the other hand, the "son" or "wanderer," moves over the body.
[3] Dull, Harold, *Watsu: Freeing the Body in Water,* Harbin Springs Publications, Middletown, Calif., 1993, p. 90.

Further Reading
Dull, Harold, *Introduction to Watsu—Freeing the Body in Water,* Harbin Springs Publications, Middletown, Calif., 1993. This easy-to-follow, photographed guide clearly describes the Watsu technique and its contraindications.

Wengrow's Synergy a respectful, balanced and progressive bodywork system that realigns the body in gravity, along its natural vertical axis. The state of one's MYOFASCIAL/structural balance or imbalance also reflects one's emotional state. Wengrow's Synergy respects these aspects of a person in a way that enhances their interplay. This system also recognizes the importance of individual volition and involvement in the healing process.

This system consists of 10 sessions that are intended to result in greater sense of well-being, better posture, less tension, long-term pain relief, more energy, increased creativity and greater physical and emotional flexibility.

Wengrow's Synergy is reported to be a minimally uncomfortable structural/neuromuscular bodywork, since vital to its bodywork philosophy is the recognition that effective bodywork depends upon a partnership relationship between client and practitioner. To this end, practitioners use techniques that encourage the client's participation in their healing process.

Developed by Florida massage therapist Vicki Wengrow, Wengrow's Synergy is an outgrowth of SOMA NEUROMUSCULAR INTEGRATION and ROLFING. The work proceeds from the surface of the body toward deeper levels. It moves from the relief of specific, local areas of contraction and displacement in the first seven sessions to the reorganization of the relationship between major segments of the body in the last three.

The work varies in its effects on people. Many individuals undergo a spontaneous **integration** process for at least a year after their sessions are completed, as their improved balance manifests itself throughout the body, especially if a conscious effort is made to replace old habits with healthier choices.

Y

The yin/yang theory one of the theories of CHINESE MEDICINE that explains relationships, patterns and the processes of natural change in the universe.[1] It is based on the construct of polar opposites, or complements, called yin and yang.

This theory regards all things as part of the whole. As such, nothing can exist on its own. Yin and yang, therefore, contain the possibility of opposite and change. Harmony between these elements represents optimum health, while an imbalance results in disease.

Yin represents the female, short, soft, controlling, passive, dark, cold, winter, the moon, downwardness, inwardness, nonverbal and emotional. The Chinese character for yin originally meant "shady side of the slope."

Yang, or "the sunny side of the slope," represents the male, tall, hard, aggressive, active, light, hot, summer, the sun, upwardness, outwardness, verbal and logical.[2]

Chinese medical tradition further expanded on this concept of duality by developing the five principles of yin and yang. The first principle explains that all things in the universe have a yin aspect and a yang aspect, which exist in relation to each other. For instance, time is divided into night and day; species are male or female; up has its opposite in down, and vice versa; temperatures are either hot or cold, etc.

The front of the body is considered to be yin, while the back is yang; the upper part is more yang as the lower half is more yin. External physical features (i.e., skin, hair) are more yang than the internal organs, which are more yin. Illnesses may also be categorized as either yang or yin. Those illnesses that manifest in symptoms of weakness, slowness, coldness and underactivity are yin. Yang illnesses are described as forceful, hot and overactive.

Secondly, any yin or yang aspect can be further divided into yin and yang. In other words, each category also contains within it, another yin and yang designation. This phenomenon divides infinitely. Relatively speaking, heat, for example, is yang, but can be divided into boiling (yang) or tepid (yin).

The third principle recognizes that the opposite aspects of yin and yang create each other and depend upon each other for definition. When speaking of a 24 hour period, for example, it cannot be defined without regards to day or night, A.M. or P.M.

The fourth principle recognizes that yin and yang control and balance each other. For instance, an aggressive nature may attract a passive one.

Finally, yin and yang transform each other, which is the source of all change. These changes can be balanced and harmonious, as in the change of seasons, or abrupt and unbalanced, such as a break-up of a relationship.[3]

Another theory of Chinese Medicine, the **Eight Principle Patterns of Differentiation,** enables a physician to ascertain and differentiate a patient's symptoms. This principle is made up of four pairs of opposites, although yin/yang are the dominant forces because of their total nature: yin/yang; interior/exterior; deficiency/excess; and cold/hot.

The MERIDIAN system of Chinese medicine, or energy pathways, are involved in moving QI and blood and regulating yin and yang. It is composed of 12 regular meridians, six yin and six yang.

The ancient Taoists believed that change and transformation are the only constants in the universe, and that yin and yang, which produce each other, actually are each other.[4]

Notes
[1] Another system of categorizing is the five element theory. According to this concept, all things in nature, including the human being, can be classified according to either wood, fire, earth, metal or water and all of their inherent relationships.

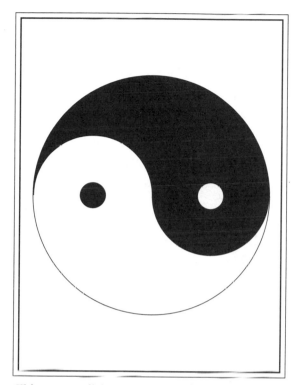

Chinese medicine explains the relationships, rhythms and patterns of natural change in the universe according to the yin/yang theory. These symbols depict the continuing flow of opposing characteristics, each unable to exist without the other.

[2] Kaptchuk, Ted J., O.M.D., *The Web That Has No Weaver,* Congdon and Weed, N.Y., 1983, p. 8.

[3] Ibid., pp. 8–12.

[4] Ibid., p. 139.

Further Reading

Connelly, Dianne M., *All Sickness Is Home Sickness,* Center for Traditional Acupuncture, Columbia, Md., 1987. This book offers a clear discussion of Chinese medicine, yin and yang, Chinese and Taoist philosophies and explanations of their complex theories. The author has written a concise, easy-to-use guide on an intricate subject.

Kaptchuk, Ted J., O.M.D., *The Web That Has No Weaver,* Congdon and Weed, N.Y., 1983. This book is considered by many to be one of the finest explanations of Chinese medicine and its complex theories. Illustrates depict the meridian system and the relationships of yin/yang, the five elements and Eight Principles of Differentiation. All other theories are clearly described.

yoga an ancient Indian Vedic philosophy and exercise system, which promotes physical/emotional/mental/spiritual balance and growth. Yoga developed in India almost 5,000 years ago. The word comes from Sanskrit, meaning to "yoke" or "join together," and the overall goal is to join the human soul with the universal energy. Yoga science has two aspects—physical and spiritual.[1]

The first written account of yoga was found in the *Yoga Sutras,* partially credited to an Indian physician and Sanskrit scholar named Patanjali. Legend says that he went into the mountains to meditate and came back with a vision of yoga.

In addition to the yoga postures, or *asanas,* to maintain health, yoga emphasizes the importance of PRANA (life's vital energy) and *pranayama,* breathing exercises. According to the yogis and practitioners of yoga, breathing is the physical manifestation of life's vital energy. The postures should always be practiced with deep, diaphragmatic breathing.

Another element of yoga is MEDITATION. This tranquil state alleviates stress, lowers blood pressure and often provides an opportunity for introspection and possibly, enlightenment.

There are many different forms of yoga, which modify mental activity, control breathing and realize God, but perhaps the most popular form is **hatha yoga.** *Ha* means "sun," while *that* translates to "moon." Hatha yoga emphasizes postures and movements, along with deep breathing, for the purpose of stretching, toning and general health. One of the most important teachings in yoga philosophy is the proper care of the body under the intelligent control of the mind.[2]

Yoga is divided into four forms, which seek to gain enlightenment, or realization of the **Brahman,** the absolute. **Karma yoga** is the path of action, which removes impurities of the mind through righteous living and service. **Bhakti yoga** is the path of devotion and love, which develops the heart. **Raja yoga** is the science of mental mastery through meditation. It is further

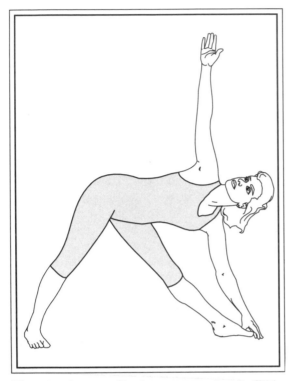

The triangle pose of hatha yoga stretches the limbs and the spine. The asanas, or postures, of hatha yoga emphasize deep breathing, stretching, toning, flexibility and promote general health.

subdivided into **mantra yoga, Kundalini yoga** and **hatha yoga. Inana yoga** is the path of knowledge, which brings awareness and intellect.

These different paths of yoga are merely various ways for an individual to reach the highest level. They are not mutually exclusive—one form may be the primary yoga practice, while an additional form may hasten the progress.

Traditionally, there are eight parts in yogic culture:

Yama, is ethics
Niyama are religious observances
Asanas are the postures of hatha yoga
Pranayama are breathing exercises
Pratyahara is the withdrawal of sense from objects

Dharana is concentration
Dhyana is meditation
Samadhi refers to superconsciousness, or enlightenment.[3]

Kriya yoga emphasizes the cleansing and purification of the body, including the respiratory system, mouth, esophagus, stomach, eyes and intestines. Exercises and internal washings help in the purification process.

Hatha yoga, or the practice of postures, emphasizes increased circulation and intake of oxygen. Yogic exercises concentrate on the flexibility of the spinal column and other joints. According to the *Yoga Sutras,* there are over 840,000 *asanas,* or postures. Out of those, fewer than 100 are traditionally practiced.[4] These *asanas* can be further divided into meditative poses, including the **lotus pose** (*padmasan—*crossed leg pose), *siddhasan* (adept's pose), *swastikasan* (ankle lock pose) and *sukasan* (easy pose) and cultural postures. The meditative poses are important during breathing exercises and meditation.

A session of yoga, which can last from as little as 15 minutes to several hours, generally begins and ends with the **corpse pose**—*savasan,* laying on the back, eye closed, palms up, legs open. This pose is designed to center the body and bring awareness to the breathing.

The **sun exercises,** or *soorya namaskar,* is designed to increase spinal flexibility, correct breathing and increase circulation. It is a 12-position exercise, which should be repeated 12 times daily.

All *asanas* promote a steady flow of *prana* throughout the body.

Notes
[1] Vishnudevananda, Swami, *The Complete Illustrated Book of Yoga,* Pollet Books, N.Y., 1972, p. 19.
[2] Ibid., pp. 12–13.
[3] Ibid., p. 69.
[4] Ibid., p. 69.

Further Reading
Hittleman, Richard, *Yoga for Health,* Ballantine Books, N.Y., 1985. This book provides a health program based

on basic hatha yoga postures, nutrition, recipes, meditation and philosophy. Introductions for each posture include its benefits and author's comments.

Iyengar, B.K.S., *Light on Yoga,* Schocke, N.Y., 1994. With over 600 photographs, this popular book provides information on hatha yoga postures and breathing exercises.

Samskriti, and Veda, *Hatha Yoga Manual I,* Himalayan International Institute of Yoga, Honesdale, Pa., 1977. This popular manual clearly explains the postures of hatha yoga. There are 80 photographs.

Samskriti, and Franks, Judith, *Hatha Yoga, Manual II,* Himalayan Institute of Yoga, Honesdale, Pa., 1978. This advanced sequel to the first manual includes meditative postures, breathing exercises, *bundhas* (locks), *mudras* (seals) and cleansing exercises. There are 80 photographs in this book.

Silva, Mira, and Mehta, Shyam, *Yoga the Iyengar Way,* Knopf, N.Y., 1990. With over 100 basic posture illustrations, this concise book provides information on hatha yoga, breathing exercises, philosophy, meditation, sample lessons and programs for select problems.

Vishnudevananda, Swami, *The Complete Illustrated Book of Yoga,* Pollet Books, N.Y., 1972. A complete yoga program, including 146 photographs of yoga *asanas,* are provided in this book. Diet, breathing, cleansing and philosophy are also discussed.

Z

Zen shiatsu is a form of SHIATSU, the ancient Japanese ACUPRESSURE massage system, based on treating the MERIDIAN SYSTEM rather than select acu-points, or TSUBOS.

This system was developed by Shizuto Masunaga. Masunaga's mother was one of the first students of Tamai Tempaku, who revitalized shiatsu in Japan during the early 1900s. Masunaga began his own study of shiatsu after graduating from Kyoto University with a degree in psychology.

After studying shiatsu for 10 years, Masunaga began to cultivate his own theories based on the energetic structure of the human body. Zen shiatsu is a fusion of ancient theories and personal exploration.

Masunaga's work concentrates on balancing the *ki* (life's vital energy) flow throughout the meridian system. He is credited with developing an extended set of meridians particular to his style, as well as an intricate system of abdominal and back diagnosis.[1]

Note
[1] Dubitsky, Carl, O.B.T., L.M.T., "History of Shiatsu/Amma," *Massage Therapy Journal*, 1992, p. 3.

Further Reading
Masunaga, Shizuto, *Zen Imagery Exercises: Meridian Exercises for Wholesome Living*, Japan Publications, N.Y., 1987. Masunaga describes the meridian theory and functions and the principles and importance of proper breathing. Exercises combined with imagery are given to stimulate and tone specific meridians. *Qi* energy circulation exercises are also provided.
————, *Zen Shiatsu*, Japan Publications, Tokyo, 1977. This book describes advanced clinical and technological explanations of Zen shiatsu. It is a very thorough, illustrated text.

Zero Balancing® a hands-on system that unifies the Western theories of anatomy and structure with Eastern theories of energy. The goal of the work is to balance these two concepts and promote physical, emotional, mental and spiritual health. Zero Balancing is the dynamic result of the merging of body and mind, where structure and energy meet.

Zero Balancing recognizes three energy levels within the body: the **vertical life flow, internal energy flow** and the **background energy field.**

The VERTICAL ENERGY FLOW connects us to nature. In this energy level, the skeletal system is regarded as the center. Three energy pathways connect vertically with the skeletal system, enabling the practitioner to work with energy and structure as a cohesive unit. The **main,** or **central** channel, flows through the skull, down the midline of the body and ends in the feet. The main central flow conducts the strongest energy currents. This is the aspect of the skeletal system that is the most grounded, vertical and the major integrating flow. It is also referred to as the **universal life flow.**

The **second vertical channel** flows through the shoulders to the transverse processes of the vertebrae and reconnects with the main channel in the pelvis. The **third vertical channel** flows through the shoulders and out to the arms.

The internal energy flows are within the body and allow us to function as an individual ecosystem. These channels are affected by the act of walking and the voluntary muscle movements within the body and are further subdivided into three levels: **deep, middle** and **superficial.** In the **deepest** level, the act of walking creates an uninterrupted, three-dimensional figure-8 pattern. This energy integrates the whole person. The **middle** level, which involves the SOFT TISSUES of the body, corresponds to the 14 regular MERIDIANS of Chinese medicine and the internal organs of structural anatomy. The last, and most **superficial** level of internal energy flow, lies just under the skin and is given the Chinese name *wei chi.* This is an insular layer of vibration, which buffers us from external influences.

The background field is a formless, vibratory energy, which penetrates inward and expands outward. This field is sensitive to the stimuli of the moment, responds to emotions and allows us to take life's changes in stride.

Dr. Fritz Frederick Smith, osteopath (1955) medical doctor (1961), acupuncturist and fellow in the Chinese College of Acupuncture, Rolfer and yoga student, came from a family of health practitioners. During the 1970s, he developed his theory of Zero Balancing, a fusion of Eastern and Western healing theories, named after an early client who claimed to be "zero balanced" after a treatment.

The work of Zero Balancing is specifically done on the **foundation and semifoundation joints** and on tissues of the body that are holding blocked energy.[1] The session moves sequentially from the lower portion of the body to the upper. Zero Balancing uses the principle of fulcrums to effect changes in the tissues and is directed at the interface between energy and structure. Specifically, the practitioner creates a fulcrum, or balancing point, through the use of gentle pressure and stationary holding, which gives the client time to orient, release and balance around the point. As the client responds to the fulcrum, he or she may enter a **working state,** indicating that changes are taking place. The practitioner often observes the person's subtle **working signs,** which include changes of the breath pattern, involuntary eyelid and eyeball movements and muscular releases.

The client remains clothed during the half-hour session. With the alignment of the musculoskeletal system, many symptoms of muscle pain, joint immobility and outlet syndromes disappear. With the release of tissue-held vibration, emotional and psychological tensions are freed along with a lessening of the signs of stress. With the clearing of energy fields, a sense of clarity, vibrancy and enhanced well-being ensue.

Note

[1] Lauterstein, David, "What Is Zero Balancing?," *Massage Therapy Journal,* Vol. 33, No. 1, Winter 1994. There are specific articulations in the body, known as **foundation joints** and **semifoundation joints,** which are primarily involved in balance, absorption and conduction of energy in the body, and which are characterized by small ranges of motion. These joints are considered to be of prime energetic significance. They include: the sacroiliac joint (the juncture of the sacrum and ilium), intervertebral joints (between the vertebrae of the spine), costovertebral (rib and vertebrae articulations) and intratarsal (foot) and intracarpal (hand) joints.

Further Reading

Smith, Frederick, Dr., M.D., *Inner Bridges: A Guide to Energy, Movement and Body Structure,* Humanics New Age, Atlanta, Ga., 1986. Dr. Smith combines the Eastern concepts of QI energy, acupuncture channels and chakras with Western theories of anatomy and physiology to create an energy system for bodyworkers. This book is a comprehensive overview of energy systems and their applications.

zone therapy the basis of FOOT and HAND REFLEXOLOGY, the science of balancing the body by stimulating specific points on the extremities.

In 1913, Dr. William Fitzgerald of Hartford, Connecticut, observed that pressure on specific areas of the body produced an anesthetic effect in a corresponding part. This interrelationship is the basis of zone therapy.

Dr. Fitzgerald had many colleagues who were proponents of his theory, including Dr. Joseph Shelby Riley who wrote *Zone Therapy Simplified* in 1919.

Advances were made in the zone therapy theory in the 1930s by one of Dr. Riley's assistants, Eunice Ingham. She has been credited with developing the more refined system of foot reflexology.

In zone therapy, the body is divided into 10 equal longitudinal zones, five on each side, from the top of the head to the tips of each toe. Each finger and toe fall into one zone (i.e. the right thumb is in the same zone as the right big toe).

An exception are the big toes. In addition to representing specific zones, they each correspond to half of the head and the four smaller toes. The smaller toes represent the head and the neck region in finer terms.

Reflex points, which run throughout the zones, pass through the body within the same zones. Any tension, blockage or congestion in any part of the zone will affect the entire zone, from top to bottom. To relieve the congestion, direct pressure on any part of the zone will affect

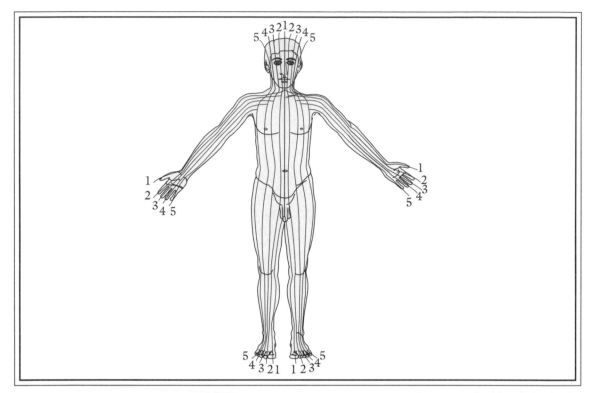

In zone therapy, the body is divided into 10 equal longitudinal zones, five on each side of the body. Reflex points, which run throughout the zones, pass through the body within the same zones. Direct pressure on any part of the zone will affect the entire zone.

that longitudinal line. Most commonly, however, points on the hands and feet are stimulated to elicit relief.

Manipulation on any injured or affected part should be avoided. Direct pressure on varicose veins, phlebitis (inflammation of a vein), limb or joint injuries is contraindicated. In zone therapy, alternate points along the same zone can be stimulated.

Referral areas are different parts of the body that relate to each other within the same zone. When an area must be avoided, referral areas can be used in its place. A tenderness will often be present in the referral area, indicating another equally effective area to work. For example, a broken right wrist, which cannot be worked on directly, can be reached by pressure on the referred area of the right ankle.

Zone therapy can be self-administered or performed by a practitioner. Daily self-treatments for 10 to 15 minutes on sensitive areas can relieve blockages along a zone and promote optimum health.

APPENDIX I
RESOURCE LIST

A Alpha Calm Therapy

Hal Brickman, C.S.W.
135 East 50 Street
New York, NY 10022
(800) 433-8622

Acupressure

Gautama Institute for the Oriental Healing
  Arts
1223 Rodman Street
Philadelphia, PA 19147
(215) 985-4466

Acupuncture

American Association of Acupuncture and
  Oriental Medicine
4101 Lake Boone Trail
Raleigh, NC 27607
(919) 787-5181

American Foundation of Traditional Chinese
  Medicine
1280 Columbus Avenue, Suite 302
San Francisco, CA 94133
(415) 776-0502

International Foundation of Oriental Medicine
42–62 Kissena Boulevard
Flushing, NY 11355
(718) 321-8642

National Acupuncture and Oriental Medicine
  Alliance
638 Prospect Avenue
Hartford, CT 06105-4298
(203) 586-7509   FAX (203) 586-7550

Pacific Institute of Oriental Medicine
915 Broadway, Third Floor
New York, NY 10010-7108
(212) 982-3456   FAX (212) 982-6514

Tri-State Institute of Traditional Chinese
  Acupuncture
80 Eighth Avenue
New York, NY 10011
(212) 242-2255

Alchemia Synergy

DoveStar Alchemian Institute
50 Whitehall Road
Hooksett, NH 03106-2104
(603) 669-9497   FAX (603) 625-1919

Alexander Technique

American Center for the Alexander Technique
129 West 67 Street
New York, NY 10023
(212) 799-0468

North American Society of the Teachers of
  Alexander Technique
PO Box 3992
Champaign, IL 61826
(217) 359-3529

AMMA Therapy

New Center for Wholistic Health
6801 Jericho Turnpike
Syosset, NY 11791-4465
(516) 364-0808

Applied Kinesiology

BioKinesiology Institute
5432 Highway 227
Trail, OR 97541
(503) 878-2080

International College of Applied Kinesiology,
  USA
PO Box 905
Lawrence, KS 66044
(913) 542-1801

Applied Physiology

International Institute of Applied Physiology
3014 East Michigan Street
Tucson, AZ 85714
(602) 889-3075

Appropriate Touch

Bob Yoder, L.M.T.
130 Mulberry Street, #8
New York, NY 10013
(212) 925-7824

Aromatherapy

American Society for Phytotherapy and
   Aromatherapy International
PO Box 3679
South Pasadena, CA 91031
(818) 457-1742

Aromatherapy Institute of Research
PO Box 2354
Fair Oaks, CA 95628
(916) 965-7546

Flower Essence Society
PO Box 459
Nevada City, CA 95959
(916) 265-9163   (800) 548-0075

National Association for Holistic
   Aromatherapy
PO Box 17622
Boulder, CO 80308-7622
(303) 444-0533

Pacific Institute of Aromatherapy
PO Box 606
San Raphael, CA 94915
(415) 459-3998

Aston-Patterning

Aston-Patterning
PO Box 3568
Incline Village, NV 89450
(702) 831-8228

Autogenic Training

International Committee for Autogenic
   Training
101 Harley Street
London, W1N 1DF
England

Avatar

Star's Edge International
237 North Westmonte Drive
Altamonte Springs, FL 32714
(407) 788-3090

Ayurvedic Medicine

Ayurvedic Institute
PO Box 23445
Albuquerque, NM 87192-1445
(505) 291-9698

Bartenieff Fundamentals

Laban/Bartenieff Institute of Movement
   Studies
11 East Fourth Street, Third Floor
New York, NY 10003
(212) 477-4299

Benjamin System of Muscular Therapy

Muscular Therapy Institute
122 Rindge Avenue
Cambridge, MA 01240
(617) 576-1300

Bioenergetics

Institute for Bioenergetics and Gestalt
1307 University Avenue
Berkeley, CA 94702
(415) 849-0101

Biofeedback

American Association of Biofeedback Clinicians
2424 Dempster
Des Plaines, IL 60016
(312) 827-0440

Association for Applied Psychophysiology and
   Biofeedback
10200 West 44 Avenue, Suite 304
Wheat Ridge, CO 80033
(303) 422-8436

Biofeedback Institute of Los Angeles
3710 South Robertson Boulevard, Suite 216
Culver City, CA 90232
(213) 933-9451

Biofeedback Therapist Training Institute
1826 University Boulevard West
Jacksonville, FL 32217
(904) 737-5821

Biofeedback Training Associates
Dr. Philip Brotman
255 West 98 Street
New York, NY 10025
(212) 222-5665

Body-Centered Transformation

The Hendricks Institute
409 East Bijou
Colorado Springs, CO 80903
(719) 632-0772   (800) 688-0772

Body-Enlightenment

Somantra Institute of Body-Enlightenment
Harbin Hot Springs
PO Box 570
Middletown, CA 95461
(707) 987-3801   FAX (707) 987-9638

Body-Mind Centering

The School for Body-Mind Centering
189 Pond View Drive
Amherst, MA 01002
(413) 256-8615   FAX (413) 256-8239

Bodymind Integration

11081 Missouri Avenue
West Los Angeles, CA 90025
(213) 473-5737

Body Mind Integrative Therapy

Somatic Therapy Institute
546 Harke Road, Suite B
Santa Fe, NM 87501
(505) 983-9695

Bodywork for the Childbearing Year

National Association of Pregnancy Massage
   Therapists
PO Box 81453
Atlanta, GA 30341

Somatic Learning Associates
Kate Jordan and Carole Osborne-Sheets
8950 Villa La Jolla Drive, Suite 2162
La Jolla, CA 92037
(619) 748-8827   FAX (619) 457-3615

Body Wraps

Doctor Wilkinson's Hot Springs
1507 Lincoln Avenue
Calistoga, CA 94515
(707) 942-4102

Life Force International
PO Box 1980
Spring Valley, CA 91979-1980
(619) 660-1270

Breath Therapy

Diamond Light School of Massage and
   Healing Arts
PO Box 5443
Mill Valley, CA 94942
(415) 454-6651

Breema

The Institute for Health Improvement
6076 Claremont Avenue
Oakland, CA 94618
(510) 428-0937

Barbara Brennan Healing Science

The Barbara Brennan School of Healing
PO Box 2005
Easthampton, NY 11937
(516) 329-0951   FAX (516) 324-9745

Cayce/Reilly Massage

Association for Research and Enlightenment
Edgar Cayce Foundation
PO Box 595
Virginia Beach, VA 23451
(804) 428-3588

A.R.E. Clinic
4018 North 40 Street
Phoenix, AZ 85018
(602) 955-0551

Chair Massage

Skilled Touch Institute of Chair Massage
584 Castro Street, Suite 555
San Francisco, CA 94114
(415) 621-6817   FAX (415) 621-1260

Chiropractic

American Chiropractic Association
1701 Clarendon Boulevard
Arlington, VA 22209

International Chiropractic Association
1110 North Glebe Road, Suite 1000
Arlington, VA 22201
(703) 528-5000

National Directory of Chiropractic
PO Box 10056
Olathe, KS 66051
(800) 888-7914

World Chiropractic Alliance
2950 North Dobson Road, Suite 1
Chandler, AZ 85224
(602) 786-9235 (800) 347-1011

Chua Ka

Arica Institute, Inc.
134 Elk Avenue
New Rochelle, NY 10804-4213
(914) 632-4895

Color Therapy

Dinshah Health Society
100 Dinshah Drive
Malaga, NJ 08328
(609) 692-4686

Constitutional Massage

Phoenix School of Holistic Health
6610 Harwin, Suite 256
Houston, TX 77036
(713) 974-5976   FAX (713) 266-6740

CORE Bodywork

Core Institute
School of Massage Therapy and Structural
   Bodywork
223 West Carolina Street
Tallahassee, FL 32301
(904) 222-8673

Core Energetics

Institute of Core Energetics
115 East 23 Street
New York, NY 10010
(212) 982-9637

CranioSacral Therapy

Colorado Cranial Institute
466 Marine Street
Boulder, CO 80302
(303) 447-2760

The Cranial Academy
1140 East Eighth Street
Meridian, ID 83642
(208) 888-1201

Upledger Institute
11211 Prosperity Farms Road
Palm Beach Gardens, FL 33410-3487
(407) 622-4334

Crystal Healing

Lifestream Associates
70 Sable Court
Winter Springs, FL 32708
(407) 699-1672

Cupping

Pacific Institute of Oriental Studies
915 Broadway
New York, NY 10010
(212) 982-3456   FAX (212) 982-6514

Tri-State School of Traditional Chinese
   Acupuncture
80 Eighth Avenue
New York, NY 10011
(212) 332-0787

Dance Injury Massage

Thomas McCracken, L.M.T.
148 Columbus Avenue
New York, NY 10023
(212) 799-1256

Dance Therapy

American Dance Therapy Association
2000 Century Plaza, Suite 108
Columbia, MD 21044
(410) 997-4040

Creative Arts Therapies
251 West 51 Street
New York, NY 10019
(212) 246-3113

Deep Massage

The Lauterstein-Conway Massage School
213 South Lamar, Suite 101
Austin, TX 78704
(512) 474-1852

Drama Therapy

Creative Arts Therapies
251 West 51 Street
New York, NY 10019
(212) 246-3113

National Association for Drama Therapy
19 Edwards Street
New Haven, CT 06511
(203) 498-1515

Ear Therapy

American Academy of Reflexology
606 East Magnolia Boulevard, Suite B
Burbank, CA 91501
(818) 841-7741

Pacific Institute of Oriental Studies
915 Broadway
New York, NY 10010
(212) 982-3456   FAX (212) 982-6514

Tri-State School of Traditional Chinese
   Acupuncture
80 Eighth Avenue
New York, NY 10011
(212) 332-0787

Egoscue Method

T.H.E. Clinic
2775 Via De La Valle
Del Mar, CA 92014
(619) 755-1075   (800) 995-8434

Embodyment Training

PO Box 1089
Great Barrington, MA 01230
(413) 528-1031

Emotional-Kinesthetic Psychotherapy

3 Central Avenue
Newton, MA 02160
(617) 332-7262   FAX (617) 965-7846

Emotional Release

Diamond Light School of Massage and
    Healing Arts
PO Box 5443
Mill Valley, CA 94942
(415) 454-6651

James Hyman
11255 SW 67 Avenue
Miami, FL 33156
(305) 926-6420   (800) 700-6420

Energy Bio-Field Work

The Barbara Brennan School of Healing
PO Box 2005
Easthampton, NY 11937
(516) 329-0951   FAX (516) 324-9745

Ericksonian Hypnotherapy

New York Training Institute for
    Neuro-Linguistic Programming
145 Sixth Avenue
New York, NY 10013
(212) 647-1660

Esalen Massage

Esalen Institute
Highway 1
Big Sur, CA 93920
(408) 667-3000

Etheric Release

DoveStar Alchemian Institute
50 Whitehall Road
Hooksett, NH 03106-2104
(603) 669-9497   FAX (603) 625-1919

Eye-Robics

Vision Training Institute
11303 Meadow View Road
El Cajon, CA 92020
(619) 440-5224

Fascial Kinetics

Dalby Massage Therapy Centre for Fascial
    Kinetics
7 New Street
PO Box 745
Dalby Q 4405, Australia
(076) 62-3702   FAX (076) 62-3656

Larry Loving
Seminar Network International
518 North Federal Highway
Lake Worth, FL 33460
(407) 582-5349   (800) 882-0903

Fascial Mobilization

Upledger Institute
1121 Prosperity Farms Road
Palm Beach Gardens, FL 33410-3487
(407) 622-4334

Feldenkrais Method

Feldenkrais Guild
PO Box 489
Albany, OR 97321-0143
(503) 926-0981

Five Element Shiatsu

Cindy Banker, B.A.
47 Jamaica Street
Jamaica Plains, MA 02130
(617) 522-0251   FAX (617) 522-7492

Robbee Fian
C.O.P.E. Acupuncture and Shiatsu Center
484 West 43 Street, Suite 29E
New York, NY 10036
(212) 564-5324

Focusing

Focusing Institute
29 South La Salle, Suite 1195
Chicago, IL 60603
(312) 629-0500

Joan Klagsbrun
173 Mt. Auburn Street
Watertown, MA 02172
(617) 924-8515

G-Jo Acupressure

G-Jo Institute
4950 SW 70 Avenue
Davie, FL 33314

Geriatric Massage

Day-Break Geriatric Massage Project
PO Box 1629
Guerneville, CA 95446
(707) 869-9628

Gestalt Therapy

Cynthia Cook
80 East 11 Street
New York, NY 10003
(212) 477-3225

Gestalt Center for Psychotherapy and Training
510 East 89 Street
New York, NY 10128
(212) 879-3669

Guided Imagery

Academy for Guided Imagery
PO Box 2070
Mill Valley, CA 94942
(800) 726-2070   FAX (415) 389-9342

American Imagery Association
4016 Third Avenue
San Diego, CA 92103-9814
(619) 298-7502

International Imagery Association
PO Box 1046
Bronx, NY 10471
(718) 423-9200

Haelan Work

Janet Quinn, Ph.D., R.N.
University of Colorado School of Nursing
4200 East Ninth Avenue
Denver, CO 80262
(303) 270-4271

Hakomi Integrative Somatics

Hakomi Institute
PO Box 1873
Boulder, CO 80306
(303) 443-6209

Hand Reflexology

American Academy of Reflexology
606 East Magnolia Boulevard, Suite B
Burbank, CA 91501
(818) 841-7741

American Reflexology Certification Board and
    Information Service
PO Box 246654
Sacramento, CA 95824
(916) 455-5381

Hanna Somatic Education

Novato Institute for Somatic Research and
    Training & Somatics Society
1516 Grant Avenue, Suite 212
Novato, CA 94945
(415) 892-0617

Hellerwork

406 Berry Street
Mt. Shasta, CA 96067
(916) 926-2500   (800) 392-3900

HEMME APPROACH

Spring Valley Lane
Route 2 Box 260A
Bonifay, FL 32425
(904) 547-9320

Hoffman Quadrinity Process

Hoffman Institute
223 San Anselmo Avenue, No. 4
San Anselmo, CA 94960
(415) 485-5220

Holotropic Breathwork

Grof Transpersonal Training
38 Miller Avenue, Suite 158
Mill Valley, CA 94941
(415) 721-9891

Hoshino Therapy

Hoshino Therapy Clinic of Miami, Inc.
814 Ponce de Leon, Suite 417
Miami, FL 33134
(305) 444-9984

Hypnotherapy

Academy of Scientific Hynoptherapy
PO Box 12041
San Diego, CA 92112
(619) 427-6225

American Association of Professional
    Hypnotherapists
PO Box 29
Boones Mill, VA 24065
(703) 334-3035

American Guild of Hypnotherapists
2200 Veterans Boulevard
New Orleans, LA 70062
(504) 468-3213

American Psychological Association
Division 30
750 First Street, NE
Washington, DC 20002-4242
(202) 336-5500

National Society of Hypnotherapists
2175 NW 86, Suite 6A
Des Moines, IA 50325
(515) 270-2280

Ice Therapy

Harold Packman, L.M.T.
PO Box 3
Whitestone, NY 11357
(718) 746-4669

Infant Massage

Infant Massage Northwest
PO Box 16374
10434 SE Lincoln Court
Portland, OR 97216
(503) 253-8482

International Association of Infant Massage
    Instructors
2350 Bowen Road
PO Box 438
Elma, NY 14059-0438
(716) 652-9789

Integrative Acupressure

The New England Institute for Integrative
    Acupressure
PO Box 496
Haydenville, MA 01039
(413) 268-0338

Integrative Eclectic Shiatsu

Nippon Shiatsu Daigaku
PO Box 34
Putney, VT 05346
(802) 387-5594

Integrative Psychotherapy

Joel Ziff
31 Jefferson Street
Newton, MA 02158
(617) 965-3932

Iridology

Bernard Jensen International
24360 Old Wagon Road
Escondido, CA 92027
(619) 749-2727

National Iridology Research Association
PO Box 33637
Seattle, WA 98133
(206) 363-5980

Jin Shin Acutouch

International Professional School of Bodywork
1366 Hornblend Street
San Diego, CA 92109
(619) 272-4142

Jin Shin Do

Jin Shin Do Foundation for Bodymind
  Acupressure
366 California Avenue, Suite 16
Palo Alto, CA 94306
(415) 328-1811

Jin Shin Jyutsu

Jin Shin Jyutsu, Inc.
8719 East San Alberto
Scottsdale, AZ 85258
(602) 998-9331

Johrei

Johrei Fellowship, National Headquarters
1971 West 190 Street, Suite 280
Torrance, CA 90504
(310) 523-3840

Johrei Fellowship
73 Spring Street, Suite 204
New York, NY 10012
(212) 343-1842

Ki-Shiatsu

Susan Krieger
306 West 18 Street
New York, NY 10011
(212) 242-4217   FAX (212) 242-0391

Kripalu Bodywork

Kripalu Center
PO Box 793
Lenox, MA 01240
(413) 448-3400

Kriya Massage

DoveStar Alchemian Institute
50 Whitehall Road
Hooksett, NH 03106-2104
(603) 669-9497

Laban Movement Analysis

Laban/Bartenieff Institute of Movement
  Studies
11 East 4 Street, Third Floor
New York, NY 10003
(212) 477-4299

Lomi Ka'Ala Hoku

Eolani Negri
42 West 72 Street, 9B
New York, NY 10023
(212) 580-4896

Lomilomi

Aunty Margaret School of Hawaiian Lomilomi
PO Box 221
Captain Cook, HI 96704
(808) 323-2416

Lymphatic Drainage Massage

Lymphedema Services
360 East 57 Street
New York, NY 10022
(212) 688-6107

National Lymphedema Network
2211 Post Street, Suite 404
San Francisco, CA 94115
(415) 921-3186

North American Vodder Association
Lymphatic Therapy
PO Box 861
Chesterland, OH 44026
(216) 729-3258

Macrobiotic Medicine

Kushi Institute of the Berkshires
PO Box 7
Becket, MA 01223
(413) 623-5741

Macrobiotic Shiatsu

International Macrobiotic Shiatsu Society
1122 M Street
Eureka, CA 95501-2442
(707) 445-2290

Magnetic Therapy

Albert Roy Davis Research Laboratory
PO Box 665
Green Cove Springs, FL 32043
(904) 264-8564

Bio-Electric Magnetics Institute
2490 West Moana Lane
Reno, NV 89509
(702) 827-9099

Nikken Products
Westwood Place, Suite 250
10866 Wilshire Boulevard
Los Angeles, CA 90024
(310) 446-4300

Pyramid International
414 Manhattan Avenue
Hawthorne, NY 10532
(914) 769-4879

Resonance
PO Box 64
Sumterville, FL 33585
(904) 793-8748

Massage Body Mechanics

Phoenix School of Holistic Health
6610 Harwin, Suite 256
Houston, TX 77036
(713) 974-5976   FAX (713) 266-6740

Medical Massage (see Swedish Massage Resources)

Medical Orgone Therapy

The American College of Orgonomy
PO Box 490
Princeton, NJ 08542
(908) 821-1144

Meditation

Center for Spiritual Awareness
PO Box 7
Lake Rabun Road
Lakemont, GA 30552-9990

Psycho-Acoustic Technology
4536 Genoa Circle
Virginia Beach, VA 23462
(804) 456-9487

MotherMassage

Elaine Stillerman, L.M.T.
108 East 16 Street
New York, NY 10003
(212) 533-3188   FAX (212) 533-3148

Moxibustion

Pacific Institute of Oriental Studies
915 Broadway
New York, NY 10010
(212) 982-3456   FAX (212) 982-6514

Tri-State School of Traditional Chinese
  Acupuncture
80 Eighth Avenue
New York, NY 10011
(212) 332-0787

Muscle Energy Work

Upledger Institute
11211 Prosperity Farms Road
Palm Beach Gardens, FL 33410-3487
(407) 622-4334

Music Therapy

American Association for Music Therapy
PO Box 80012
Valley Forge, PA 19484
(610) 265-4006   FAX (610) 265-1011

Creative Arts Therapies
251 West 51 Street
New York, NY 10019
(212) 246-3113

National Association for Music Therapy
8455 Colesville Road, Suite 930
Silver Spring, MD 20910
(301) 589-3300

Myofascial Release

Myofascial Release Centers
10 South Leopard Road, Suite One
Paoli, PA 19301
(610) 644-0136   (800)-FASCIAL
  FAX (610) 644-1662

Naprapathy

Chicago National College of Naprapathy
3330 North Milwaukee Avenue
Chicago, IL 60641
(312) 282-2686

Neural Organization Technique

Dr. Annalee Kitay
904 Pleasant Valley
West Orange, NJ 07052
(201) 325-0065

NeuroCellular Repatterning

Wellness Institute for Personal Transformation
8300 Rock Springs Road
Penryn, CA 95663

Neuro-Linguistic Programming

New York Training Institute for
  Neuro-Linguistic Programming
145 Sixth Avenue
New York, NY 10013
(212) 647-1660

Neuromuscular Reprogramming

Alive and Well! Institute of Conscious
  Bodywork, Inc.
100 Shaw Drive
San Anselmo, CA 94960
(415) 258-0402

Ohashiatsu

Ohashi Institute
12 West 27 Street
New York, NY 10001
(212) 684-4189/90   (800) 810-4190
  FAX (212) 447-5819

Okazaki Restorative Massage

Brian Fennen
PO Box 1001
Calistoga, CA 94515
(707) 942-9380

Ortho-Bionomy

PO Box 1974-70
Berkeley, CA 94701

Osteopathic Medicine

American Academy of Osteopathy
3500 De Pauw Boulevard, Suite 1080
Indianapolis, IN 46268
(317) 879-1881

American Osteopathic Association
142 East Ontario Street
Chicago, IL 60611
(312) 280-5800   FAX (312) 280-3860

Parma Training Program

Vincent Parmentola, L.M.T., C.S.P.
PO Box 1324
Boca Raton, FL 33429
(407) 997-8839

Past Life Regression

Association for Past Life Research and Therapy
PO Box 20151
Riverside, CA 92516
(714) 784-1570

Pesso Boyden System Psychomotor

Psychomotor Institute
60 Western Avenue
Cambridge, MA 02139
(617) 354-1044

Thérèse Pfrimmer Method of Deep Muscle Therapy

Alexandria School of Scientific
  Therapeutics
PO Box 287
Alexandria, IN 46001
(312) 724-7745

Pennsylvania School of Muscle Therapy
994 C Old Eagle School Road, Suite 1005
Wayne, PA 19087
(610) 687-0888

Thérèse C. Pfrimmer International Association
  of Deep Muscle Therapists, Inc.
105 Woodland Lane
Norristown, PA 19403
(215) 666-7088

Phoenix Rising Yoga Therapy

PO Box 819
Housatonic, MA 01236
(413) 274-0265

Physical Therapy

American Physical Therapy Association
1111 North Fairfax Street
Alexandria, VA 22314
(703) 684-2782

The Pilates Method

2121 Broadway, Suite 201
New York, NY 10023
(212) 875-0189   (800) 474-5283
    FAX (212) 769-2368

Polarity Therapy

American Polarity Therapy Association
2888 Bluff Street, Suite 149
Boulder, CO 80301
(303) 545-2080

Postural Integration

International Center for Release and
  Integration
450 Hillside Avenue
Mill Valley, CA 94941
(415) 383-4017

Pranic Healing

Center for Pranic Healing
Madison Square Station
Box 1737
New York, NY 10159
(212) 769-8721

American Institute of Asian Studies
PO Box 1605
Chino, CA 91708
(909) 465-0967

Process Acupressure

Process Acupressure Association
2621 Willowbrook Lane, Suite 104
Aptos, CA 95003
(408) 476-7721   FAX (408) 462-6662

Bonnie Prudden Myotherapy

7800 East Speedway
Tucson, AZ 85710
(520) 529-3979   FAX (520) 722-6311

Pulse Reading

Pacific Institute of Oriental Studies
915 Broadway
New York, NY 10010
(212) 982-3456   FAX (212) 982-6514

Tri-State School of Traditional Chinese
   Acupuncture
80 Eighth Avenue
New York, NY 10011
(212) 332-0787

The Radiance Technique

The Radiance Technique Association
   International, Inc.
PO Box 40570
St. Petersburg, FL 33743-0570
(813) 392-9278

RADIX

RADIX Instructors Institute
6300 Ridglea Place, Suite 1212
Ft. Worth, TX 76116-5738
(817) 738-3638

Rebirthing

Loving Relationships Training International
PO Box 1465
Washington, CT 06793
(800) 468-5578

Rebirthing Institute and Inspiration University
Mail Route 3, Box 88
Afton, VA 22920
(703) 885-0551

Reflexology

American Academy of Reflexology
606 East Magnolia Boulevard, Suite B
Burbank, CA 91501
(818) 841-7741

American Reflexology Certification Board and
   Information Service
PO Box 246654
Sacramento, CA 95824
(916) 455-5381

Foot Reflexology Awareness Foundation
PO Box 7622
Mission Hills, CA 91346-7622
(818) 361-0528

International Institute of Reflexology
PO Box 12642
St. Petersburg, FL 33733-3642
(813) 343-4811

Reiki

Loving Touch Center
172 Madison Avenue, Suite 208
New York, NY 10016
(212) 725-4930

Reiki Alliance
PO Box 41
Cataldo, ID 83810
(208) 682-3535   FAX (208) 682-4848

Reiki Healing Institute
1239 San Dieguito Drive
Encinitas, CA 92024

Relational Dialogue

Neal Katz
3 Central Avenue
Newton, MA 02160
(617) 332-7262

Release Work

11255 SW 67 Avenue
Miami, FL 33156
(305) 926-6420   (800) 700-6420

Resonant Kinesiology

41 Main Street
Burlington, VT 05401
(802) 860-2814

Rolfing

Rolf Institute of Structural Integration
PO Box 1868
Boulder, CO 80306-1868
(303) 449-5903   (800) 499-5978
    FAX (303) 449-5978

Rosen Method of Bodywork and Movement

Rosen Center Northeast
5337 College Avenue, Suite 255
Oakland, CA 94618
(510) 653-9113

Rosen Center West
825 Bancroft Way
Berkeley, CA 94710
(510) 644-4166

Rubenfeld Synergy Method

Rubenfeld Center
115 Waverly Place
New York, NY 10011
(212) 254-5100   FAX (212) 254-1174

Russian Massage

Kuroshova Institute for Studies in Physical
    Medicine
PO Box 6246
Rock Island, RI 61204
(309) 786-4888   (800) 791-9248

Sacro-Occipital Technique
(see Chiropractic Resources)

Safe Touch

Safe Touch Seminars
55 Ford's Landing
43 Mast Road Extension
Dover, NH 03820-4574
(603) 749-4780

Sensory Awareness

Box 1314 Star Route
Muir Beach, CA 94965

Charlotte Selver Foundation, Inc.
32 Cedars Road
Caldwell, NJ 07006
(201) 226-2202

Service Through Touch

41 Carl Street, Apt. C
San Francisco, CA 94117
(415) 564-1750

SHEN

International SHEN Therapy Association
3213 West Wheeler Street, #202
Seattle, WA 98199
(206) 298-9468

Shiatsu

American Oriental Bodywork Therapy
    Association

Shintaido

Shintaido of America
PO Box 22622
San Francisco, CA 94122
(415) 731-9364

Soma Neuromuscular Integration

Soma Institute of Neuro Muscular Integration
730 Klink Street
Buckley, WA 98321
(206) 829-1025

Somatic Psychotherapy

Association for Humanistic Psychology
45 Franklin Street, Suite 315
San Francisco, CA 94102
(415) 864-8850

Massachusetts Association of Body Oriented
   Psychotherapists and Counseling
   Bodyworkers
PO Box 410
Cambridge, MA 02140
(617) 576-9766

Massachusetts Coalition of Somatic
   Practitioners
2 Traymore Street
Cambridge, MA 02140
(617) 497-7278

Somatics

California Institute of Integral Studies
765 Ashbury Street
San Francisco, CA 94117
(415) 753-6100

SomatoEmotional Release

Upledger Institute
11211 Prosperity Farms Road
Palm Beach Gardens, FL 33410-3487
(407) 622-4334

Sound Healing

Diamond Light School of Massage and
   Healing Arts
PO Box 5443
Mill Valley, CA 94942
(415) 454-6651

Spinal Touch Treatment

Shawn Mossell, L.M.T.
1185 Wilmette Avenue
Wilmette, IL 60091
(708) 256-7708   (708) 491-0468

Spirit Releasement Therapy

Hypnosis and Neuro-Linguistic Programming
   Counseling Center
1799 Akron-Peninsula Road
Akron, OH 44313
(216) 923-5240

Center for Human Relations
William I. Baldwin, Ph.D.
PO Box 4061
Enterprise, FL 32725

Spiritual Healing

Jewish Association of Spiritual Healers
Florence M. Horn
106 Cabrini Boulevard
New York, NY 10033
(212) 928-4275

National Federation of Spiritual Healers
Old Manor Farm Studio, Church Street
Sunbury-On-Thames
Middlesex, TW106RG, England
(0932) 78-3164

Spiritual Frontiers Fellowship
3310 Baring Street
Philadelphia, PA 19104
(215) 222-1991

World Federation of Healing
33 The Park, Kingswood
Bristol, B5154BL, England

Sports Massage (see the Swedish Massage Resources)

International Sports Massage Federation and
   Training Institute
2156 Newport Boulevard
Costa Mesa, CA 92627
(714) 642-0735

St. John Neuromuscular Therapy

St. John Neuromuscular Pain Relief Institute
10950 72 Street, Suite 101
Largo, FL 34647
(813) 541-1900

Swedish Massage

American Alliance of Massage Professionals
3108 Route 10 West
Denville, NJ 07834
(201) 989-8941

American Massage Therapy Association
820 Davis Street #100
Evanston, IL 60201-4444
(708) 864-0123   FAX (708) 864-1178

Associated Bodywork and Massage
  Professionals
28677 Buffalo Park Road
Evergreen, CO 80439-7347
(303) 674-8478   FAX (303) 674-0859

California Coalition of Somatic Practices
PO Box 5611
San Mateo, CA 94402-0611   (415) 637-1233

International Massage Associates
3000 Connecticut Avenue, NW, Suite 102
Washington, DC 20008
(202) 387-6555   FAX (202) 332-0531

International Myomassethics Federation, Inc.
3732 East Carpenter Avenue
Cudahy, WI 53110
(800) 433-4463

National Association of Bodyworkers in
  Religious Service
7603 Forsyth Boulevard, Suite 214
Clayton, MO 63105

National Association of Nurse Massage
  Therapists
147 Windward Drive
Osprey, FL 34229
(813) 966-6288

National Certification Board for Therapeutic
  Massage and Bodywork
PO Box 1080
Evanston, IL 60204-1080
(708) 864-0774   FAX (708) 864-1178

New York State Society of Medical Massage
  Therapists, Inc.
PO Box 826
Glenwood Landing, NY 11547
(212) 697-7668

Nurse Healers Professional Association, Inc.
175 Fifth Avenue, Suite 2755
New York, NY 10011

Tai Chi Chuan

A Taste of China
111 Shirley Street
Winchester, VA 22601

Northeastern Tai Chi Chuan Association
10 West 18 Street
New York, NY 10011
(212) 741-1922

Tantsu

Worldwide Aquatic Bodywork Association
Harbin Hot Springs
PO Box 570
Middletown, CA 95461
(707) 987-3801   FAX (707) 987-9638

Thai Massage

American Oriental Bodywork Therapy
  Association
Glendale Executive Campus, Suite 510
1000 White Horse Road
Voorhees, NJ 08043
(609) 782-1616

International Professional School of Bodywork
1366 Hornblend Street
San Diego, CA 92109
(619) 542-0884   FAX (619) 542-0949

New Jersey School of Massage
3699 Route 46
Parsippany, NJ 07054
(201) 263-2229

Therapeutic Touch

Nurse Healers Association, Inc.
175 Fifth Avenue, Suite 2755
New York, NY 10011

Tongue Diagnosis

Pacific Institute of Oriental Studies
915 Broadway
New York, NY 10010
(212) 982-3456   FAX (212) 982-6514

Tri-State School of Traditional Chinese
  Acupuncture
80 Eighth Avenue
New York, NY 10011
(212) 332-0787

Touch For Health

Touch For Health Association
6955 Fernhill Drive, Suite 2
Malibu, CA 90265
(310) 457-8342   (800) 466-8342
  FAX (310) 457-9267

Touch For Health Foundation
4400 Coldwater Canyon Avenue, Suite 202
Studio City, CA 91604-1480
(818) 798-7893

Trager

Trager Institute
33 Millwood
Mill Valley, CA 94941-1891
(415) 388-2688   FAX (415) 388-2710

Transpersonal Bodywork and Psychology

Grof Transpersonal Training
20 Sunnywide Avenue, A-314
Mill Valley, CA 94941
(415) 383-8779

The Center for Transpersonal Body/Mind
  Studies
51 Upland Avenue
Metuchen, NJ 08840
(908) 548-8579

Trauma Touch Therapy

Colorado School of Healing Arts
7655 West Mississippi, Suite 100
Lakewood, CO 80226
(303) 986-2320

Trigger Point Therapy

National Association of Trigger Point
  Myotherapists
2600 South Parker Road, Suite 1–214
Aurora, CO 80014
(303) 368-1408

Tsubo Point Therapy (see Shiatsu Resources)

Tui-Na

American Oriental Bodywork Therapy
  Association
Glendale Executive Campus, Suite 510
1000 White Horse Road
Voorhees, NJ 08043
(609) 782-1616

Pacific Institute of Oriental Studies
915 Broadway
New York, NY 10010
(212) 982-3456   FAX (212) 982-6514

Taoist Institute of Los Angeles
10632 Burbank Boulevard
North Hollywood, CA 91601
(818) 760-4219

Taoist Sanctuary of San Diego
4229 Park Boulevard
San Diego, CA 92103
(619) 692-1155

UNTIE

Arnold Hermelin, L.M.T.
Route 2, Box 647
Sumnerland, FL 33042
(305) 745-2450

Vibrational Healing Massage Therapy

World School of Massage and Advanced
  Healing Arts
401 32 Avenue
San Francisco, CA 94121
(415) 221-2533

Visceral Manipulation

Upledger Institute
11211 Prosperity Farms Road
Palm Beach Gardens, FL 33410-3487
(407) 622-4334

Jean Pierre Barral
24 Rue Humbert II
Grenoble, France 38000

Wassertanzen (see Watsu Resource)

Watsu

Worldwide Aquatic Bodywork Association
Harbin Hot Springs
PO Box 570
Middletown, CA 95461
(707) 987-3801   FAX (707) 987-9638

Wengrow's Synergy

Vicki Wengrow
721 Stockton Street
Jacksonville, FL 32204
(904) 388-3635

Yoga

American Yoga Association
3130 Mayfield Road, W-301

Cleveland Heights, OH 44118
(216) 371-0078

American Yoga Association
513 South Orange Avenue
Sarasota, FL 34236

Zen Shiatsu

American Oriental Bodywork Therapy
    Association
Glendale Executive Campus, Suite 510
1000 White Horse Road
Voorhees, NJ 08043
(609) 782-1616

Zero Balancing

Zero Balancing Association
PO Box 1727
Capitola, CA 95010
(408) 476-0665

Zone Therapy (see Reflexology Resources)

APPENDIX II
BOARDS OF MASSAGE—UNITED STATES AND CANADA

The following states and provinces require a license to practice massage therapy. If your state is not listed, check with the local government authorities to find out about education requirements.

Alaska

(The state has a business license requirement)
Department of Commerce and Economic
  Development
Business Licensing Section
PO Box 110806
Juneau, AK 99811-0806
(907) 465-2550

Arkansas (500 hours)

State Board of Massage Therapy
PO Box 34163
Little Rock, AK 72203-4163
(510) 682-9170

Connecticut (500 hours)

Department of Public Health and Addiction
  Services
410 Capitol Avenue
Hartford, CT 06134
(203) 509-7566

Delaware (500 hours)

Department of Administrative Services
Division of Professional Regulation
Commission on Adult Entertainment
  Establishments
PO Box 1401
Dover, DE 19903
(302) 739-4522

Florida (500 hours)

Department of Professional Regulation
Board of Massage
1940 North Monroe Street
Tallahassee, FL 32399-0774
(904) 488-6021

Hawaii (570 hours)

Department of Commerce and Consumer
  Affairs
State Board of Massage
PO Box 3469
1010 Richards Street
Honolulu, HI 96801
(808) 586-3000

Iowa (500 hours—certification required)

Bureau of Professional Licensure
Department of Public Health
Lucas State Office Building, 4 Floor
Des Moines, IA 50319
(515) 281-4422

Louisiana (500 hours)

Louisiana Department of Health and Hospitals
Board of Massage Therapy
(504) 658-8941

Maine (certification required)

Commissioner of Professional and Financial
  Regulations
35 State House Station
Augusta, ME 04333
(207) 624-8603

Nebraska (1,000 hours)

Department of Health
Board of Massage
State Office Building
PO Box 95007
Lincoln, NE 68509-5007
(402) 471-2115

New Hampshire (750 hours)

Department of Health
Bureau of Health Facilities
6 Hazen Drive
Concord, NH 03301-6527
(603) 271-4592

New Mexico (650 hours)

New Mexico Regulation and Licensing
    Department
Massage Therapy Board
PO Box 25101
Santa Fe, NM 87504
(505) 827-7013

New York (500 hours)

State Board of Massage
Cultural Education Center
Room 3041
Albany, NY 12230
(518) 474-3866

North Dakota (500 hours)

Board of Massage
22 Fremont Drive
Fargo, ND 58103
(701) 237-4036

Ohio (600 hours)

State Medical Board
Massage Licensing Division
77 South High Street, 17 Floor
Columbus, OH 43266-0315
(614) 466-3934

Oregon (330 hours)

Board of Massage Technicians
800 NE Oregon Street
Portland, OR 97232
(503) 731-4064

Rhode Island (500 hours)

Division of Professional Regulation
Department of Health
3 Capitol Hill, Room 104
Providence, RI 02908-5097
(401) 277-2827

Tennessee (500 hours)

Department of Health Related Boards
283 Plus Park Boulevard
Nashville, TN 37247-1010
(615) 367-6393

Texas (300 hours)

Texas Department of Health
Massage Therapy Registration
1100 West 49 Street
Austin, TX 78756-3199
(512) 834-6616

Utah (600 or 1,000 hours)

Division of Occupational and Professional
    Licensing
160 East 300 South
PO Box 45802
Salt Lake City, UT 84145
(801) 530-6628

Washington (500 hours)

Washington Department of Health
Board of Massage
1300 Quince Street
Mail Stop 7869
Olympia, WA 98504-7869
(360) 586-6351

Canada

British Columbia

Association of Physiotherapists and Massage
  Practitioners of B.C.
103–1089 West Broadway
Vancouver, B.C., V6H 1E5
(604) 736-3404

Ontario

Board of Directors of Masseurs
1867 Yonge Street, Suite 810
Toronto, Ontario M4S 1Y5
(416) 489-2626

BIBLIOGRAPHY

Academy for Guided Imagery, "What is Guided Imagery?" brochure, Mill Valley, Calif., 1993.

Academy of Traditional Chinese Medicine, *An Outline of Chinese Acupuncture,* Beijing: Foreign Languages Press, 1975.

Achterberg, Jeanne, Ph.D., *Imagery in Healing: Shamanism and Modern Medicine,* Boston: Shambala Publications, 1985.

Achterberg, Jeanne, Ph.D.; Dossey, Barbara, R.N., M.S., F.A.A.N.; Kolkmeier, Leslie, R.N., M.Ed., *Rituals of Healing—Using Imagery for Health and Wellness,* New York: Bantam Books, 1994.

Ahmad, Sager, "The Eye Tells the Story," *New Straits Times,* Peninsular Malaysia, September 26, 1991.

Alexander, F.M., *The Alexander Technique: The Essential Writings of F. Matthais Alexander,* New York: Carol Publishing Group, 1989.

Alexander, F. Matthais, *The Use of Self,* Long Beach, Calif.: Centerline Press, 1986.

Amber, Reuben B., Dr., *Color Therapy,* New York: Samuel Weiser, 1964.

American Academy of Osteopathy, "Osteopathic Medicine: A Distinctive Branch of Mainstream Medical Care" brochure, Indianapolis, Ind.: American Academy of Osteopathy, no date.

American Association for Music Therapy brochure, Valley Forge, Pa.: 1994.

American Center for the Alexander Technique, Inc., "The Alexander Technique," New York: 1988.

American Massage Therapy Association, "A Guide to Massage Therapy in America," Evanston, Ill.: A.M.T.A., 1989.

American Oriental Bodywork Therapy Association, AOBTA Bulletin, Vol. 1, No. 3, 1992.

American Osteopathic Association, "Osteopathic Medicine," Chicago, Ill.: 1991.

American Physical Therapy Association, "A Historical Perspective," Alexandria, Va: A.P.T.A., 1994.

———, "Taking Care of Your Back," Alexandria, Va.: A.P.T.A., 1990.

American Society of Clinical Hypnosis Press catalogue, Des Plaines, Iowa: 1994.

Anavy, Regina Sigal, "Thai Massage," *Massage and Bodywork Magazine,* Vol. 1, Issue 5, 1986.

Angelo, Jack, "Spiritual Healing: Energy Medicine for Today," *Health Essentials,* London: no date.

Angelo, Jean Marie, "Healing Ourselves with Hands of Light," *Yoga Journal,* May/June 1993.

Aoki, Hiroyuki, *Shintaido,* San Francisco: Shintaido of America, 1982.

"Aroma Care—So Far," *Original Swiss Aromatics,* San Rafael, Calif.: 1991.

Arthritis Foundation Speakers' Bureau, "New Treatment Studied for Arthritis," *Arthritis Observer,* Vol. 44, No. 3, Winter 1992.

Ashley, Martin, J.D., L.M.T., *Massage: A Career at Your Fingertips,* Barrytown, N.Y.: Station Hill Press, 1992.

"Aston Movement," Upledger Institute brochure, Upledger Institute, Palm Beach Gardens, Fla.: no date.

Aston Training Center, "Aston-Patterning," Incline Village, Nev.: 1987.

Atlanta School of Massage, "Untie: A Pain Relief Alternative," Atlanta, Ga.: no date.

Auteroche, B., et al., *Acupuncture and Moxibustion—A Guide to Clinical Practice,* New York: Churchill Livingstone, 1992.

Bacon, Theresa, "Healing is a Form of Learning—The Resonant Kinesiology Training Program," *Massage,* Issue No. 40, November/December 1992.

Baek, Sung, *Classical Moxibustion—Skills in Contemporary Clinical Practice,* Boulder, Colo.: Blue Poppy Press, 1990.

Baloti, Lawrence D., *Massage Techniques,* New York: Perigree Books, Putnam Publications, 1986.

Baniel, Anat, "Feldenkrais® Somatic Education Accredited Professional Training Programs," Albany, Oreg.: The Feldenkrais Guild, no date.

Barasch, Marc Ian, "The Amazing Power of Visualization," *Natural Health,* July/August 1994.

Barnes, John F., P.T., "Myofascial Release: An Introduction for the Patient," *Physical Therapy Forum,* October 3, 1988.

———, "The Elasto-Collagenous Complex," *Physical Therapy Forum,* April 25, 1988.

———, "Myofascial Release," *Physical Therapy Forum,* September 16, 1987.

———, "MFR Techniques—The Psoas: The Myofascial Release Approach," *Physical Therapy Forum,* October 28, 1992.

Barry, William, "Constitutional Massage," Houston, Tex.: Phoenix School of Holistic Health, 1994.

Basic Massage Manual, New York: Swedish Institute, 1994.

Bauer, Cathryn, *Acupressure for Women,* Freedom, Calif.: Crossing Press, 1987.

———, *Acupressure for Everybody,* New York: Owl Books, 1991.

Becker, Robert O., M.D., *Cross Currents,* Los Angeles: Jeremy P. Tarcher, Inc., 1990.

Becker, Robert O., M.D., and Selden, Gary, *The Body Electric,* New York: Quill, 1985.

Behnke, Elizabeth A., "Sensory Awareness and Phenomenology: A Convergence of Traditions," Newsletter of the Study Project in Phenomenology of the Body, 1989.

Benjamin, Ben E., Ph.D., *Are You Tense? The Benjamin System of Muscular Therapy,* New York: Pantheon Books, 1978.

Bensoussam, Allan, *The Vital Meridian,* New York: Churchill Livingstone, 1991.

Biofeedback Training Client Information Paper, Wheat Ridge, Colo.: Association for Applied Psychophysiology and Biofeedback, 1993.

Biokinesiology Institute, *Muscle Testing Your Way to Health Using Emotions, Nutrition and Massage,* Shady Cove, Oreg.: 1982.

Bird, Jane, "Autogenic Training," *General Practitioner,* London: January 21, 1994.

Bischko, Johannes, M.D., *Introduction to Acupuncture,* Heidelberg: Haug Publications, 1978.

Blate, Michael, "G-Jo Acupressure Points," *Massage and Bodywork Magazine,* Vol. 1, Issue 5, 1986.

Bodian, Stephan, "At the Speed of Life: An Interview with Gay and Kathryn Hendricks," *Yoga Journal,* January/February 1994.

Bodymind Institute, "Bodymind Integration" brochure, West Los Angeles, Calif.: Bodymind Institute, no date.

Bogardus, Stephen, "Aunty Margaret Revisited," *Massage and Healing Arts Magazine,* Vol. 1, Issue 6, 1986.

Borg, Susan Gallagher, "The Resonant Kinesiology Training Program," *I.S.S.S.E.E.M.,* Vol. 4, No. 1, no date.

Borner, Russ, L.M.T., "On-Site Massage Comes of Age," *Hands On,* Vol. V, No. 4, Winter 1989.

Bourdiol, Rene J., Dr., *Auriculo-Somatology,* Moulins-lès-Metz, France: Maisonneuve, 1983.

Brennan, Barbara, *Hands of Light: A Guide to Healing through the Human Energy Field,* New York: Bantam Books, 1988.

Barbara Brennan School of Healing, News Release, no date.

British Association for Autogenic Training and Therapy, "Autogenic Training" brochure, Watford, England: 1993.

Brown, Lonny J., Ph.D., "Training Good Hands—with Heart at Cambridge's Muscular Therapy Institute," *Whole Health Network,* no date.

Brown, Sarida, "The Four Dimensions: Barbara Brennan in Interview Part II," *Caduceus,* Issue 22, 1993.

———, "Healing through the Human Energy Field—Barbara Brennan in Interview—Pts. I & II," *Caduceus,* Issues 21 & 22, 1994.

Budzynski, Thomas, "Brain Lateralization and Re-scripting," *Somatics,* Spring/Summer 1981.

Burmeister, David, and Landon, Michou, "Jin Shin Jyutsu," *Massage and Bodywork Quarterly,* Fall 1992.

Burton, Dierdre, "Zero Balancing," *International Journal of Alternative and Complementary Medicine,* March 1992.

———, "Zero Balancing: The Art of Balancing the Dynamic Relationship Between a Person's Energy and Their Body Structure," *International Journal of Alternative and Complementary Medicine,* March 1992.

Butler, Kurt, *A Consumer's Guide to Alternative Medicine,* Buffalo, N.Y.: Prometheus Books, 1992.

Calvert, Judi, and Flatley, David, "Mantak Chia on Chi Nei Tsang: Internal Organ Massage," *Massage Magazine,* January/February 1992.

Calvert, Robert, "Judith Aston: Developer of Aston-Patterning Bodywork," *Massage Magazine,* October/November 1988.

———, "John Barnes—Parts I & II," *Massage,* No. 41, January/February 1993.

———, "Lymphatics: The Body's Drainage System," *Massage and Bodywork Magazine,* Vol. 1, Issue 5, 1986.

———, "An Interview with Joseph Heller," *Massage Magazine,* Issue 19, April/May 1989.

———, "John Barnes: Founder of Myofascial Release," *Massage,* Issue 41, January/February 1993.

———, *International Massage and Bodywork Resource Guide,* Davis, Calif.: Noah Publications Co., 1991.

———, "Wataru Ohashi," *Massage,* No. 48, March/April 1994.

Calvert, Robert, and Calvert, Judi, "Interview with Marion Rosen, Founder of the Rosen Method

Bodywork and Gloria Hessellund, Rosen Practitioner," *Massage Magazine,* July/August 1991.

Campbell, Editha, "Balancing Life's Energies: The Gentle Art of Jin Shin Jyutsu," *Insight Network,* Issue 9, January–March 1994.

Cantu, Robert I., M.M.Sc., P.T., M.T.C., and Grodin, Alan J., P.T., M.T.C., *Myofascial Manipulation: Theory and Clinical Application,* Gaithersburg, Md.: Aspen Publications Co., 1992.

Carethers, Michael, Dr., "Health Promotion in the Elderly," *American Family Physician,* May 1992.

Carruthers, Malcolm, Dr., "Autogenic Training," London: *General Practitioner,* July 1982.

Carter, Mildred, *Hand Reflexology: Key to Perfect Health,* West Nyack, N.Y.: Parker Publications Co., 1975.

———, *Helping Yourself with Foot Reflexology,* West Nyack, N.Y.: Parker Publications Co., 1969.

Castleman, Michael, "The Healing Power of Music," *Natural Health,* September/October 1994.

Center for Gestalt Somatics brochure, New York: 1994.

Cerney, J.V., D.C., *Acupuncture without Needles,* West Nyack, N.Y.: Parker Publications, 1974.

Chaitow, Leon, N.D., D.O., *Acupuncture Treatment of Pain,* Rochester, Vt.: Healing Arts Press, 1976.

Chan, Pedro, *Finger Acupressure,* New York: Ballantine Books, 1974.

Chang, Stephen Thomas, Dr., *The Complete Book of Acupuncture,* Berkeley, Calif.: Celestial Arts, 1976.

Chen, Ze-lin, M.D., and Chen, Mei-Fang, M.D., *A Comprehensive Guide to Chinese Herbal Medicine,* Long Beach, Calif.: Oriental Healing Arts Institute, 1992.

Chia, Mantak, *Chi Self Massage: The Taoist Way of Rejuvenation,* Huntington, N.Y.: Healing Tao Books, 1986.

Chia, Mantak and Chia, Maneewan, *Chi Nei Tsang: Internal Organ Chi Massage,* Huntington, N.Y.: Healing Tao Books, 1990.

Cherry, Nina, "Hakomi Mindful Self-Observation, " 1988.

Chopra, Deepak, M.D., *Perfect Health: The Complete Mind/Body Guide,* New York: Random House, 1991.

Clark, Barbara, *Jin Shin Acutouch: The Tai Chi of Healing Arts,* San Diego, Calif.: Clark Publishing Co., 1987.

Cohen, Bonnie Bainbridge, *Sensing, Feeling and Action: The Experiential Anatomy of Body-Mind Centering,* Northampton, Mass.: Contact Editions, 1993.

Colorado School of Healing Arts, "Trauma Touch Therapy" brochure, Lakewood, Colo.: 1994.

Connelly, Diane M., Ph.D., M.Ac., *Traditional Acupuncture: The Law of the Five Elements,* Columbia, Md.: The Center for Traditional Acupuncture, 1979.

Connelly, Michael, "Tibetan Massage with Lobsang Rapgay," *Massage,* Issue No. 25, May/June, 1990.

Connor, Danny, *QiGong: Chinese Moevment and Meditation for Health,* York Beach, Maine: Samuel Weiser, 1992.

Cook, Jennifer, "Body Ease," *Self Magazine,* December 1985.

Corcon, Archimedes, M.D., "Principles and Practice of Classical Chinese Acupuncture," Burlingame, Calif.: *The Best of Health World,* Health World Magazine Inc., 1993.

Core Institute, "CORE Bodywork: A Myofascial Approach to Structural Integration" brochure, Tallhassee, Fla.: Core Institute School of Massage Therapy and Structural Bodywork, no date.

———, "Core Massage" brochure, Tallahassee, Fla.: Core Institute School of Massage Therapy and Structural Bodywork, no date.

Coseo, Marc, *The Acupressure Warm-Up for Athletic Preparation and Injury,* Brookline, Mass.: Paradigm Books, 1992.

Cousins, Norman, *Head First: The Biology of Hope and the Healing Power of the Human Spirit,* New York: Penguin Books, 1988.

Cramer, Patricia A., *Vibrational Healing Massage Therapy,* San Francisco: Vibrational Healing Massage Therapy Association, 1993.

Daglish, W.E., *Diet, Massage and Hydrotherapy,* Mokelumne Hill, Calif.: Health Research, 1961.

Danzan Ryu Seifukujitsu Institute, "Okazaki Restorative Massage" brochure, Calistoga, Calif.: 1994.

Davis, Patricia, *Aromatherapy—An A to Z,* Beekman Publications, Woodstock, N.Y.: 1991.

Day, Leslie, "Infant Massage," *Massage and Bodywork Magazine,* Vol. 1, Issue 5, 1986.

Dean, Judy, *Cellulite Control,* San Diego, Calif.: Judy Dean and Mueller College of Holistic Studies, 1988.

DeFino, Theresa, "The Miracle Worker—Tomezo Hoshino's Healing Hands Speak Distinctive Body Language," *Sun-Sentinel,* September 27, 1992.

De Jarnette, Major Bertrand, D.C., *The Philosophy, Art, and Science of Sacro Occipital Technic,* Nebraska City, Nebr.: Major Bertrand De Jarnette, 1967.

Denmei, Shudo, trans. Brown, Stephen, *Introduction to Meridian Therapy,* Seattle: Eastland Press, 1983.

Dennis, Larry, "Watch That Back!" *Golf Digest,* February 1991.

Despard, *Text-Book of Massage and Remedial Gymnastics,* no date.

Dossey, Larry, M.D., *Healing Words: The Power of Prayer and the Practice of Medicine,* New York: HarperCollins, 1993.

———, *Space, Time and Medicine,* Boston: Shambala Publications, 1985.

Dubitsky, Carl, O.B.T., L.M.T., "History of Shiatsu Anma," *Massage Therapy Journal,* October/November 1992.

Dudley, Michael Kioni, "Man, Gods and Nature," Na Kane Oka Malo, Waipahu, HI.: 1990.

Dull, Harold, *Watsu Freeing the Body in Water,* Middletown, Calif.: Harbon Hot Springs, 1993.

Dunkin, Mary Anne, "Putting the Reins on Pain," *Arthritis Today,* March/April 1990.

Durckheim, Karl Fried, *Hara: The Vital Center of Man,* New York: Samuel Weiser, Inc., 1962.

Durling, Bob, "What Is Rebirthing?" *Inspire,* Vol. 1, Issue 1, May/June 1993.

Ebner, Maria, *Connective Tissue Massage: Theory and Therapeutic Application,* Huntington, N.Y.: Robert E. Krieger Publications, 1962.

———, *Connective Tissue Massage,* Baltimore, Md.: The William Wilkins Co., 1962.

Egoscue, Pete, "The Egoscue Method," Del Mar, Calif.: T.H.E. Clinic, no date.

Egoscue, Pete, with Gittines, Roger, *The Egoscue Method of Health through Motion,* New York: HarperCollins, 1992.

Eisenberg, David M., M.D., et al., "Unconventional Medicine in the United States," *New England Journal of Medicine,* Vol. 328, No. 4, January 1993.

Elden, Harry R., Ph.D.; Wyrick, Dana L.; Brown, William N.; and Guarino, John F., "In Class: Massage and Lymphology." *Massage Magazine,* Issue 16, October/November 1988.

Electrotherapy, compiled by Benitah, Lise, P.T., L.M.T., Fort Lauderdale, Fla.: American Institute for Massage Therapy, no date.

"Elsa Gindler," Muir Beach, Calif.: Charlotte Selver Foundation, 1978.

Epstein, Gerald, M.D., *Healing Visualizations: Creating Health through Imagery,* New York: Bantam Books, 1989.

Esalen Institute, "Esalen Massage," Big Sur, Calif.: no date.

Family Guide to Natural Healing: How to Stay Healthy the Natural Way, Pleasantville, N.Y.: Reader's Digest Association, 1993.

Fein, Esther B., "Gaps in Geriatric Medicine Alarm Health Professionals," *New York Times,* May 16, 1994.

Feit, Richard, and Zmiewski, Paul, *Acumoxa Therapy: Reference and Study Guide,* Vol. I & II, Brookline, Mass.: Paradigm Books, 1990.

Feitis, Rosemary, *Ida Rolf Talks about Rolfing and Physical Reality,* Boulder, Colo.: The Rolf Institute, 1978.

The Feldenkrais Guild®, "The Feldenkrais Method®," Albany, Oreg.: 1993.

Fennen, Brian, L.Ac., "Okazaki's Restorative Massage," *Kiai Echo,* Spring 1994.

Field, Tiffany, Ph.D., et al., "Massage Reduces Anxiety in Child and Adolescent Psychiatric Patients," *Journal of the American Academy of Child and Adolescent Psychiatry,* Vol. 31, No. 1, January 1992.

Fischer-Rizzi, Susanne, *Complete Aromatherapy Handbook—Essential Oils and Radiant Health,* New York: Sterling Publications Co., 1990.

Flocco, William, "Foot, Hand, Ear Reflexology for a Healthy, Vital Life," in *The Whole Person,* August 1993.

Forester, A., *Clayton's Electrotherapy,* London: Bailliere Tindall Publishing Company, 1981.

Frawley, David, *Ayurvedic Healing,* Sandy, Utah: Passage Press, 1989.

Frohse, Franz; Brodel, Max; Schlossberg, Leon, *Atlas of Human Anatomy,* New York: Barnes and Noble Books, 1961.

Gach, Michael Reed, *Acupressure, Potent Points,* New York: Bantam Books, 1990.

Gach, Michael Reed, and Marco, Carolyn, *Acu-Yoga,* Tokyo: Japan Publications, 1981.

Gan, Carole F., "Massage: A Hands-on Therapy," *Grolier, Inc. Encyclopedia, Health and Medicine Annual,* 1992.

Gelb, Michael, *Body Learning: An Introduction to Alexander Technique,* New York: Henry Holt & Co., 1987.

German Therapology, Inc., "Spinal Touch Treatment," Salt Lake City: German Therapology, Inc., no date.

Gibson, Roberta, "The Role of Bodywork in Recovery from Trauma," Lakewood, Colo.: no date.

Goddard, Lisa, "Oh, My Aching Back," *The News,* December 15, 1992.

Gold, Rick, Dr., "Traditional Thailand Medical Massage," San Diego, Calif.: The International Professional School of Bodywork, no date.

Golden, Stephanie, "Body-Mind Centering," *Yoga Journal,* September/October 1993.

Gonzalez, David, "Tending the Spirit as Well as the Body," *New York Times,* September 7, 1994.

Goodell, Caroline, "Rosen Method Bodywork," *Journey Magazine,* April 1992.

Gould, Dave, "The Back Fixer," *Golf Digest,* no date.

Greene, Alice, Dr., "Autogenic Training—A Psychotherapeutic Resource in Chronic Illness," London: no date.

Grimm, Ellen, "Beat: Tai Chi Helps Elderly Find Balance," *Natural Health,* November/December 1994.

Grof, Stanslav, and Grof, Christina, "Grof Transpersonal Training" brochure, Mill Valley, Calif.: no date.

Hakomi Institute catalogue, Boulder, Colo.: 1992.

——— , "Hakomi Integrative Somatics," Boulder, Colo.: no date.

"Hanging Loose," *Harper & Queens Magazine,* London: September 1980.

Heinrich, Steve, P.T., "Learning to Let Go—The Role of SomatoEmotional Release in Clinical Treatment," *Physical Therapy Forum,* Vol. VIII, No. 24, 1989.

——— , "Enlightened Movement," *Massage Therapy Journal,* Winter 1993.

Heline, Corinne, *Healing and Regeneration through Color,* Santa Barbara, Calif.: J.F. Rowney Press, 1943.

Heller, Joseph and Hanson, Jan, *Hellerwork: The Client's Handbook,* Mount Shasta, Calif.: 1993.

Hermelin, Arnold, L.M.T., "Untie: A Pain Relief Alternative," Key West, Fla.: no date.

Higgins, Donna, "UM [Upper Merion] School Teaches Unique Muscle Therapy Method," *King of Prussia Courier/Suburban,* March 8, 1989.

Higgins, Melissa, "Mary Burmeister, Master of Jin Shin Jyutsu," *Yoga Journal,* March/April 1988.

Hodgkinson, Liz, "In Training for Relaxation," *The Times,* London: October 13, 1988.

Hoffman Institute, "Hoffman Quadrinity Process" brochure, San Anselmo, Calif.: 1993.

——— , *The Hoffman Quadrinity Process,* Oakland, Calif.: 1991.

Hopkins, Carol Lee, "Incorporating Reiki Healing into Massage," *Intra Myomassethics Forum,* Vol. 21, No. 2, March 1994.

Hoshino Therapy Clinic, "Hoshino Therapy," Miami: no date.

——— , "Growing (Old) Pains," *Boca Raton Magazine,* March/April 1992.

Hughes, Howard; Brown, Barry W.; Lawlis, G. Frank; Fulton, James E., Jr., "Treatment of Acne Vulgaris by Biofeedback Relaxation and Cognitive Imagery," *Journal of Psychosomatic Research,* Vol. 27, No. 3, Great Britain: Pergamon Press, Ltd., 1983.

Hui, Jia Li, and Xiang, Jia Zhao, *Pointing Therapy: A Chinese Traditional Therapeutic Skill,* Beijing, China: Technology Press, 1987.

Hurly, John L., Dr., "Figures Don't Lie," Bio-Mechanics brochure, 1937.

Hyman, James, "Emotional Freedom," *Inner Self,* April 1994.

Ichazo, Oscar, *Arica Theory and Practice,* New Rochelle, N.Y.: Arica Institute, 1972.

Ingham, Eunice D., *Stories Feet Can Tell,* Rochester, N.Y.: Eunice Ingham, 1938.

Insight Meditation Society Vipassana Retreat Schedule, Barre, Mass.: 1994.

Institute for Health Improvement, "The Breema Touch," Oakland, Calif.: 1992.

International College of Applied Kinesiology—USA, "An Historical Overview of Applied Kinesiology," Lawrence, Kans.: no date.

International College of Applied Kinesiology—USA, "Applied Kinesiology Status Statement," Lawrence, Kans.: 1992.

International Macrobiotic Shiatsu Society, "Macrobiotic Shiatsu," Eureka, Calif.: International Macrobiotic Shiatsu Society, 1990.

International Professional School of Bodywork, "Nuad Bo-Rarn—The Art of Traditional Medical Massage of Thailand," San Diego, Calif.: IPSB, no date.

International Professional School of Bodywork, "Thailand Massage," San Diego, Calif.: IPSB, no date.

International SHEN Therapy Association, "SHEN: Physio-Emotional Release Therapy," Edmonds, Wash.: no date.

Jacobs, Miriam, M.S., "Massage for the Relief of Pain: Anatomical and Physiological Considerations," *The Physical Therapy Review,* Vol. 40, No. 2, 1960.

Jensen, Bernard, D.C., N.D., *The Science and Practice of Iridology,* Provo, Utah: Bi-World Publications Inc., 1952.

Jewish Association of Spiritual Healers, "L'Chaim:

To Life!'' New York: March 1994.

―――, Articles of Constitution, New York: March 1993.

Jin Shin Do Foundation for Bodymind Acupressure, "Directory of Authorized Teachers and Registered Acupressurists,'' Palo Alto, Calif.: Jin Shin Do Foundation, no date.

Johrei Fellowship, "Johrei Fellowship'' brochure, New York: no date.

Joy, M. Brugh, M.D., *Joy's Way—A Map for the Transformational Journey,* New York: Putnam, 1979.

Juhan, Deane, "The Physiology of Hook-Up: How TRAGER Works,'' Keynote address, Sixth International TRAGER Conference, San Diego, Calif.: September 1992.

―――, "The Trager Approach: A Comprehensive Introduction,'' Mill Valley, Calif.: Trager Institute, 1993.

Junying, Geng and Zhihong, Su, *Practical Traditional Chinese Medicine and Pharmacology—Basic Theories and Principles Vol. I,* Beijing: New World Press, 1990.

Kain, Kathy and Berns, Jim, "Ortho-Bionomy: A Manual of Practice,'' Berkeley, Calif.: Russell Publishing Co., 1992.

Kaptchuk, Ted J., O.M.D., *The Web That Has No Weaver,* New York: Congdon and Weed, 1983.

Kastner, Mark L., Ac., Dipl. Ac., and Burroughs, Hugh, *Alternative Healing,* La Mesa, Calif.: Halcyon Publications, 1993.

Keider, Norma S., "Spirit Releasement Therapy'' brochure, Akron, Ohio: no date.

Kendall, Henry O., P.T.; Kendall, Florence P., P.T.; Wadsworth, Gladsy E., P.T., *Muscles: Testing and Function,* Baltimore: Williams & Wilkins, 1971.

Kisner, Carolyn Dieball, M.S., and Taslitz, Norman, Ph.D., "Connective Tissue Massage: Influence of the Introductory Treatment on Autonomic Functions,'' *Physical Therapy,* Vol. 48, No. 2, no date.

Kitay, Annalee, Dr., "N.O.T.—Neural Organization Technique,'' *Relevant Times,* March/April 1993.

―――, "Neural Organization Technique—Healing Through Applied Neurology,'' West Orange, N.J.: no date.

Knapp, Miland E., M.D., "Massage,'' *Physical Medicine and Rehabilitation,* Vol. 44, July 1968.

Knaster, Mirka, "Thomas Hanna: Mind Over Movement,'' *East West: The Journal of Natural Healing and Living,* February 1989.

Koren, Tedd, Dr., D.C., "TMJ Syndrome/Dysfunction'' brochure, Koren Publications, Inc.,

1991.

―――, "Why Should I Go to a Chiropractor?'' brochure, Philadelphia: Koren Publications Inc., 1991.

―――, "Your Natural Healing Ability'' brochure, Philadelphia: Koren Publications Inc., 1988.

―――, "Retracing—What Is It?'' brochure, Philadelphia: Koren Publications Inc., 1990.

―――, "Sports, Athletics and Chiropractic'' brochure, Philadelphia: Koren Publications Inc., 1990.

Kotzsch, Ronald, "Hoshino Therapy—Nothing Can Surpass the Hands,'' *East West Magazine,* December 1988.

Kousaleos, George, "A Myofascial Approach to Soft-Tissue Therapies,'' Tallahassee, Fla.: Core Institute, no date.

Krames Communications, "Physical Therapy: Improving Movement and Function,'' Daly City, Calif.: 1984.

Kresge, Carol A., C.I., R.M.T., "Massage and Sports,'' *The Massage Journal,* April 1985.

Kripalu Center, "The Kripalu Experience,'' Lenox, Mass.: Kripalu Center, 1993.

Kumins, Noel, "A Revolution in King of Prussia,'' Main Line Living, Vol. 1, No. 11.

Kunz, Kevin, and Kunz, Barbara, *The Complete Guide to Foot Reflexology,* Albuquerque, N.Mex.: Reflexology Research Project, 1980.

Kurashova Institute for Studies in Physical Medicine, General Information—Russian Massage, Rock Island, Ill.: no date.

Kurashova Institute for Studies in Physical Medicine, "Russian Massage'' brochure, Rock Island, R.I.: 1994.

Kurshova Institute for Studies in Physical Medicine, Newsletter, Vol. 5, Issue 1, 1994.

Kurz, W., M.D., et al., "Effect of Manual Lymph Drainage Massage on Urinary Excretion of Neurohormones and Minerals in Chronic Lymphedema,'' *Angology,* Vol. 29, No. 764, 1978.

Laban/Bartenieff Institute of Movement Studies, Inc., brochure, New York: 1994.

Lad, Vasant, *Ayurveda, the Science of Healing,* Sante Fe, N.Mex.: Lotus Press, 1985.

Lauterstein, David, "What Is Zero Balancing?'' *Massage Therapy Journal,* Vol. 33, No. 1, Winter 1994.

Law, Donald, *A Guide to Alternative Medicine,* Garden City, N.Y.: Dolphin Books, 1976.

Lawson, Carol, "Doo-Wop, Doo-Wop, Scalpel, Scalpel,'' *New York Times,* October 5, 1994.

Leflet, David H., *HEMME Approach to Soft-Tissue Therapy,* Bonifay, Fla.: HEMME Approach Publications, 1992.

_____, *HEMME Approach to Managing Low Back Pain,* Bonifay, Fla.: HEMME Approach Publications, 1994.

Leviton, Richard, "Moving with Milton Trager," *East West Journal,* January 1988.

Liebowitz, Judith, and Connington, Bill, *The Alexander Technique,* New York: Harper Perennial Books, 1990.

Life Magazine, "Why We Pray," New York: March 1993.

Loderus, Ronayne, "Hawaiian Shamanism and the Aloha Way," no date.

Loving Touch Center, *Reiki: First Degree,* New York: Loving Touch Center, no date.

Loving, Larry, "Introducing Fascial Kinetics" brochure, Lake Worth, Fla.: no date.

Low, Jeffrey, "The Modern Therapies—Aston-Patterning," *Massage Magazine,* October/November 1988.

Lowen, Alexander, M.D., *Bioenergetics,* New York: Penguin Books, 1976.

_____, "Thoughts on Bioenergetic Analysis," The International Institute for Bioenergetic Analysis NY, Newsletter, Vol. 12, No. 2, Spring 1992.

Lymphedema Services, P.C., "Complete Decongestive Physiotherapy: An Innovative and Logical Approach to Lymphedema," New York: Lymphedema Services, P.C., 1991.

Maciocia, Giovanni, *Tongue Diagnosis in Chinese Medicine,* Seattle: Eastland Press, 1987.

_____, *The Foundations of Chinese Medicine: A Comprehensive Text to Acupuncturists and Herbalists,* Edinburgh: Churchill Livingstone, 1989.

Maffetone, Philip, Dr., "The Missing Piece in Alternative Health Care," Lawrence, Kans.: International College of Applied Kinesiology—USA, no date.

Mandel, Bill, "Sniffing Out Aromatherapy," *San Francisco Examiner,* November 2, 1983.

Manheim, Carol J., M.Sc., P.T., and Lavett, Diane K., Ph.D., *The Myofascial Release Manual,* Thorofare, N.J.: Slack, Inc., 1989.

Mann, Casey, "Supporting Pregnancy with Bodywork for the Childbearing Year," no date.

Mann, Felix, *Acupuncture,* New York: Vintage Books, 1973.

Mantell, Matthew E., "Applied Kinesiology: A New Drive for Total Health," Lawrence, Kans.: no date.

Marcus, Paul, M.D., *Thorson's Introduction Guide to Acupuncture,* New York: HarperCollins, 1984.

Markowitz, Dan, "Old Fitness Plan Finds a New Clientele," *The New York Times,* January 9, 1994.

Marks, Linda, "Psychotherapy That Includes the Body: A Consumer's Guide to Somatic Psychotherapy," Boston, 1995.

Martin, Arthur, "The History of NeuroCellular Repatterning," Penryn, Calif.: The Institute for Personal Transformation, revised 1993.

Masunaga, Shizuto, *Zen Shiatsu,* New York: Japan Press, 1990.

Matsumoto, Kiiko, and Birch, Stephen, *Five Elements and Ten Stems,* Brookline, Mass.: Paradigm Publications, 1983.

_____, *Hara Diagnosis,* Brookline, Mass.: Paradigm Books, 1988.

Matusow, Vajra, "Laying on of Hands," Mill Valley, Calif.: Diamond Light School of Massage and Healing Arts, 1994.

_____, "Healing With Sound," Mill Valley, Calif.: Diamond Light School of Massage and Healing Arts, 1994.

Mayo Clinic Health Letter, "Massage," May 1993.

McClellan, Samuel, "New England Institute for Integrative Acupressure" brochure, Haydenville, Mass.: 1994.

McKechnie, Alasdair A.; Wilson, Florence; Watson, Nan; and Scott, David, "Anxiety States: A Preliminary Report of the Value of Connective Tissue Massage," *Journal of Psychosomatic Research,* Vol. 27, No. 2, 1983.

Meagher, Jack, and Boughton, Pat, *Sports Massage,* Garden City, N.Y.: Dolphin Books, 1980.

Mennell, J.B., *Massage: Its Principles and Practice,* Philadelphia: Blakiston Co., 1920.

Miesler, Dietrich, M.A., "Geriatric and Regular Massage—How Do They Differ?" Day-Break Yearbook, Guerneville, Calif.: 1994.

_____, "Geriatric Massage the Day-Break Way," Evergreen, Colo.: *Massage and Bodywork Quarterly,* Association of Bodywork and Massage Professionals, Fall 1993.

_____, "Geriatric Massage—Why Doesn't Everybody Do It?" Day-Break Yearbook, Guerneville, Calif.: 1994.

Miller, Leslie, "Healthful Benefits of Massage Gaining Attention," *USA Today,* October 15, 1992.

_____, "Reassuring Music to Have Surgery By," *USA Today,* September 6, 1994.

Mitsui, Mieko, "Reiki," New York: no date.

_____ , "The Radiance Technique" brochure, New York: no date.

Montgomery, Kate, "Sports Touch: The Athletic Ritual," *Massage,* Issue No. 25, May/June, 1990.

Moor, Fred B., B.A., M.D., Peterson, Stella, B.S., R.N., et al., *Manual of Hydrotherapy and Massage,* Boise, Idaho: Pacific Press Publishing Association, 1964.

Mower, Melissa B., "Zhenya Kurashova Wine: Russian Clinical Massage—The Kurashova Method," *Massage,* Issue No. 43, May/June, 1993.

Muscular Therapy Institute, Inc., brochure, Cambridge, Mass.: no date.

Myofascial Release Treatment Center brochure, Paoli, P.A.: no date.

Nambiar, Shanty, "More Than a Massage," *The Boston Globe,* July 20, 1992.

Namikoshi, Tokujiro, *Shiatsu: Health and Vitality at Your Fingertips,* Tokyo: Japan Publications, 1969.

National Association for Music Therapy, Inc., "Music Therapy" brochure, Silver Spring, Md.: no date.

Negri, Folani, "Lomi Ha'a Mauli Ola," personal interview, November 1993.

Netherby, Margaret, and Wilson, Robin J., "Ortho-Bionomy and Michi," *Massage and Bodywork Magazine,* Vol. 1, Issue 5, 1986.

Neubert, Robert, "Reiki—The Radiance Technique," *New Realities,* March/April 1987.

Newman, Tim "Zero Balancing," South West Connection, August/November 1993.

New York Times, "Study Finds That Weight Training Can Benefit the Very Old," June 23, 1994.

New York Times, "As Americans Age, Arthritis Increases, Too," *June 24, 1994.*

New York Training Institute for NLP brochure, New York: 1995.

Nikken, "Total Wellness Naturally," brochure, Los Angeles, Calif.: no date.

Nippon Shiatsu Daigaku, Course Outline, Putney, Vt.: no date.

Nolte, Marcia, "Soma Institute," Miami: no date.

Norman, Laura, *Feet First,* New York: Fireside, 1988.

NurrieStearns, Mary, "Rediscover Your Essence," Lotus, *Journal for Personal Transformation,* Spring 1994.

Nurse Healers—Professional Associates, "Therapeutic Touch: The Krieger-Kunz Model" brochure, New York: no date.

O'Donovan, J.B., Dr., "Autogenic Training—A Ne-glected Therapeutic Resource," British Association for Autogenic Training and Therapy, Watford, England: no date.

The Ohashi Institute, "Ohashiatsu: A Healing Method of Touch for Peace," New York: no date.

_____ , "1995 Ohashiatsu Program" brochure, New York: 1994.

Ohashi, Wataru, *Do-It-Yourself Shiatsu,* New York: E.P. Dutton, 1976.

Oleson, Terry, Ph.D., and Flocco, William, "Randomized Controlled Study of Premenstrual Symptoms Treated with Ear, Hand and Foot Reflexology," *Obstetrics and Gynecology,* Vol. 82, No. 6, December 1993.

On-Site Enterprises, "Advantages of On-Site Massage," Boulder, Colo.: 1990.

Original Swiss Aromatics, "Inside Aromatherapy," Newsletter of Original Swiss Aromatics and Pacific Institute of Aromatherapy, San Rafael, Calif.: 1993.

O'Sullivan, William, "The Gift of Touch," *Common Boundary,* May/June 1994.

Ouseley, S. G. J., *The Power of the Rays,* Essex, England: L.N. Fowler and Co., Ltd., 1951.

Painter, Jack, *Postural Integration: Transformation of the Whole Self,* Mill Valley, Calif.: International Center for Release and Integration, 1986.

Palmer, David, "Researching Massage in the Workplace," *The Bodywork Entrepreneur,* 1989.

Palmer, Harry, *Creativism: The Art of Living Deliberately,* Longwood, Fla.: 1987.

Parker Chiropractic Research Foundation, "Spinal Curvature" brochure, Parker Chiropractic Research Foundation, 1973.

_____ , "If You Wear Out Your Body, Where Are You Going to Live?" brochure, Parker Chiropractic Research Foundation, 1992.

Parmentola, Vincent, R.M.T., C.S.P., "Parma Training," Boca Raton, Fla.: April 1994.

_____ , "Parma Symmetry" brochure, Boca Raton, Fla.: no date.

Pati, Kumar, Dr., "Basic Therapies of Ayurvedic Medicine," Burlingame, Calif.: The Best of Health World, Health World Magazine, 1993.

Pavek, Richard Rainbow, *Handbook of SHEN,* Sausalito, Calif.: The SHEN Therapy Institute, 1987.

Pelletier, Kenneth R., *Mind As Healer, Mind As Slayer,* New York: Delta Books, 1992.

Pemberton, R., and Scull, C.W., "Massage," *Handbook of Medical Physics,* Chicago, Ill.: Year Book

Publications, 1984.

Perlman, Jeff, "Learn the Healing Touch," *Delray Times,* Delray Beach, Fla.: October 24, 1994.

Perls, Frederick S., M.D., Ph.D., *Gestalt Therapy Verbatim,* New York: Bantam, 1969.

Peterson, Gary, "Polarity Therapy," American Polarity Therapy Association, Boulder, Colo.: 1994.

Pfrimmer, Thérèse C., *Muscles—Your Invisible Bonds,* Blyth, Ontario: Blyth Printing, 1970.

Thérèse C. Pfrimmer International Association of Deep Muscle Therapists brochure, Norristown, Pa.: no date.

Pharus the Egyptian, *The Zonery System,* Mokelumne Hill, Calif.: Health Research, 1926.

Phipps, Toshiko, "Integrative/Eclectic Shiatsu," American Oriental Bodywork Therapy Association Education Program, no date.

Phoenix Rising brochure, Housatonic, Mass.: no date.

Pilates Studio, "The Pilates Method" brochure, New York: 1994.

Porter, Arnold, "The Two Eyes of Jin Shin Do," Heartwood: *Journal of Experience, Expression and Odyssey,* Vol. VII, No. 4, September/October 1988.

Prevention Magazine Health Books, *Hands-On Healing: Massage Remedies for Hundreds of Health Problems,* Emmaus, Pa.: Rodale Press, 1989.

Price, Kathie, "Japanese Art Lets Fingers Do Healing," *The Arizona Public,* February 13, 1993.

Prudden, Bonnie, *Pain Erasure: The Bonnie Prudden Way,* New York: Ballantine Books, 1980.

Quale, Kamala, and Smith, Becky, "Acupressure News," Palo Alto, Calif.: Jin Shin Do Foundation for Body-mind Acupressure, Vol. 10, 1993.

Quinn, Janet, Ph.D,. R.N., F.A.A.N., "Haelen Work" brochure, Boulder, Colo.: The Center For Human Caring Group Practice, no date.

Raheem, Aminah, Ph.D., *Process Acupressure I,* Capitola, Calif.: Aminah Raheem, 1991.

———, *Soul Return,* Lower Lake, Calif.: Aslan Publications, 1987.

Ray, Barbara, Ph.D., *The "Reiki" Factor in the Radiance Technique,* St. Petersburgh, Fla.: Radiance Associates, 1983.

Rebirthers Association of New York, "What Is Rebirthing?" New York: no date.

Reilly, Harold, Dr., and Brod, Ruth Hagy, *The Edgar Cayce Handbook for Health through Drugless Therapy,* New York: Jove Publications, 1975.

Rendel, Peter, *Introduction to the Chakras,* New York: Samuel Weiser, 1974.

Resonant Kinesiology Training Program brochure, Burlington, Vt.: no date.

Richardson, Nancy, R.P.T., "Aston-Patterning," *Physical Therapy Forum,* Vol. VI, No. 43, October 28, 1987.

Riley, Joe Shelby, Dr., *Zone Reflexology,* Mokelumne Hill, Calif.: Health Research, 1961.

Roche, Mary Alice, "Sensory Awareness—The Basic Connection," Newsletter to the Study Project in Phenomenology of the Body, 1989.

———, "Sensory Awareness," personal interview, February 1994.

Rolf Institute, "Rolfing and Rolfing Movement Integration" brochure, Boulder, Colo.: 1991.

Rosen, Marion, and Brenner, Sue, *The Rosen Method of Movement,* Berkeley, Calif.: North Atlantic Books, 1991.

Rosen, Sidney, ed., *My Voice Will Go with You: The Teaching Tales of Milton H. Erickson,* New York: W.W. Norton & Company, 1982.

Rosenfeld, Albert, "Teaching the Body How to Program the Brain is Moshe's 'Miracle'," *Smithsonian Magazine,* January 1981.

Rossi, Joanne, "Cross-Cultural Healing and Energy-Based Bodywork," *Holistic Living,* no date.

Rossi, Ernest L. and Check, David B., *Mind-Body Therapy: Methods of Ideodynamic Healing in Hypnosis,* New York: W.W. Norton & Co., 1988.

Rubenfeld, Ilana, "Beginner's Hands: Twenty-Five Years of Simple Rubenfeld Synergy—The Birth of a Therapy," *Somatics,* Spring/Summer 1988.

———, "Ushering in a Century of Integration," *Somatics,* Autumn/Winter 1990–91.

———, "Rubenfeld Synergy Method," brochure, New York: 1988/1991.

Ruch, Meredith Gould, Ph.D., "Release Your Body's Healing Wisdom," *Changes,* June 1993.

———, "Phoenix Rising Yoga Therapy," *Yoga Journal,* July/August 1992.

Safe Touch Seminars, Ltd., brochure, Dover, N.H.: 1994.

Schneiderman, Ian, F.R., C.P., M.R., *Medical Acupuncture,* Hong Kong: Mayfair Medical Supplies, 1988.

School for Body-Mind Centering, "Certification Program in Body-Mind Centering" catalogue, Amherst, Mass.: 1990.

School of Shiatsu and Massage catalogue, Middletown, Calif.: Harbin Hot Springs, 1994.

Schreiber, Jon, Dr., *Touching the Mountain: The*

Self-Breema Handbook, Oakland, Calif.: California Health Publications, 1989.

Schwartz, Mike, "Massage," *The Press-Enterprise,* April 6, 1993.

Scorboria, Francine M., "Hypnosis Seen Key to Boy Seeing," *Journal of Hypnosis,* September 1993.

Scull, C. Wesler, Ph.D., "Massage: Physiologic Basis," Archives Physical Medicine, No. 26, March 1945.

Seedman, Barry, "Hypnosis: Key to Unlocking Our Minds" brochure, New York: The Hypnosis Institute, no date.

Seem, Mark, Ph.D., *Acupuncture Imaging,* Rochester, Vt.: Healing Arts Press, 1990.

———, *Acupuncture Energetics,* Rochester, Vt.: Healing Arts Press, 1987.

Selver, Charlotte, "Sensory Awareness and Total Functioning," General Semantics Bulletin, Nos. 20, 21, 1957.

———, "Sensory Awareness," Muir Beach, Calif.: Sensory Awareness Foundation, 1989.

Serizawa, Katsusuke, *Effective Tsubo Therapy: Simple and Natural Relief without Drugs,* Tokyo: Japan Publications, 1984.

———, *Tsubo—Vital Points for Oriental Therapy,* Tokyo: Japan Publications, 1976.

Shanghai College of Traditional Medicine—O'Connor, John and Bensky, Dan, *Acupuncture—A Comprehensive Text,* Seattle: Eastland Press, 1981.

Share International, "Chiropractic Questions and Answers," Ft. Worth, Tex.: Share International Inc., no date.

Shealy, C. Norman, M.D., Ph.D., and Myss, Carolyn M., M.A., *The Creation of Health: The Emotional, Psychological and Spiritual Responses That Promote Health and Healing,* Walpole, N.H.: Stillpoint Publications, 1988.

Shenandoah Taijiquan Center brochure, Winchester, Va.: 1994.

Shintaido of America, Newsletter, San Francisco: Fall 1991.

———, "A New Art of Movement and Life Expressions," San Francisco: 1994.

Siegel, Bernie S., M.D., *Peace, Love and Healing—Bodymind Communication and the Path to Self-Healing: An Exploration,* New York: HarperCollins, 1989.

———, *Love, Medicine and Miracles: Lessons Learned About Self-Healing from a Surgeon's Experience with Exceptional Patients,* New York: HarperCollins, 1990.

Smith, Fritz Frederick, M.D., *Inner Bridges,* Atlanta, Ga.: Humanics New Age, 1986.

Smith, Irene, *Bodywork for People with HIV Infection,* San Francisco: Service Through Touch, 1994.

Sobel, David S., M.D., M.P.H., "Childbirth: Emotional Support in Labor Reduces C-Sections and Shortens Labor," Los Altos, Calif.: Mental Medicine Update, The Center for Health Sciences, 1993.

Sohn, Tina and Finando, Donna, *Amma—The Ancient Art of Oriental Healing,* Rochester, Vt.: Healing Arts Press, 1988.

Soma Institute of Neuromuscular Integration brochure, Buckley, Wash.: 1994.

SOMA Practitioners Association, "SOMA Neuromuscular Integration" brochure, Miami: no date.

Somatic Learning Associates, "Bodywork for the Childbearing Year" brochure, La Jolla, Calif.: no date.

Somatic Therapy Institute, "A Body/Mind Integrative Therapy" brochure, Santa Fe, N.Mex.: Somatic Therapy Institute, 1993.

Sorsi, "Enter the Powerful World of SOT" brochure, Prairie Village, Kans.: no date.

Stearns, Ann Kaiser, *How to Live Through Loss,* Chicago, Ill.: Thomas More Press, 1984.

Stein, A., "Comprehensive Family Therapy," The Psychotherapy Handbook, New York: New American Library, 1980.

Stevens, Chris, *Alternative Health: Alexander Technique,* Boston, Mass.: MacDonald Optima, 1988.

Stillerman, Elaine, L.M.T., *MotherMassage: A Handbook for Relieving the Discomforts of Pregnancy,* New York: Delacorte Press, 1992.

———, "MotherMassage: Massage during Pregnancy," *Massage Therapy Journal,* Summer 1994.

St. John, Paul, L.M.T., "Five Physiological Principles That Explain Pain in Mechanisms," Palm Beach Gardens, Fla.: St. John Neuromuscular Pain Relief Institute, no date.

Sturgess, Russell, "Fascial Kinetics" brochure, 1993.

Stux, Gabriel, and Pomeranz, Bruce, *Acupuncture Textbook and Atlas,* Heidelberg: Springer Verlag, 1987.

———, *Basics of Acupuncture,* Heidelberg: Springer Verlag, 1988.

Swedish Institute, *Energetic Shiatsu: A Manual,* New York: Swedish Institute, 1988.

Swirsky, Joan, "Magnetic Therapy to Relieve Arthritis Pain," *New York Times,* January 17, 1993.

Systems DC, "Temporo-Mandibular Joint" brochure, Pueblo, Colo.: 1981.

Taber, Jerriann J., Ph.D., "Eye-Robics" pamphlet, El Cajon, Calif.: Vision Training Institute, no date.

_____ , *Eye-Robics: The Natural Alternative to Glasses, Contacts or Surgery,* San Diego, Calif.: Eye-Care Publications Co., 1986.

Tai-Chi Center, "Tai-Chi Chuan: Body and Mind in Harmony," Winchester, Va.: The Tai-Chi Center, 1981.

Tappan, Frances M., *Healing Massage Technique: A Study of Eastern and Western Methods,* New York: Reston Publishing Co., 1980.

Teeguarden, Iona Marsaa, *Acupressure Way of Health: Jin Shin Do,* New York: Japan Publications, 1978.

_____ , "Jin Shin Do," Palo Alto, Calif.: Jin Shin Do Foundation, no date.

_____ , "Body-Mind Acupressure: Jin Shin Do," Palo Alto, Calif.: 1983.

_____ , *The Joy of Feeling: Jin Shin Do Bodymind Acupressure,* New York: Japan Publications, 1987.

Thie, John F., D.C., and Marks, Mary, *Touch For Health,* Marina del Ray, Calif.: DeVorss & Co. Publishers, 1973.

Thompson, Clem W., *Manual of Structural Kinesiology,* 11th ed., St. Louis, Mo.: *Times Mirror*/Mosby College Publications, 1989.

Thompson, Roberta Gibson, with Smith, Chris, "Trauma Touch Therapy," Lakewood, Colo.: no date.

Tisserand, Maggie, *Aromatherapy for Women,* New York: Thorson's Publications, 1985.

Tisserand, Robert B., *The Art of Aromatherapy,* New York: Destiny Books, 1977.

"To Find a Way to Age in Health," *Insight, April 10, 1989.*

Tortora, Gerald J., and Anagnostakos, Nicholas P., *Principles of Anatomy and Physiology,* 3d ed., New York: Harper and Row, 1981.

Trager Institute, *The Trager Journal Vol. I,* Mill Valley, Calif.: Trager Institute, Fall 1988.

_____ , *The Trager Journal Vol. II,* Mill Valley, Calif.: Trager Institute, Fall 1987.

Tuckerman, Belle, "Saving Face: Facial Fitness," *Massage,* Issue 41, January/February 1993.

Upledger Institute, Comprehensive brochure, Palm Beach Gardens, Fla.: 1994.

_____ , "CranioSacral Therapy I" brochure, Palm Beach Gardens, Fla.: no date.

_____ , "Discover the CranioSacral System" brochure, Palm Beach Gardens, Fla.: Upledger Institute, 1988.

_____ , "Fascial Mobilization" brochure, Palm Beach Gardens, Fla.: no date.

_____ , "Muscle Energy Workshop, Health Care Workshop" brochure, Palm Beach Gardens, Fla.: Upledger Institute, 1994.

_____ , "Process Acupressure" brochure, Palm Beach Gardens, Fla.: no date.

Upledger, John E., Dr., D. O., and Vrederoogd, J. D., *Craniosacral Therapy,* Seattle, Eastland Press, 1983.

_____ , "The Therapeutic Value of the Craniosacral System," Palm Beach Gardens, Fla.: Upledger Institute, no date.

Veith, Ilza, trans., *Huangdi Nei Jing* (The Yellow Emperor's Classic of Internal Medicine), Berkeley, Calif.: University of California Press, 1949.

Vishnudevananda, Swami, *The Complete Illustrated Book of Yoga,* New York: Pocket Books, 1972.

Wagenheim, Jeff, "Body Rebuilder," *New Age Journal,* November/December 1989.

Wale, J.O., C.S.M.M.G., ed., *Tidy's Massage and Remedial Exercises,* Bristol, England: John Wright & Sons, Ltd., 1968.

Walther, David S., *Applied Kinesiology: Basic Procedures and Muscle Testing, Vol. I,* Pueblo, Colo.: SDC Systems DC, 1981.

_____ , *Applied Kinesiology: Synopsis,* Pueblo, Colo.: SDC Systems DC, 1988.

Weiner, Barbara, "Deep Emotional Release: Interview with James Hyman," *New Lifestyles,* no date.

Wells, Valerie, *The Joy of Visualization,* San Francisco: Chronicle Books, 1990.

Wengrow, Vicki L., M.A., L.M.T., "Wengrow's Synergy" brochure, Jacksonville, Fla.: no date.

_____ , "Theory and Background of Wengrow's Synergy," research paper, Jacksonville, Fla.: no date.

Wester, William C., II, Ed.D., A.B.P.H., "Questions and Answers about Clinical Hypnosis," Columbus, Ohio: Ohio Psychology Publications, Inc., 1982.

Williams, Kelly L., "Muscle Sense," Greensboro, N.C.: *USAir Magazine,* Pace Communications, Inc., November 1991.

Wiltse, Patricia, "Lymphatic and Visceral Massage" brochure, San Anselmo, Calif.: 1994.

Wine, Zhenya Kurashova, "Russian Sports Massage: Post-Event Massage," *Massage,* Issue No. 41, January/February 1993.

Witt, Phil, "Trager Psychological Integration," *Whirlpool,* Summer 1986.

Wolfe, Honora Lee, "China," *Massage and Bodywork Magazine,* Vol. 1, Issue 4, 1986.

Wooten, Sandra, "Rosen Method," *Massage Magazine,* Issue 44, July/August 1993.

Worsley, J.R., *Traditional Chinese Acupuncture—Vol. I–II,* London: College of Traditional Acupuncture, 1990.

Wyrick, Dana, R.M.T., "European Manual Lymph Drainage," Dallas, Tex.: Body Therapy, October/November 1994.

_____ , "Dr. Vodder's Manual Lymph Drainage," *Ontario Massage Therapist Association Newsletter,* April/May 1988.

Xiangtong, Zhang, ed., *Research on Acupuncture, Moxibustion and Anesthesia,* Beijing: Science Press, 1986.

Xinnong, Cheng, *An Outline of Chinese Acupuncture,* Beijing: Foreign Languages Press, 1975.

_____ , *Chinese Acupuncture,* Beijing: Foreign Languages Press, 1987.

Yamamoto, Shizuko, *Barefoot Shiatsu,* Tokyo: Japan Publications, 1979.

Yamamoto, Shizuko and McCarthy, Patrick, *Whole Health Shiatsu,* New York: Japan Publications, 1993.

_____ , *The Shiatsu Handbook,* Eureka, Calif.: Turning Point Publications, 1986.

Yates, John, Ph.D., *A Physician's Guide to Therapeutic Massage: Its Physiological Effects and Their Application to Treatment,* Vancouver, B.C.: Massage Therapists' Association of British Columbia, 1990.

Yu-min, Chuang, Dr., *The Historical Development of Acupuncture,* Long Beach, Calif.: Oriental Healing Arts, 1982.

Zeiger, Sam, "Blue Light Flotation," New York: no date.

Zerinsky, Sidney S., Ph.D., *Handbook of Swedish Massage,* New York: Swedish Institute, 1982.

_____ , *Introduction to Pathology for the Massage Practitioner,* New York: Swedish Institute, 1985.

Zero Balancing Association, "Zero Balancing," Capitola, Calif.: no date.

THE CHRONOLOGICAL DEVELOPMENT OF THE BODYWORK SYSTEMS
(All dates are approximate)

3000–2500 B.C.	Acupressure	1600–1700	
	Acupuncture		
	Amma	1700–1800	Hypnotherapy
	Aromatherapy		
	Chi Nei Tsang	1800–1900	Chiropractic
	Color Therapy		Occupational Therapy
	Cupping		Osteopathic Medicine
	Dō-In		Reiki rediscovered
	Ear Therapy		Russian Massage
	Five Element Theory		Swedish Massage
	Hydrotherapy		introduced to Europe
	Laying on of Hands		
	Meditation	1900–1910	Jin Shin Acutouch
	Moxibustion		rediscovered
	Pointing Therapy		Naprapathy
	Pulse Reading		Radionics
	Shiatsu		Spiritual Healing
	Spiritual Healing		introduced in United
	Tai Chi Chuan		States
	Tongue Diagnosis		
	Tui-Na	1910–1920	Connective Tissue Massage
			Foot Reflexology
2500–2000	Ayurvedic Medicine		rediscovered
	Chakra Balancing		Hand Reflexology
	Classic Massage		rediscovered
	Reflexology		McMillan Massage
	Thai Massage		Technique
	Tibetan Massage		Mennell Massage
	Yoga		Technique
			Zen Shiatsu
2000–1000	Lomilomi		Zone Therapy
	Reiki		
		1920–1930	Autogenic Training
1000 B.C.–0	Breath Therapy		Bates Method of Vision
			Training
A.D. 0–1500	Magnetic Therapy		Bindegewebsmassage
	Music Therapy		Cayce/Reilly Massage
	Qigong		Cyriax Massage
			Hoffa Massage Technique
1500–1600	Breema		Physical Therapy

The Pilates Method
Sacro-Occipital Technique
Sensory Awareness

1930–1940   Alexander Technique
Aura Therapy
Hoshino Therapy
Johrei
Laban Movement Analysis
Lymphatic Drainage
  Massage
Medical Orgone Therapy
Okazaki Restorative
  Massage
Polarity Therapy
Trager

1940–1950   Macrobiotic Medicine
Thérèse Pfrimmer Method
  of Deep Muscle Therapy
Shiatsu introduced in
  United States

1950–1960   Applied Kinesiology
Bartenieff Fundamentals
Bioenergetics
Biofeedback
Core Energetics
Flotation
Gestalt Therapy
Iridology
Pesso Boyden System
  Psychomotor
Rolfing
The Rosen Method of
  Bodywork and
  Movement
Spray and Stretch
  Technique
Trigger Point Therapy

1960–1970   Barefoot Shiatsu
Body-Mind Centering
Barbara Brennan Healing
  Science
Dance Therapy

Dō-In introduced in
  United States
Egoscue Method
Esalen Massage
Feldenkrais Method
Hanna Somatic Education
Hoffman Quadrinity
  Process
Integrative Eclectic Shiatsu
Jin Shin Do
Jin Shin Jyutsu introduced
  in United States
Kinesiology
Macrobiotic Shiatsu
Myofascial Release
Ohashiatsu
Ortho-Bionomy
PNF Stretches
Past Life Regression
Postural Integration
The Radiance Technique
Rebirthing
Rubenfield Synergy
  Method
Shintaido
Soma Neuromuscular
  Integration
SomatoEmotional Release
St. John Neuromuscular
  Therapy
Strain-Counterstrain
  Therapy
Therapeutic Touch
Touch For Health
Zero Balancing

1970–1980   Acu-Yoga
Alchemia Heart Breath
Alchemia Synergy
Applied Physiology
Aston-Patterning
Benjamin System of
  Muscular Therapy
Chua Ka
CranioSacral Therapy
Drama Therapy

Embodyment Training
Ericksonian Hypnotherapy
Eye-Robics
Five Element Shiatsu
G-Jo Acupressure
Guided Imagery
Hakomi Integrated
 Somatics
Hellerwork
Holotropic Breathwork
Infant Massage
Integrative Acupressure
Ki-Shiatsu
Kripalu Bodywork
Kriya Massage
Lomilomi introduced to
 the West
Neural Organization
 Technique
NeuroCellular Repatterning
Neuro-Linguistic
 Programming
NeuroMuscular
 Reprogramming
Parma Training Program
Phoenix Rising Yoga
 Therapy
Bonnie Prudden
 Myotherapy
RADIX
Release Work
Resonant Kinesiology
Russian Massage introduced
 in United States
Safe Touch
Service Through Touch
SHEN
Somatic Psychotherapy
Sôtai
Spinal Touch Treatment
Spiritual Releasement
 Therapy
Sports Massage
Tantsu

1980–1990

Transpersonal Bodywork
 and Psychology
Trauma Touch Therapy
UNTIE
Vibrational Healing
 Massage Therapy
Visceral Manipulation
Wassertanzen
Watsu
Wengrow's Synergy

A Alpha Calm Therapy
Appropriate Touch
Avatar
Body-Centered
 Transformation
Body-Enlightenment
Bodymind Integration
Body Mind Integrative
 Therapy
Bodywork for the
 Childbearing Year
Chair Massage
CORE Body Work
Dance Injury Massage
Emotional-Kinesthetic
 Psychotherapy
Facial Massage
Fascial Kinetics
Focusing
Geriatric Massage
Gravitational Release
Haēlan Work
HEMME APPROACH
Integrative Psychotherapy
LooyenWork
Massage Body Mechanics
MotherMassage
Pranic Healing
Process Acupressure
Relational Dialogue

1990–2000

Constitutional Massage
Deep Massage

INDEX

This index is designed to be used in conjunction with the extensive A-to-Z encyclopedia entries. Page references to titles, names and terms that have their own encyclopedia entry are **boldfaced** below; for additional references, see their text entries. Other titles, names and terms that are not the subjects of the A-to-Z entries are generally given fuller citations here. *Italicized* page references indicate illustrations.

A

Alpha Calm Therapy, **1**
  resources, 265
abduction (joint
  movement), 189
Abrams, Albert, 188–89
Abrams Generator, 189
absent healing, in color
  therapy, 60
absolute template body. *See*
  divine template body
abuse
  Body Mind Integrative
    Therapy, 40
  emotional-kinesthetic
    psychotherapy, 85
  Safe Touch approach, 204
  sexual. *See* sexual abuse
  Trauma Touch Therapy,
    242–43
Academy for Guided
  Imagery (Mill Valley,
  Calif.), 103
accidents. *See* trauma
acetylcholine, 219
acquired *chi*, 51
actinotherapy, **1**
acu-points, **1**
  acupressure use of, 2
  Jin Shin Do Bodymind
    Acupressure use of, 133
acupressure, **1–3**, *4*
  acu-yoga use of, 8
  chair massage use of, 48
  cumulative effects, 2
  facial massage, 89

g-jo, 98
  Integrative, **126**
  Jin Shin Do Bodymind,
    131–34, *132*, 273
  process, 182–83
  resources, 265
  self-administration, 2, *3*
  Tibetan massage, 235–36
  Touch for Health
    technique, 239
  trigger point therapy, 245
  tsubo point therapy, 246
acupuncture, **3–8**
  acu points, 1
  AMMA Therapy and, 12
  applications, 7
  in Ayurvedic medicine,
    28–29
  bladder meridian, 37
  chakra balancing, 51
  channels, 5–6
  cupping technique, 72
  ear therapy, 77, *78*, 79
  face-lifts, 89
  fascia role, 161
  gallbladder meridian, 98
  governing vessel meridian,
    101, *102*
  hand therapy and, 119
  heart constrictor meridian,
    112
  heart meridian, 112
  kidney meridian, 137
  large intestine meridian,
    139
  lesser chakras and, 49
  liver meridian, 140

lung meridian, 142
  meridian treatment
    points, 154
  moxibustion and, 158
  needle, 4, *4*, 6–7
  NeuroCellular
    Repatterning, 163
  resources, 265
  small intestine meridian,
    213
  spleen meridian, 218
  stomach meridian, 222
  triple heater, 245
acu-yoga, **8–9**
  addictions, and A Alpha
    Calm Therapy, 1
  adduction (joint
    movement), 189
  adhesions, friction stroke
    impact on, 97
  adipose tissue, 62
  adjustment, 239
  adolescents, and Hawaiian
    massage, 140
  adrenals
    associated muscle, 16
    root chakra link, 49
  aged. *See* elderly
  aggregative *qi*, 55
  Agyan (god), 50
  ahita (harmful life), 28
  ah shui points, 12
  AIDS. *See* HIV infection
  ukusha, 140
  akido, 148
  Alaska, 283
  alchemia heart breath, **9**

Alchemical Synergy and,
    10
  Alchemical Synergy, **9–10**
    alchemia heart breath, 9
    etheric release, 87
    Kriya Massage
      component, 138
    resources, 265
  Alexander, Frederick
    Mathias, 10–11, 31, 215
  Alexander the Great, 225
  Alexander Technique,
    10–12, 31, 194, 199
    resources, 265
  Alexandria School of
    Scientific Therapeutics
    (Va.), 174
  alignment, **12**
    Alexander Technique, 11
    chiropractic methods,
      56–57
    CORE Bodywork, 65–66
    Parma Symmetry, 170
    Pilates Method, 176
    Sôtai, 215
    Zero Balancing work, 263
    See also misalignment
  Alive and Well! Institute of
    Conscious BodyWork (San
    Anselmo, Calif.), 165
  allergies, 20
  allopathic medicine, 58
  alpha motor nerves, 226
  alpha waves,
    electroencephalograph
    measurement of, 36